Vascular Imaging

Editor

CHRISTOPHER J. FRANÇOIS

RADIOLOGIC CLINICS
OF NORTH AMERICA

www.radiologic.theclinics.com

Consulting Editor
FRANK H. MILLER

July 2020 • Volume 58 • Number 4

ELSEVIER

1600 John F. Kennedy Boulevard ● Suite 1800 ● Philadelphia, Pennsylvania, 19103-2899

http://www.theclinics.com

RADIOLOGIC CLINICS OF NORTH AMERICA Volume 58, Number 4
July 2020 ISSN 0033-8389, ISBN 13: 978-0-323-72074-8

Editor: John Vassallo (j.vassallo@elsevier.com)
Developmental Editor: Donald Mumford

Radiologic Clinics of North America (ISSN 0033-8389) is published bimonthly by Elsevier Inc., 360 Park Avenue South, New York, NY 10010-1710. Months of issue are January, March, May, July, September, and November. Periodicals postage paid at New York, NY and additional mailing offices. Subscription prices are USD 513 per year for US individuals, USD 980 per year for US institutions, USD 100 per year for US students and residents, USD 594 per year for Canadian individuals, USD 1253 per year for Canadian institutions, USD 703 per year for international individuals, USD 1253 per year for international institutions, USD 100 per year for Canadian students/residents, and USD 315 per year for international students/residents. To receive student and resident rate, orders must be accompanied by name of affiliated institution, date of term and the signature of program/residency coordinatior on institution letterhead. Orders will be billed at individual rate until proof of status is received. Foreign air speed delivery is included in all *Clinics* subscription prices. All prices are subject to change without notice. **POSTMASTER:** Send address changes to *Radiologic Clinics of North America*, Elsevier Health Sciences Division, Subscription Customer Service, 3251 Riverport Lane, Maryland Heights, MO63043. **Customer Service: Telephone: 1-800-654-2452** (U.S. and Canada); **1-314-447-8871** (outside U.S. and Canada). **Fax: 1-314-447-8029. E-mail: journalscustomerservice-usa@elsevier.com (for print support); journalsonlinesupport-usa@elsevier.com (for online support).**

Reprints. For copies of 100 or more of articles in this publication, please contact the Commercial Reprints Department, Elsevier Inc., 360 Park Avenue South, New York, New York 10010-1710. Tel.: +1-212-633-3874; Fax: +1-212-633-3820; E-mail: reprints@elsevier.com.

Radiologic Clinics of North America also published in Greek Paschalidis Medical Publications, Athens, Greece.

Radiologic Clinics of North America is covered in *MEDLINE/PubMed (Index Medicus), EMBASE/Excerpta Medica, Current Contents/Life Sciences, Current Contents/Clinical Medicine, RSNA Index to Imaging Literature, BIOSIS, Science Citation Index,* and *ISI/BIOMED.*

Contributors

CONSULTING EDITOR

FRANK H. MILLER, MD, FACR
Lee F. Rogers MD Professor of Medical
Education, Chief, Body Imaging Section and
Fellowship Program, Medical Director, MRI,
Department of Radiology, Northwestern
Memorial Hospital, Northwestern University
Feinberg School of Medicine, Chicago, Illinois,
USA

EDITOR

CHRISTOPHER J. FRANÇOIS, MD
Professor, Department of Radiology, University
of Wisconsin-Madison, Madison, Wisconsin,
USA

AUTHORS

GERHARD ADAM, MD
Head, Department of Diagnostic and
Interventional Radiology and Nuclear
Medicine, University Medical Center Hamburg-
Eppendorf, Hamburg, Germany

BRADLEY D. ALLEN, MD, MS
Department of Radiology, Northwestern
University Feinberg School of Medicine,
Chicago, Illinois, USA

JOAO AMARAL, MD
Department of Diagnostic Imaging, The
Hospital for Sick Children and Medical
Imaging, University of Toronto, Division of
Image Guided Therapy (IGT), Department of
Diagnostic Imaging, The Hospital for Sick
Children, Toronto, Ontario, Canada

PETER BANNAS, MD
Senior Medical Doctor, Department of
Diagnostic and Interventional Radiology and
Nuclear Medicine, University Medical Center
Hamburg-Eppendorf, Hamburg, Germany

ARASH BEDAYAT, MD
Clinical Assistant Professor, Department of
Radiological Sciences, Thoracic and
Diagnostic Cardiovascular Imaging, David
Geffen School Medicine, University of
California, Los Angeles (UCLA), Los Angeles,
California, USA

NICHOLAS S. BURRIS, MD
Assistant Professor of Radiology, University of
Michigan, Frankel Cardiovascular Center, Ann
Arbor, Michigan, USA

HAMID CHALIAN, MD
Clinical Assistant Professor, Department of
Radiology, Cardiothoracic Imaging, Duke
University Medical Center, Durham, North
Carolina, USA

GOVIND B. CHAVHAN, MD, DABR
Department of Diagnostic Imaging, The
Hospital for Sick Children and Medical
Imaging, University of Toronto, Toronto,
Ontario, Canada

JEREMY D. COLLINS, MD, FSIR
Senior Associate Consultant, Department of
Radiology, Mayo Clinic, Rochester, Minnesota,
USA

CHRISTOPHER J. FRANÇOIS, MD
Professor, Department of Radiology, University
of Wisconsin-Madison, Madison, Wisconsin,
USA

JULIO GARCIA, PhD
Assistant Professor, Department of Radiology
and Cardiac Sciences, Cumming School of
Medicine, Libin Cardiovascular Institute of
Alberta, Alberta Children's Hospital Research
Institute, University of Calgary, Calgary,
Alberta, Canada

LORI MANKOWSKI GETTLE, MD, MBA
Assistant Professor of Radiology, Chief of
Ultrasound, University of Wisconsin-Madison,
Madison, Wisconsin, USA

MARY-LOUISE C. GREER, MD
Department of Diagnostic Imaging, The
Hospital for Sick Children and Medical
Imaging, University of Toronto, Toronto,
Ontario, Canada

LARS GROSSE-WORTMANN, MD
Department of Diagnostic Imaging, The
Hospital for Sick Children and Medical
Imaging, Division of Cardiology, Department of
Paediatrics, The Hospital for Sick Children,
University of Toronto, Toronto, Ontario,
Canada

MICHAEL R. HAROWICZ, MD
Diagnostic Radiology Resident, Russell H.
Morgan Department of Radiology and
Radiological Science, Johns Hopkins School of
Medicine, Johns Hopkins Hospital, Baltimore,
Maryland, USA

ALI FATEHI HASSANABAD, MD
Clinical Fellow, Department of Cardiac
Sciences, Cumming School of Medicine,
University of Calgary, Calgary, Alberta, Canada

CAMERON HASSANI, MD
Clinical Assistant Professor, Department of
Radiological Sciences, Thoracic and
Diagnostic Cardiovascular Imaging, David

Geffen School Medicine, University of
California, Los Angeles (UCLA), Los Angeles,
California, USA

AMIRA HUSSEIN, MD
Department of Radiology, Johns Hopkins
Hospital, Baltimore, Maryland, USA

FATEMEHSADAT JAMALIDINAN, PhD
Postdoctoral Research Associate,
Departments of Radiology and Cardiac
Sciences, Cumming School of Medicine,
University of Calgary, Calgary, Alberta, Canada

KIMBERLY G. KALLIANOS, MD
Assistant Professor of Clinical Radiology,
Department of Radiology and Biomedical
Imaging, University of California, San
Francisco, San Francisco, California, USA

PEGAH KHOSHPOURI, MD
Research Fellow, Department of Radiology,
Thoracic Imaging, Duke University Medical
Center, Durham, North Carolina, USA

CHRISTOPHER Z. LAM, MD
Department of Diagnostic Imaging, The
Hospital for Sick Children and Medical
Imaging, University of Toronto, Toronto,
Ontario, Canada

ALEXANDER LENZ, MD
Resident, Department of Diagnostic and
Interventional Radiology and Nuclear
Medicine, University Medical Center Hamburg-
Eppendorf, Hamburg, Germany

NAGINA MALGURIA, MD
Department of Radiology, Johns Hopkins
Hospital, Baltimore, Maryland, USA

ASHLEY E. PROSPER, MD
Clinical Assistant Professor, Department of
Radiological Sciences, Thoracic and
Diagnostic Cardiovascular Imaging, David
Geffen School Medicine, University of
California, Los Angeles (UCLA), Los Angeles,
California, USA

**PRABHAKAR RAJIAH, MBBS, MD, FRCR,
FSCMR**
Department of Radiology, Mayo Clinic,
Rochester, Minnesota, USA

MARGARITA V. REVZIN, MD, MS, FSRU, FAIUM
Associate Professor of Diagnostic Radiology, Department of Radiology and Biomedical Imaging, Yale School of Medicine, Yale New Haven Hospital, New Haven, Connecticut, USA

STEFAN G. RUEHM, MD
Professor, Department of Radiological Sciences, Thoracic and Diagnostic Cardiovascular Imaging, David Geffen School Medicine, University of California, Los Angeles (UCLA), Los Angeles, California, USA

MARK L. SCHIEBLER, MD
Department of Radiology, University of Wisconsin-Madison School of Medicine and Public Health, Madison, Wisconsin, USA

AMAR SHAH, MD, MPA
Associate Professor, Department of Radiology, Donald and Barbara Zucker School of Medicine at Hofstra/Northwell, Manhasset, New York, USA

MICHAEL TEMPLE, MD
Department of Diagnostic Imaging, The Hospital for Sick Children and Medical Imaging, University of Toronto, Division of Image Guided Therapy (IGT), Department of Diagnostic Imaging, The Hospital for Sick Children, Toronto, Ontario, Canada

JULIUS MATTHIAS WEINRICH, MD
Resident, Department of Diagnostic and Interventional Radiology and Nuclear Medicine, University Medical Center Hamburg-Eppendorf, Hamburg, Germany

STEFAN L. ZIMMERMAN, MD
Associate Professor, Russell H. Morgan Department of Radiology and Radiological Science, Johns Hopkins School of Medicine, Johns Hopkins Hospital, Baltimore, Maryland, USA

Contents

There are several vascular ultrasound technologies that are useful in challenging diagnostic situations. New vascular ultrasound applications include directional power Doppler ultrasound, contrast-enhanced ultrasound, B-flow imaging, microvascular imaging, 3-dimensional vascular ultrasound, intravascular ultrasound, photoacoustic imaging, and vascular elastography. All these techniques are complementary to Doppler ultrasound and provide greater ability to visualize small vessels, have higher sensitivity to detect slow flow, and better assess vascular wall and lumen while overcoming limitations color Doppler. The ultimate goal of these technologies is to make ultrasound competitive with computed tomography and magnetic resonance imaging for vascular imaging.

Computed tomography angiography (CTA) has become a mainstay for the imaging of vascular diseases, because of high accuracy, availability, and rapid turnaround time. High-quality CTA images can now be routinely obtained with high isotropic spatial resolution and temporal resolution. Advances in CTA have focused on improving the image quality, increasing the acquisition speed, eliminating artifacts, and reducing the doses of radiation and iodinated contrast media. Dual-energy computed tomography provides material composition capabilities that can be used for characterizing lesions, optimizing contrast, decreasing artifact, and reducing radiation dose. Deep learning techniques can be used for classification, segmentation, quantification, and image enhancement.

Dynamic contrast-enhanced magnetic resonance lymphangiography is a novel technique to image central conducting lymphatics. It is performed by injecting contrast into groin lymph nodes and following passage of contrast through lymphatic system using T1-weighted MR images. Currently, it has been successfully applied to image and plan treatment of thoracic duct pathologies, lymphatic leaks, and other lymphatic abnormalities such as plastic bronchitis. It is useful in the assessment of chylothorax and chyloperitoneum. Its role in other areas such as intestinal lymphangiectasia and a variety of lymphatic anomalies is likely to increase.

Pulmonary vascular assessment commonly relies on computed tomography angiography (CTA), but continued advances in magnetic resonance angiography have allowed pulmonary magnetic resonance angiography (pMRA) to become a reasonable alternative to CTA without exposing patients to ionizing radiation. pMRA allows the evaluation of pulmonary vascular anatomy, hemodynamic physiology, lung parenchymal perfusion, and (optionally) right and left ventricular function with a single examination. This article discusses pMRA techniques and artifacts; performance in commonly encountered pulmonary vascular diseases, specifically pulmonary embolism and pulmonary hypertension; and recent advances in both contrast-enhanced and noncontrast pMRA.

High-quality aortic imaging plays a central role in the management of patients with thoracic aortic aneurysm. Computed tomography angiography and magnetic resonance angiography are the most commonly used techniques for thoracic aortic aneurysm diagnosis and imaging surveillance, with each having unique strengths and limitations that should be weighed when deciding patient-specific applications. To ensure optimal patient care, imagers must be familiar with potential sources of artifact and measurement error, and dedicate effort to ensure high-quality and reproducible aortic measurements are generated. This review summarizes the imaging evaluation and underlying pathology relevant to the diagnosis of thoracic aortic aneurysm.

Preoperative assessment with computed tomography (CT) is critical before transcatheter interventions for structural heart disease. CT provides information for device selection, device sizing, and vascular access approach. The interpreting radiologist must have knowledge of appropriate CT protocols, how and where to obtain the important measurements, and know additional imaging characteristics that are important to describe for optimal support of the interventionalist. CT is the modality of choice for pre-operative evaluation in patients undergoing transcatheter aortic valve replacement and left atrial appendage occlusion, and is also useful before transcatheter mitral valve replacement, which is an ongoing area of research.

Blood flow through the heart and great vessels is sensitive to time and multiple velocity directions. The assessment of its three-dimensional nature has been limited. Recent advances in magnetic resonance imaging (MRI) allow the comprehensive visualization and quantification of in vivo flow dynamics using four-dimensional (4D)-flow MRI. In addition, the technique provides the opportunity to obtain advanced hemodynamic measures. This article introduces 4D-flow MRI as it is currently used for blood flow visualization and quantification of cardiac hemodynamic parameters. It discusses its advantages relative to other flow MRI techniques and describes its potential clinical applications.

Julius Matthias Weinrich, Alexander Lenz, Gerhard Adam, Christopher J. François, and Peter Bannas

Vasculitides are a complex group of diseases sharing the defining feature of inflamed vessel walls. Vasculitides can be classified depending on the size of the predominantly affected vessels. Modern cross-sectional imaging methods have become a cornerstone in the diagnosis of vasculitis and may help in narrowing down differential diagnoses. This review presents the most important imaging modalities and typical findings in large and medium size vasculitis, implementing current imaging recommendations.

Arash Bedayat, Cameron Hassani, Ashley E. Prosper, Hamid Chalian, Pegah Khoshpouri, and Stefan G. Ruehm

Noninvasive imaging of the vascular renal system is a common request in diagnostic radiology. Typical indications include suspected renovascular hypertension, vasculitis, neoplasm, vascular malformation, and structural diseases of the kidney. Profound knowledge of the renal anatomy, including vascular supply and variants, is mandatory for radiologists and allows for optimized protocolling and interpretation of imaging studies. Besides renal ultrasound, computed tomography and MR imaging are commonly requested cross-sectional studies for renal and renal vascular imaging. This article discusses basic renal vascular anatomy, common imaging findings, and current and potential future imaging protocols for various renovascular pathologic conditions.

Jeremy D. Collins

MR angiography is a flexible imaging technique enabling morphologic assessment of mesenteric arterial and venous vasculature. Conventional gadolinium-based contrast media and ferumoxytol are used as contrast agents. Ferumoxytol, an intravenous iron replacement therapy approved by the US Food and Drug Administration for iron deficiency anemia, is an effective and well tolerated blood pool contrast agent. The addition of 4D flow MR imaging enables a functional assessment of the arterial and venous vasculature; when coupled with a meal challenge, the severity of mesenteric arterial stenosis is well appreciated. Noncontrast MR angiographic techniques are useful for evaluating suspected mesenteric ischemia.

Amira Hussein and Nagina Malguria

Recent advances in imaging have allowed a better understanding of imaging features and classification of vascular anomalies. This article focuses on imaging of vascular malformations; describes the updated classification system and clinical and imaging characteristics of the different subtypes; and discusses the associated syndromes, differential diagnosis, and available treatment options, including the role of imaging in management.

A variety of nonatherosclerotic diseases affect the arteries of the pelvis and lower extremities. Chronic repetitive traumatic conditions, such as popliteal entrapment and external iliac artery fibroelastosis, vasculitis and connective tissue diseases, and noninflammatory vascular diseases, are a few of the more commonly encountered nonatherosclerotic peripheral vascular diseases. Ultrasound, computed tomography angiography, and magnetic resonance angiography are essential in the initial assessment and management of patients with peripheral vascular disease.

PROGRAM OBJECTIVE

The objective of the *Radiologic Clinics of North America* is to keep practicing radiologists and radiology residents up to date with current clinical practice in radiology by providing timely articles reviewing the state of the art in patient care.

TARGET AUDIENCE

Practicing radiologists, radiology residents, and other healthcare professionals who provide patient care utilizing radiologic findings.

LEARNING OBJECTIVES

Upon completion of this activity, participants will be able to:

1. Describe important emerging applications for MR imaging that may be used for assessing various vascular disease states such as vasculitis, mesenteric ischemia, renal vascular disease, vascular malformations, and nonatherosclerotic peripheral vascular disease.
2. Discuss recent innovations in non-invasive vascular imaging, including new applications for ultrasound, computed tomography angiography, and magnetic resonance angiography.
3. Recognize best practices on appropriate imaging for the management and treatment of cardiovascular disease.

ACCREDITATION

The Elsevier Office of Continuing Medical Education (EOCME) is accredited by the Accreditation Council for Continuing Medical Education (ACCME) to provide continuing medical education for physicians.

The EOCME designates this journal-based CME activity for a maximum of 12 *AMA PRA Category 1 Credit*(s)™. Physicians should claim only the credit commensurate with the extent of their participation in the activity.

All other healthcare professionals requesting continuing education credit for this enduring material will be issued a certificate of participation.

DISCLOSURE OF CONFLICTS OF INTEREST

The EOCME assesses conflict of interest with its instructors, faculty, planners, and other individuals who are in a position to control the content of CME activities. All relevant conflicts of interest that are identified are thoroughly vetted by EOCME for fair balance, scientific objectivity, and patient care recommendations. EOCME is committed to providing its learners with CME activities that promote improvements or quality in healthcare and not a specific proprietary business or a commercial interest.

The planning committee, staff, authors and editors listed below have identified no financial relationships or relationships to products or devices they or their spouse/life partner have with commercial interest related to the content of this CME activity:

Gerhard Adam, MD; Bradley D. Allen, MD, MS; Joao Amaral, MD; Peter Bannas, MD; Arash Bedayat, MD; Nicholas S. Burris, MD; Hamid Chalian, MD; Govind B. Chavhan, MD, DABR; Jeremy D. Collins, MD, FSIR; Christopher J. François, MD; Julio Garcia, PhD; Lori Mankowski Gettle, MD, MBA; Mary-Louise C. Greer, MD; Lars Grosse-Wortmann, MD; Michael R. Harowicz, MD; Ali Fatehi Hassanabad, MD; Cameron Hassani, MD; Amira Hussein, MD; Fatemehsadat Jamalidinan, PhD; Kimberly G. Kallianos, MD; Marilu Kelly, MSN, RN, CNE, CHCP; Pegah Khoshpouri, MD; Pradeep Kuttysankaran; Christopher Z. Lam, MD; Alexander Lenz, MD; Nagina Malguria, MD; Ashley E. Prosper, MD; Prabhakar Rajiah, MBBS, MD, FRCR, FSCMR; Margarita V. Revzin, MD, MS, FSRU, FAIUM; Stefan G. Ruehm, MD; Amar Shah, MD, MPA; Michael Temple, MD; John Vassallo; Julius Matthias Weinrich, MD; Stefan L. Zimmerman, MD.

The planning committee, staff, authors and editors listed below have identified financial relationships or relationships to products or devices they or their spouse/life partner have with commercial interest related to the content of this CME activity:

Mark L. Schiebler, MD: owns stock in Healthmyne and Stemina Biomarker Discovery, Inc.

UNAPPROVED/OFF-LABEL USE DISCLOSURE

The EOCME requires CME faculty to disclose to the participants:

1. When products or procedures being discussed are off-label, unlabelled, experimental, and/or investigational (not US Food and Drug Administration [FDA] approved); and
2. Any limitations on the information presented, such as data that are preliminary or that represent ongoing research, interim analyses, and/or unsupported opinions. Faculty may discuss information about pharmaceutical agents that is outside of FDA-approved labelling. This information is intended solely for CME and is not intended to promote off-label use of these medications. If you have any questions, contact the medical affairs department of the manufacturer for the most recent prescribing information.

TO ENROLL

To enroll in the *Radiologic Clinics of North America* Continuing Medical Education program, call customer service at 1-800-654-2452 or sign up online at http://www.theclinics.com/home/cme. The CME program is available to subscribers for an additional annual fee of USD 330.00.

METHOD OF PARTICIPATION

In order to claim credit, participants must complete the following:

1. Complete enrolment as indicated above.
2. Read the activity.
3. Complete the CME Test and Evaluation. Participants must achieve a score of 70% on the test. All CME Tests and Evaluations must be completed online.

CME INQUIRIES/SPECIAL NEEDS

For all CME inquiries or special needs, please contact elsevierCME@elsevier.com.

RADIOLOGIC CLINICS OF NORTH AMERICA

RELATED SERIES

Magnetic Resonance Imaging Clinics
Neuroimaging Clinics
PET Clinics

THE CLINICS ARE AVAILABLE ONLINE!
Access your subscription at:
www.theclinics.com

RADIOLOGIC CLINICS OF NORTH AMERICA

Preface
Recent Innovations in Vascular Imaging

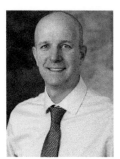

Christopher J. François, MD
Editor

In this issue of *Radiologic Clinics of North America*, readers discover recent innovations in noninvasive vascular imaging, including new applications for ultrasound, computed tomography angiography, and magnetic resonance angiography. The articles on pulmonary vascular disease and magnetic resonance lymphangiography introduce readers to important emerging applications for MR imaging. As minimally invasive and endovascular approaches to treating cardiovascular disease become more mainstream, it is critical that physicians become up to date on the appropriate imaging that is a part of the management, particularly in patients with structural heart disease and thoracic aortic disease. Other areas where substantial changes have occurred in assessing vascular disease include vasculitis, mesenteric ischemia, renal vascular disease, vascular malformations, and nonatherosclerotic peripheral vascular disease.

Christopher J. François, MD
Department of Radiology
University of Wisconsin
600 Highland Avenue
Madison, WI 53792, USA

E-mail address:
cfrancois@uwhealth.org

Radiol Clin N Am 58 (2020) xv
https://doi.org/10.1016/j.rcl.2020.04.001
0033-8389/20/© 2020 Published by Elsevier Inc.

Innovations in Vascular Ultrasound

Lori Mankowski Gettle, MD, MBA[a],*, Margarita V. Revzin, MD, MS, FSRU, FAIUM[b]

KEYWORDS

- Vascular ultrasound • Contrast-enhanced ultrasound • B-flow ultrasound • Doppler ultrasound
- Microvascular imaging • Microflow imaging • 3-D vascular ultrasound • Intravascular ultrasound

KEY POINTS

- Innovative vascular ultrasound technologies offer improved visualization of small vessels and higher sensitivity to slow flow.
- Just as in Doppler ultrasound, image optimization and recognition of artifacts are key to accurate interpretation.
- New vascular ultrasound techniques continue to develop and will have more applications with additional research and experience.
- Contrast-enhanced ultrasound requires an intravenous line for administration.

INTRODUCTION

Ultrasound (US) is a powerful tool for evaluating vasculature because it provides valuable information regarding blood flow and vessel morphology. The benefits of US are well recognized, including portability, availability, cost-effectiveness, and lack of ionizing radiation. Challenges common to all US technologies are limited penetration in bariatric patients, poor acoustic windows, and user dependence. Because of its importance in vascular imaging, there have been many recent innovative advances in US techniques meant to improve the diagnostic capability of US.

Doppler US—including its 3 main modes: color Doppler, spectral Doppler, and conventional power Doppler—has been a part of most US examinations for more than 40 years and its advantages and challenges are well documented. Color Doppler US (CDUS) provides information about flow, including direction of flow within a selected box superimposed on the gray-scale US image and mean blood flow velocity. Spectral Doppler US has the added benefit of providing the absolute velocity of blood flow within a small sample gate placed in a vessel. The spectral tracing gives vital information on hemodynamic values of blood flow, such as acceleration time and peak systolic and diastolic velocities, which can be used to calculate resistive indices. Conventional power Doppler US (PDUS) is more sensitive to slow flow than color Doppler and provides detail on the strength of the Doppler signal within an area but lacks directional information. PDUS is most useful in assessing global perfusion of an organ. Although all these modes are useful in assessing and diagnosing vascular pathologies, some of their capabilities are limited, especially in the assessment of vascular beds that demonstrate very slow flow and pathologies that are associated with vascular wall and lumen.[1]

Challenging vascular systems that are difficult to evaluate using conventional Doppler modes or equivocal Doppler cases require more advanced US applications with the highest sensitivity to flow to provide more definitive and accurate diagnosis. Newly developed innovative US techniques emphasize the role of US in accurate diagnosis of

[a] University of Wisconsin – Madison, 600 Highland Avenue, E3/380, Madison, WI 53792, USA; [b] Department of Radiology and Biomedical Imaging, Yale School of Medicine, Yale New Haven Hospital, 330 Cedar Street, TE 2-214, New Haven, CT 06520, USA
* Corresponding author.
E-mail address: lmankowskigettle@uwhealth.org
Twitter: @Lori_M_Gettle (L.M.G.); @MargaritaRevzin (M.V.R.)

Radiol Clin N Am 58 (2020) 653–669
https://doi.org/10.1016/j.rcl.2020.03.002

various vascular pathologies and conditions, including assessment of atherosclerotic plaque and visualization of plaque ulceration, detection of significant endoleaks in patients post–endovascular aneurysm repair (EVAR), identification of patency of arterial and venous flow in organ transplants, and accurate diagnosis of near occlusion and its differentiation from complete occlusion of either central or peripheral arterial or venous bed. In many of aforementioned pathologic conditions, a reliable US tool is imperative in improvement of diagnostic capability of US and reliability of the imaging findings. Additionally, a safe and highly diagnostic technique is desired for screening of vascular pathologies and for offering a sensitive and robust tool for a lifetime follow-up of major vascular conditions.

Most of the advanced US vascular applications were designed with the overall goal of trouble-shooting absence of flow detection in order to avoid false-positive diagnoses of vascular occlusion and increase confidence of an interpreter to an accurate identification of vascular pathology. This article is a review of the latest innovations in vascular US with examples of their applications as well as a discussion of their strengths and weaknesses (Table 1).

IMAGE OPTIMIZATION AND AutoScan FUNCTION

With the new era of US vascular imaging, most US units are now equipped with automatic image optimization (AutoScan) capabilities. One of the most common advantages of the AutoScan function is automatic localization and identification of a vessel within the area of scanning on color Doppler and placement of the spectral gate in the center of the identified vessel. Adjustment of gain, velocity scale, wall filter, and color box also is automatic. Although this automated function is less operator dependent, in challenging cases manual override may be necessary for optimal image acquisition and correct interpretation. Therefore, knowledge of and expertise in Doppler optimization parameters remain significant and necessary to ensure the performance of high quality Doppler examinations.[1,2] In addition, just as with the traditional Doppler, image optimization is imperative when new advanced techniques and applications are used. Thus, for microvascular flow, contrast-enhanced US (CEUS), and B-flow imaging (BFI), selection of appropriate parameters, such as acoustic window, gain, zone, focus, depth, transducer choice, and in some cases angle of insonation, is critical for optimal scanning. Moreover, recognition of modern vascular application

specific artifacts and understanding of their significance as well as how to avoid them also are paramount in accurate assessment of flow.[1]

DIRECTIONAL POWER DOPPLER

Directional power Doppler is a relatively new application that is based on the conventional power Doppler mode. In addition to providing information regarding presence of slow flow and global perfusion of an organ or vascular structure, it also allows determination of flow direction (Fig. 1). This is particularly important in the field of obstetric US, where accurate assessment of vessel patency as well as flow pattern and direction have a significant impact on patient and fetal management. For example, assessment of flow direction in the umbilical cord is of critical importance in the setting of multigestation pregnancies and in the evaluation of twin-twin transfusion. Additionally, directional power Doppler plays a significant role in the assessment of neovascularity within visceral organ masses as well as when there is concern for a postintervention arteriovenous fistula in a native or transplanted visceral organ.[3,4] Directional power Doppler increases the diagnostic confidence of radiologists in the assessment of complete occlusion of key vasculature, such as the carotid and portal vein systems, also allowing for accurate differentiation of occlusion from near occlusion or stasis (as in cases of a carotid string sign or slow flow in the portal venous system). Directional PDUS, however, has limitations similar to those of conventional PDUS. For example, it does not provide an estimation of absolute or mean velocity, it is susceptible to significant motion artifact, and it is affected by the Doppler angle. A significant disadvantage is that, as in conventional power Doppler, directional PDUS cannot produce aliasing, making it difficult to quickly identify areas of potential vascular high-level stenosis. One of the differentiating features between conventional and directional power Doppler ultrasound is that conventional PDUS is independent of the angle of insonation. Utilization of a combination of new applications is becoming a trend in vascular imaging. For example, there is an interest in the use of directional power Doppler in conjunction with 3-dimensional (3-D) rendering techniques and contrast agents, which show great promise for the evaluation of vascular beds.

CONTRAST-ENHANCED ULTRASOUND

Although CEUS has been readily available in Asia and Europe, it has been slow to gain acceptance in the United States in part due to regulatory

Table 1
Comparison of vascular ultrasound technologies

Application	Pros	Cons
Color Doppler	Provides information on presence or absence of flow, direction of flow, mean flow velocity, gray-scale tissue characteristics	Absolute velocity cannot be determined. Motion outside of a vessel may be seen as flow. Color can bloom beyond the wall of the vessel. Angle dependent
Spectral Doppler	Provides information on velocity and direction of flow Provides quantitative assessment of flow (acceleration, peak systolic velocity, end diastolic velocity, etc.)	Only a small area can be assessed. Angle dependent
Conventional power Doppler	More sensitive to slow flow than color Doppler Enables global assessment of perfusion Not angle dependant	Does not provide direction of flow or velocity Sensitive to motion artifact of surrounding tissues
CEUS	No nephrotoxicity Excellent safety profile Can repeat dose Provides information on flow in microvasculature Aids in differentiating benign and malignant thrombus	Minimally invasive (intravenous) Gray-scale imaging is degraded by low mechanical index. More time consuming
B-flow	Based on gray-scale US and amplifies signal of moving blood Can subtract gray-scale background Provides information of all vessels in field of view, including small and slow-flow vessels regardless of angle	Does not provide direction of flow or velocity.
MVI	Based on PDUS Provides information on very small vessels by reducing background clutter and maintaining high frame rates	Detection of flow can be affected by adjacent high velocity and pulsating vessels. Some of the applications do not provide absolute velocity calculation.
PAI	Newly emergent molecular imaging, based on combination of thermoelastic expansion of light energy (laser) and sonographic beam production. Provides information on blood oxygen saturation and hemoglobin, capable of measuring blood velocity and detection and distribution of biomarkers; visualizes blood vessel structure and associated plaque	High resolution is at the expanse of depth of penetration. A majority of applications still are preclinical.
IVUS imaging	Provides intraluminal assessment of a vessel lumen, wall and anatomy; plaque distribution and size; allows measurement of the intravascular diameter; offers guidance for intravascular procedures, including stents and graft placement, assists in fenestration of dissection flap	No information about the outer vascular wall and adjacent structures

(continued on next page)

Table 1 *(continued)*		
Application	**Pros**	**Cons**
Elastography, strain and shear wave	Provides assessment of arterial wall elasticity Offers assessment of chronicity of blood clot	Reproducibility still varies No defined threshold values or criteria available at this time
3-D vascular imaging	Offers assessment of atherosclerotic plaque volume and intrinsic characteristics: composition, surface irregularity, size, and dimensions Improved ability to estimate flow volume and more accurate assessment of degree of stenosis	Errors in calculation of flow volume due to vascular motion and pulsation

obstacles and in part because of heavy reliance on computed tomography (CT) and magnetic resonance imaging (MRI).[5] The Food and Drug Administration only approved the use of Lumason (Bracco Diagnostics, Monroe Township, New Jersey) for characterization of liver lesions in 2016.

CEUS agents consist of gas-filled microbubbles surrounded by a supportive shell usually made of phospholipids.[6] These agents are metabolized exclusively by the liver and lungs and are not nephrotoxic, making them safe for use in patients with renal insufficiency and allergies to other contrast agents.[7] No laboratory tests are required before use. Microbubble US contrast agents have an excellent safety profile with a severe adverse reaction rate of 0.007% to 0.009%, which is comparable to that of gadolinium and superior to that of iodinated contrast agents.[8,9]

Challenges specific to CEUS include special software necessary on the machine to perform contrast-enhanced examinations. This is available on all major US vendors. An intravenous line must be placed for administration of the contrast agent and there must be an additional person available to inject the contrast. There is a learning curve to optimize CEUS imaging, which includes timing of the vascular phases after injection for imaging of masses, properly decreasing the gain before administering contrast to avoid artifactual enhancement of background tissue, and minimizing mechanical energy imparted into the area being imaged. Microbubbles are sensitive to mechanical energy and burst with increased mechanical index or continuous imaging in one place.

CEUS agents are smaller than a red blood cell and remain purely intravascular.[7,10] CEUS imaging provides dynamic, real-time imaging of vasculature

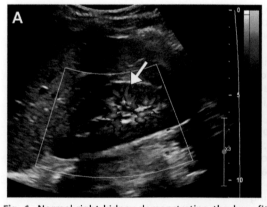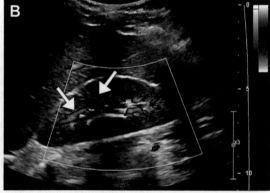

Fig. 1. Normal right kidney demonstrating the benefits of directional power Doppler ultrasound. (*A*) Conventional power Doppler ultrasound obtained in the sagittal plane provides information on global perfusion of the kidney, but lacks directional information, therefore both venous and arterial flow are displayed with the same color code (*arrow* in *A*). (*B*) Directional power Doppler provides additional information on direction of flow in this normal kidney allowing identification of venous and arterial intrarenal vasculature (*arrows* in *B*).

along with excellent spatial and temporal resolution. Because of the excellent safety profile of these contrast agents, the dose can be repeated in the same session. These characteristics makes CEUS great for vascular and microvascular imaging. Some of the vascular applications of CEUS are evaluating endoleaks in patients post-EVAR, assessment of vascular thrombus, and vessel patency.

Surveillance after Endovascular Aneurysm Repair

Approximately 70% of abdominal aortic aneurysm repairs are performed using EVAR procedures as opposed to the more invasive open technique.[11] EVARs require perpetual surveillance for graft-related complications, which occur in approximately 40% of patients within 4 years of EVAR.[12] CT angiography is considered the gold standard for surveillance, but it is expensive and uses ionizing radiation and iodinated contrast. CDUS can detect a change in the aneurysm sac diameter but is less sensitive for detection of endoleak compared with CT angiography.[13–15] A meta-analysis demonstrated a 0.72 sensitivity and 0.95 specificity of CDUS to detect an endoleak. CEUS showed a higher sensitivity of 0.91 and a slightly lower specificity of 0.89, meaning that CEUS was better to ruling in an endoleak (Fig. 2). The drawback of these techniques were that a majority of endoleaks detected were type II, which often do not require intervention as opposed to type I or III endoleaks.[16] The addition of 3-D to CEUS evaluation of the EVAR repair shows promise as being equivalent to CT angiography in detecting and classifying the type of endoleak.[17] Taken together, CEUS may be an appropriate examination for follow-up of an EVAR procedure with CTA reserved for further evaluation of suspicious findings.[17]

Challenges with this examination can include finding an appropriate acoustic window that would allow appropriate visibility of the EVAR stent graft and ultrasound beam penetration. The examination should be performed in a fasting state to limit interference by bowel gas. CEUS examination can also be challenging in bariatric patients.

Evaluation of Portal Vein Thrombus

Hepatocellular carcinoma (HCC) is the third most common cause of cancer death in the world.[18] Bland portal vein thrombus can be seen in 5% to 26% of cirrhotic livers and in up to 42% of patients with HCC.[19] Tumor in vein (also known as tumor thrombus) occurs in 10% to 60% of patients with HCC.[18] Distinguishing between bland and tumor thrombus is diagnostically important because it influences prognosis and is a contraindication to liver transplantation. Tumor thrombus can be difficult to detect by gray-scale US in the background of a heterogenous, cirrhotic liver. Slow flow in the portal vein can mimic thrombus on CDUS and, although detection of an arterial spectral Doppler tracing is 100% specific for tumor thrombus, the sensitivity is approximately only 20%.[20] In 1 study of 54 patients with known HCC and portal vein thrombus, the addition of CEUS to detect tumor in vein increased sensitivity to 88% compared with CDUS, with a sensitivity of 20%.[21] The real-time, dynamic evaluation of the portal vein with CEUS and the ability to repeat the contrast dose during examination makes this a valuable adjunct to US, which often is a part of the HCC screening program (Fig. 3).

Transplant Artery Patency

Given the small size of the hepatic artery and it main branches, accurate diagnosis of occlusion of the transplant hepatic artery may be challenging. Hepatic artery thrombosis (HAT) is the most common and one of the most devastating vascular complications in liver transplant and must be recognized early for appropriate treatment and management in order to save the graft. Part of the difficulty in diagnosing hepatic artery occlusion using conventional US is due to its close proximity to the portal vein. A known limitation of CDUS is the blooming of color beyond vascular walls, which in this case means that the flow in the larger portal vein can obscure the hepatic artery. Based on the published literature,[12,16,18,19] there is clear evidence that CEUS improves the diagnostic assessment of HAT and hepatic artery stenosis, compared with conventional US.[22–25] CEUS also has been shown to be a more optimal choice when comparing it to other imaging modalities. Thus, 1 study showed an increased sensitivity of CEUS to detect HAT compared with CT angiography, with sensitivities of 89% and 82%, respectively.[26]

Renal transplants also are well suited for evaluation by CEUS, especially because the use of iodinated contrast often is avoided to protect renal function. Vascular complications of renal transplants range from renal vein thrombosis, which happens early after transplant, to renal artery thrombosis, which is a very rare occurrence, to renal artery stenosis, which is a later but not uncommon complication occurring in approximately 3% of renal transplants.[27] Renal transplants commonly are followed with CDUS for evaluation of potential vascular complications but the gold standard remains digital subtraction angiography,

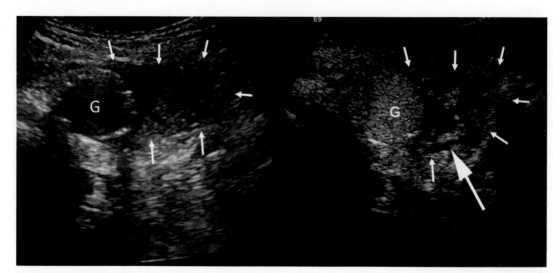

Fig. 2. Type II endoleak in a 75 year old male with prior endovascular aortic stent graft repair (EVAR). Gray scale (*left*) and contrast enhanced (*right*) ultrasound images of the aorta obtained in transverse plane demonstrate contrast opacification of the post EVAR lumen of the aorta (G) at the level of the aneurysm, findings compatible with patency of the stent graft. There is a focal area of contrast opacification (*long white arrow*) within the aneurysmal sac (*short white arrows*), likely from the lumbar artery, compatible with Type II endoleak. (Images *courtesy* of John S. Pellerito, MD, Diagnostic Radiology, Northwell Health System, Manhasset, NY.)

which is an invasive technique. CEUS can provide important information about the patency of the transplant vasculature as well as the vessel caliber and assess for the presence of arterial or venous stenosis.[28] CEUS also can be useful in detecting areas of infarct (**Fig. 4**).

Challenges with CEUS imaging of visceral organ transplants include the presence of overlying bandages obscuring a possible sonographic window or overlying drains in the early postoperative period.

B-FLOW IMAGING

BFI is a non-Doppler technology that provides real-time imaging of blood flow during gray-scale sonography.[29] BFIs are formed by using (1) coded excitation to improve blood echo sensitivity and (2) tissue equalization to reduce the relative brightness of tissue, so that both tissue and blood can be simultaneously visualized. This technique has no detrimental effect on frame rate compared with Doppler US, and because of this can be displayed in the entire field of view irrespective of direction or flow velocity. Thus the information on the display can be updated quickly and the vessel of interest can be assessed for patency even if it is located deep in the abdomen or pelvis. Because BFI is based on gray-scale US, it does not have the same limitations as CDUS and spectral Doppler US for detection of flow, such as aliasing and angle dependency. Moreover, B-flow

identifies and amplifies motion of individual blood cells as reflectors and can detect either low-flow or high-flow states without blooming, thus allowing for the simultaneous evaluation of vascular walls and enhancing the ability to identify nonocclusive thrombi. The ability of B-mode to image blood flow and tissue simultaneously allows for the display of blood flow and vessel walls with exceptional speed and clarity, which holds promise for expanding the clinical applications of US and improving early detection of peripheral vascular diseases. The benefits of B-flow do not come without some drawbacks, however, namely the inadequate sensitivity of this application to discern flow direction or velocity.[30]

Carotid Arteries and Peripheral Vascular Disease

BFI revolutionized evaluation of the carotid arteries by offering more flow-sensitive capabilities to the US examination. In contrast to Doppler sonography, which is predisposed to loss of signal due to inadvertent filtering out of a specific range of Doppler shifts that could be originating from slow flow but instead are presumed to be generated by noise and tissue vibration, BFI allows for all information from moving blood to be analyzed and displayed. Additionally, oversaturation that may be associated with color Doppler imaging, due to high gain settings, does not play role in BFI. This allows for clear visualization of the vascular wall,

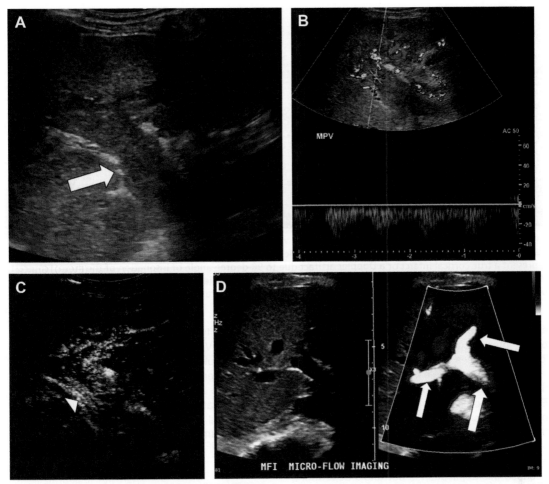

Fig. 3. Utility of Contrast-enhanced Ultrasound in diagnosis of portal vein thrombus in a 56 year old male with chronic hepatitis. (*A*) Grey scale US shows echogenic thrombus in the dilated main portal vein (*white arrow*). Note heterogeneous liver parenchyma. (*B*) Spectral Doppler image of the portal vein demonstrates a low-resistance arterial wave form, however, it is uncertain if the presence of arterial flow is attributable to tumor thrombus or contamination from the adjacent hepatic artery. (*C*) Contrast-enhanced ultrasound of the liver shows enhancement in the portal vein thrombus at 10 seconds after injection confirms tumor thrombus and increases diagnostic confidence (*arrowhead*). (*D*) Comparison dual gray scale and MFI image of the liver in a different patient demonstrates patent main portal vein and its main braches (*white arrows in D*).

clear assessment of lumen patency, and, if present, the surface of an atherosclerotic plaque (**Fig. 5**). BFI can demonstrate blood flow swirling in regions of ulceration or vessel tortuosity, a pattern of flow that should be commented on in the radiology report because it has been shown to contribute to thrombus formation.[31] Moreover, a nonocclusive thrombus within a vessel lumen can be accurately detected and not overlooked as on color Doppler. BFI has been demonstrated to be superior to CDUS in the identification of internal carotid artery dissection, with sensitivity of 94% and specificity of 94% (compared with 83% and 84%, respectively, on CDUS).[32]

A few limitations associated with BFI are worth mentioning. A substantial technical limitation of BFI is in estimating the degree of carotid artery stenosis, which usually is attributable to the presence of extensive calcified plaque in the carotid artery wall that interferes with the ability of BFI to achieve a clear sonographic window into the vessel. Another significant limitation of BFI is a display of an ill-defined vessel wall that usually is caused by excessive pulsation and resultant movement of the surrounding structures. Additionally, the sensitivity of BFI is decreased with increasing depth because of a strong dependence of BFI on signal intensity strength. This limitation is

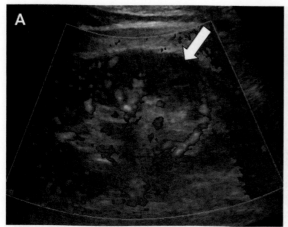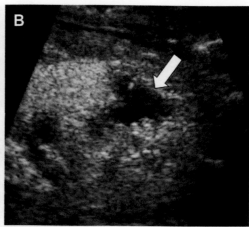

Fig. 4. Cortical focal infarct in a 48-year-old patient with renal transplant with infarct. (*A*) Power Doppler US demonstrates a peripheral, wedge-shaped hypoechoic area of absent perfusion (*white arrow*). This may either represent a true cortical infarct or a Doppler artifact due to 90-degree angle of insonation of the area of interest. (*B*) CEUS of the renal transplant obtained 5 minutes post contrast injection demonstrates focal area of absent perfusion in the renal cortex compatible with a true renal cortical infarct (*white arrow*).

especially important in the evaluation of the post-bulbar internal carotid artery, because the vessel location increases in depth as it courses cranially.

BFI plays a major role in the assessment of peripheral vascular disease. In 1 study of 60 patients, BFI was found particularly beneficial in evaluating patients with small vessels, minimal wall calcifications, multilevel stenoses, tortuous vessels, and vascular collaterals. BFI was shown to be less affected by shadowing from calcifications and, because this application is not angle dependent, it often could assess flow in vessels that could not be interrogated with color Doppler. BFI appears to have value in regions of near occlusion, where color Doppler may incorrectly suggest complete occlusion.[33] Soft tissue vibration associated with an arteriovenous fistula, known as a perivascular color bruit, is a phenomenon that can significantly exaggerate the apparent dimensions of a vascular fistula on Doppler sonography, whereas BFI correctly displays the true dimensions.[29]

Abdominal Vasculature

Because BFI amplifies the signal of moving blood cells, it is less likely to artifactually demonstrate no flow in a slow-flow vessel. This is particularly useful in assessing liver vasculature,[29,30] because BFI can be used to detect thrombus in the portal vein in the challenging setting of slow flow or cirrhosis. Transjugular intrahepatic portosystemic shunts also are well evaluated with BFI because it is free from the challenges and limitations of color Doppler (**Fig. 6**). The modality remains of limited overall utility in this setting, however, due

to its inability to determine directionality and velocity of flow. Vascular stenosis typically is diagnosed when Doppler sonography reveals a localized flow jet. Turbulence and other factors, however, also can cause localized acceleration of flow that is not associated with anatomic narrowing. BFI can be helpful in distinguishing between false-positive and true-positive cases of vascular stenosis.[29]

Transplants

Imaging of transplant organs can be challenging. The use of BFI can eliminate the challenges often encountered by CDUS, such as angle dependence, aliasing, and blooming. Because of angle dependency, CDUS can have difficulty demonstrating flow in the poles of a transplant kidney, but BFI does not have this limitation and will demonstrate all patent vessels in the field of view regardless of their direction of flow or velocity (**Fig. 7**). Also, because there is no blooming, vessel size can be measured accurately, which provides additional aid in evaluation of vascular stenosis. Moreover, BFI may be able to detect small occlusive or nonocclusive thrombi that could be obscured by oversaturation of CDUS signal.[34] In instances where there is more than 1 transplant artery, BFI can be useful in identifying the vascular anatomy. BFI also can help detect small arteriovenous malformations or pseudoaneurysms that commonly are seen in transplant organs as a sequela of prior biopsy.

Evaluation of solid organ transplants with BFI is a relatively understudied area that is bound to

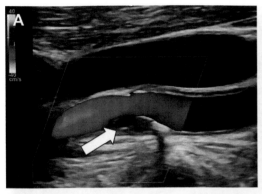
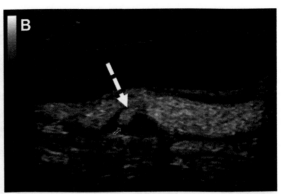

Fig. 5. Internal carotid artery plaque with plaque ulceration in a 67-year old female. (*A*) Color Doppler US obtained in long axis shows patent internal carotid artery (ICA) lumen with associated soft plaque without significant luminal stenosis. No flow is seen on CDUS within the plaque to suggest an ulceration. (*B*) B-flow imaging demonstrates flow within the carotid plaque compatible with ulceration (*dashed arrow*).

expand with greater acceptance of these new, innovative vascular US techniques. The ability of BFI to detect slow flow and relatively small vessels makes it a great adjunct imaging modality in addition to Doppler US in evaluating solid organ transplants.

MICROVASCULAR IMAGING

Microvascular imaging (MVI), microflow imaging (MFI), and superb microvascular flow imaging (SMI) are the new frontier techniques for detection of slow flow that are based on PDUS. MVI and MFI combine the direct imaging capabilities of digital microscopy with the precise control of microfluidics. They offer high-resolution images with 85% sampling efficiency, more precise sizing and counting, full morphologic detail for all subvisible particles in a sample, and the complete confidence of the interpreting radiologist to accurately identify vascular flow. They are capable of detecting flow in very small vessels with a high frame rate by suppressing motion in surrounding tissue (clutter).[1,35] The MVI, MFI, and SMI technologies can either allow overlay of a 2-dimensional (2-D) image behind the microvascular flow, thus displaying both the vascular bed and the background information (for example organ parenchyma and the intraparenchymal vessel), or may use subtraction capabilities in which only vasculature is displayed while the rest of the background signal is eliminated (2-D blending). These techniques also can offer a dual display of 2-D and subtraction images simultaneously. The ability to detect vascular flow utilizing these newer techniques is striking. MVI has excellent 2-D temporal resolution that minimizes side lobe artifacts and misregistrations and offers superb depth of beam penetration that allows evaluation of deeply located structures and vessels.

Artifact reduction capabilities can also reduce unwanted and image degrading artifacts.

SMI can be operated in 2 modes, either with color display or monochromatic. With the monochromatic option, the background signals are subtracted and only signals related to the vasculature are displayed.

Current research and work on these applications is focused on improved identification of flow direction and measurement of absolute velocities, which some of the aforementioned technologies are still lacking. An additional significant limitation relates to poor performance of these applications in the setting of high velocities. For example, when a high-velocity vessel is seen adjacent to a low-velocity vessel, detection of flow is compromised. Moreover, when the vessel is located adjacent to a larger caliber vessel that displays significant cardiac pulsation (for example the aorta or carotid artery), analysis of blood flow in the vessel of interest may be impeded by artifact generated by pulsation. In these cases, a different acoustic window may be selected that can help in separating the pulsating vessel from the vessel of interest.

Carotid Plaque and Peripheral Vascular Disease

Microflow and related imaging techniques are promising applications for differentiating stable from unstable plaque in the carotid vascular bed. Due to their ability to identify very-low-amplitude flow, these applications are able to detect microvascularity in carotid plaques, which imply that they are unstable. It recently has been established that atheromatous plaques with neovascularity are associated with instability.[36,37] Although CEUS also has been shown useful in

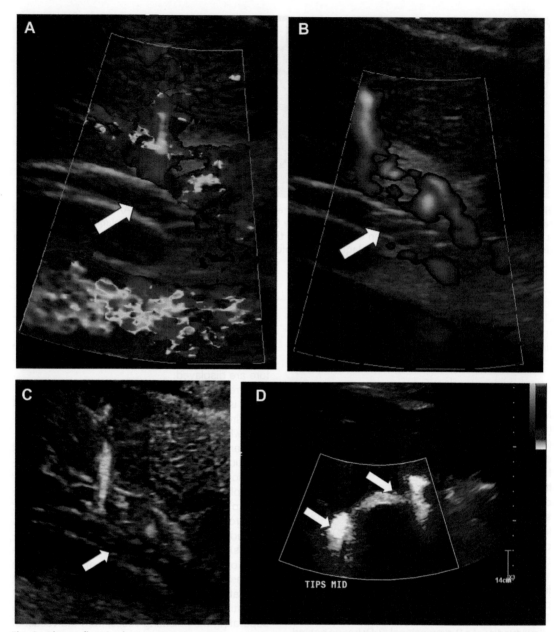

Fig. 6. Absent flow in the transjugular intrahepatic portosystemic shunt (TIPS) in a 63-year-old male 6 days post TIPS placement. (*A*) Color Doppler US obtained in a transverse plane demonstrates absent flow within the TIPS (*white arrow*). Note excessive flow outside of the TIPS in the hepatic parenchyma and its vasculature due to high gain setting and color blooming artifact. (*B*) Conventional power Doppler also shows no flow within the TIPS concerning for occlusion versus air related artifact (*white arrow*). (*C*) B-flow imaging of the TIPS demonstrates absent flow within the shunt (*white arrow*) confirming diagnosis of occlusion. Note also improved visualization of the hepatic vessels adjacent to the TIPS, which is attributable to better sensitivity to flow and absence of blooming artifact on B-flow imaging. (*D*) Comparison MFI image of the liver in a different patient obtained in transverse plane demonstrates patency of the TIPS throughout its length (*white arrows*).

detecting flow within a plaque, this technique requires placement of an intravenous line and is more time consuming. On the other hand, MVI has been shown to have 100% specificity and 63% sensitivity for detection of flow within a plaque compared with CEUS.[38]

MVI can play a significant role in evaluation of patients with peripheral arterial disease. Imaging

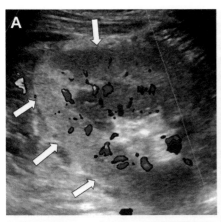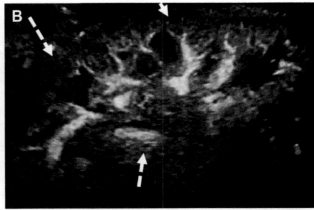

Fig. 7. Limitations of B-flow imaging in visualization of the background nonvascular structures. Early postoperative renal transplant. (A) Color Doppler US of the renal transplant obtained in transverse plane demonstrates patent intrarenal vessels and markedly heterogenous renal cortical parenchyma (*white arrows* in A). (B) B-flow image of the renal transplant shows improved visualization of the intrarenal vasculature, demonstrating interlobar and interlobular vessels, however limits in its ability to visualize gray scale background information of the heterogeneous renal parenchyma (*dashed arrows* in B), which is concerning for possible transplant rejection or infection.

findings can strongly influence management of these patients, regarding available options for operative intervention, such as angioplasty, thrombectomy, plaque removal, and stent or bypass graft placement. For example, when no flow is identified on color Doppler in a lower extremity peripheral artery, the vessel is considered occluded and intraluminal revascularization is not considered feasible. In contrast, when even minimal trickling of flow is detected in the artery of interest, the surgeon can be confident that the attempt to revascularize this artery with angioplasty will likely be successful. Therefore, the availability of sonographic applications, such as MFI and MVI, which have a very high sensitivity for flow detection, is appealing. Microflow applications may have potential in improving diagnostic accuracy and capability of flow detection and in providing a road map to guide management options for patients with PAD.

Imaging of microvascular flow also can be useful in distinguishing partial from complete occlusion when evaluating for deep vein thrombosis (**Fig. 8**).

Endoleak after Endovascular Aneurysm Repair

MVI also may offer some advantages over CDUS for detecting endoleaks after EVAR. It has been established that, depending on the severity and type of endoleak, patient management may be altered and reoperation may be required. This is true particularly if imaging identifies progression of aneurysmal sac size. Because conventional Doppler US may not detect slow flow at the level of the endoleak, this pathology may go unrecognized. MFI offers much

more sensitive slow flow detection and may improve diagnostic accuracy in the assessment of endoleaks. It also has to be taken into consideration, however, that some of the smaller endoleaks, in particular type 2 leaks (associated with the inferior mesenteric artery or lumbar arterial supply to the aneurysmal sac), do not always need to be addressed because their presence does not change the morbidity or mortality of patients post-EVAR. In 1 study of 57 patients who had undergone EVAR, 8 type II endoleaks were detected using digital subtraction angiography as the gold standard, and results were compared with CT angiography, CEUS, MVI, and CDUS. MVI was demonstrated to be more accurate than CDUS in the identification of endoleaks, with a sensitivity of 75% and a specificity of 98% compared with 63% and 93%, respectively. CEUS in this study had the best performance in detecting endoleak, with sensitivity and specificity of 100%.[39] The benefit of MVI in this setting is that it does not require an intravenous line and is less expensive and time consuming. As discussed previously, one of the limitations of MVI in evaluation of endoleak is related to its inability to accurately detect flow due to interference from cardiac pulsation in the adjacent aorta. To minimize this artifact, only the aneurysmal sac itself can be assessed for the presence of flow, while the stent graft is kept out of the image.

Native Abdominal Vasculature and Transplant Evaluation

As discussed previously, the most common complications of solid organ transplants are vascular

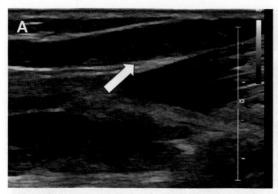
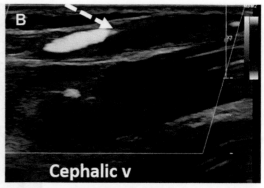

Fig. 8. Nonocclusive cephalic vein thrombosis in a 58-year-old male. (*A*) Longitudinal gray scale US image of the left upper extremity obtained at the level of the antecubital fossa demonstrates echogenic material within the distended cephalic vein (*white arrow*) compatible with likely acute/subacute superficial thrombus. (*B*) Microflow imaging (MFI) of the area of interest demonstrates flow through part of the left cephalic vein and is able to accurately diagnose the thrombus as only partially occlusive (*dashed arrow*).

complications; therefore, accurate assessment of vessels for potential occlusion or vascular compromise is paramount in graft evaluation. In patients with liver transplants, flow within the hepatic artery and its branches may be compromised either by hepatic artery occlusion or significant stenosis, and differentiation of these 2 entities plays an essential role in management of liver transplants. MVI and MFI offer detection of low amplitude flow within the liver parenchyma and improve confidence in the diagnosis of hepatic artery patency as well as overall liver perfusion.

Also, MFI and MVI potentially can improve visibility of slow flow in the hepatic veins in patients with suspected Budd-Chiari syndrome. Generally, the color Doppler diagnosis relies mainly on detection of flow in the central hepatic veins and intrahepatic inferior vena cava, due to limitations in

visualization of more peripheral branches of the hepatic venous system. The postsinusoidal type of Budd-Chiari syndrome, however, typically results from the occlusion of more peripheral hepatic veins that usually are not well seen on color Doppler imaging, and, in these instances, MFI and MVI may be able to aid in establishing an accurate diagnosis.

Renal transplants may be complicated by development of cortical infarcts due to thromboembolization, vascular stenosis, or vasospasm that may not be apparent on color Doppler imaging (due to limitation in flow visualization in the cortical vessels). MFI and MVI also may aid in identification of flow in the fine vessels of the renal cortex, thus providing a better assessment of overall transplant perfusion and viability (**Fig. 9**). Moreover, both MFI and MVI, can be used to obtain and analyze wave-

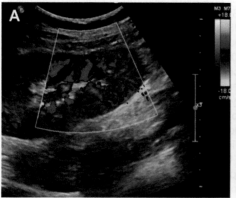
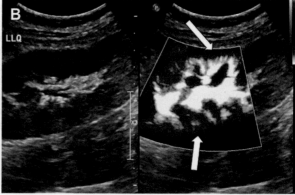

Fig. 9. Comparison of CDUS and MFI imaging in demonstration of normal renal transplant perfusion. (*A*) CDUS of the left lower quadrant (LLQ) renal transplant obtained in sagittal plane demonstrates flow within the interlobar arteries of the transplant kidney. (*B*) Dual gray scale (left) and MFI (right) images show that MFI is more sensitive for detection of slow flow and thus demonstrates improved visualization of flow in the interlobular and arcuate arteries (*white arrows in B*). Note intact corticomedullary differentiation best appreciated on gray scale image (left in *B*).

forms in the arcuate and interlobar arteries of the renal transplant.

Although Doppler US traditionally has been the first imaging modality in evaluating renal and liver transplants, its application in evaluating pancreatic transplants has not been shown to be as useful and in these cases it often is relegated to guiding biopsies in cases of rejection. Because of its ability to detect slow flow in small vessels, microvascular flow imaging shows promise in monitoring pancreatic transplants for vascular complications.[40]

DEVELOPMENTS ON THE HORIZON

There are several additional sonographic imaging applications that have a potential role in the field of advanced vascular sonography; however, they still are under investigation and are minimally utilized. These include but are not limited to photoacoustic imaging (PAI), 3-D vascular imaging, vascular elastography, intravascular US (IVUS), and applications for accurate flow volume estimation. The literature is still scarce, however, regarding their use in clinical practice.

PAI allows the delivery of light energy that is absorbed by tissues and causes a thermoelastic expansion. This expansion then generates US waves that are detected by the transducer and produce images of optical absorption contrast within tissues. PAI is a promising new technique to obtain both anatomic and functional information about the vascular bed. It can provide an insight into the plaque structure and composition by utilizing the optical contrast, which is derived from the differences in the absorption spectra of plaque components to image composition. This imaging is capable of differentiating oxygenated and deoxygenated blood flow within tissues.[41] One of the main goals for this application is to be able to determine if a cardiac or carotid plaque contains oxygenated plaque, which would imply vulnerable plaque.[42,43] Additionally, this application can aid in differentiation of chronic versus acute blood that would be of clinical significance in management of patients with deep vein thrombosis.[44] For example, if the deep vein thrombus is acute, thrombectomy by either vascular surgeons or by interventional radiologists can be performed.

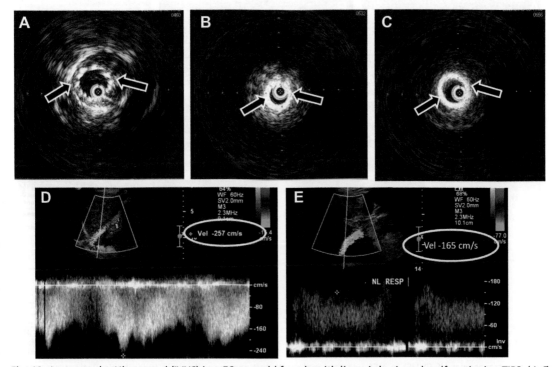

Fig. 10. Intravascular Ultrasound (IVUS) in a 56-year-old female with liver cirrhosis and malfunctioning TIPS. (A-C) IVUS images of the TIPS obtained within the lumen of the TIPS at the portal end (A), mid (B) and hepatic end (C) levels demonstrate marked narrowing of the diameter in the mid portion of the TIPs (arrows in B) when compared to luminal diameter at the portal end (arrows in A) and the hepatic end (arrows in C). (D) Corresponding Spectral Doppler US reveals high peak systolic velocities in the mid TIPS (yellow circle, velocity=240 cm/s) compatible with significant stenosis. (E) Spectral Doppler images obtained after dilatation of the TIPS reveal improvement in the PSVs in the mid TIPs (yellow circle, velocity=165 cm/s).

Moreover, this technique has a capacity to image lipids within the atheromatous plaque and target disease markers such as inflammatory cells, calcium, and more. PAI can provide a powerful prognostic marker for disease progression and, therefore, transform the management of vascular disease.[42]

Shear wave elastography (SWE) has been used mainly for detection of cancerous tumors and staging of liver fibrosis.[45] SWE, however, also may be used for the measurement of arterial wall stiffness. Additionally, Couade and colleagues[46] suggested that this method may be used for the detection of unstable (vulnerable) plaque. It has been established that SWE can provide quantitative assessment of arterial wall biomechanical properties.[46-48]

When blood clot age cannot be determined by US duplex analysis, elastography may offer a helpful adjunct. Both strain elastography and SWE are the most common techniques to age thrombus. These elastography techniques can distinguish between acute and chronic clots by characterizing tissue stiffness.[49]

Recent advances in technology and the development of 3-D US imaging software for assessment of vascular flow raise hopes for changing the current perception of US as functioning solely as a tool for screening and a noninvasive modality for evaluation of the carotid circulation. With this new technology, US not only may be comparable to but also actually may exceed the capabilities of CTA and MRA, by providing better 3-D characterization of a carotid plaque (wall irregularity, composition, size in three dimensions, and presence or absence of ulceration), more accurately measuring the degree of luminal stenosis, and most importantly by assessing flow dynamics proximal and distal to the plaque.[50-53] These factors potentially could have a significant impact on the surgical decision to intervene. The ability to accurately determine flow volume in a normal vascular segment as well as at a level of marked stenosis will completely revamp the thinking about

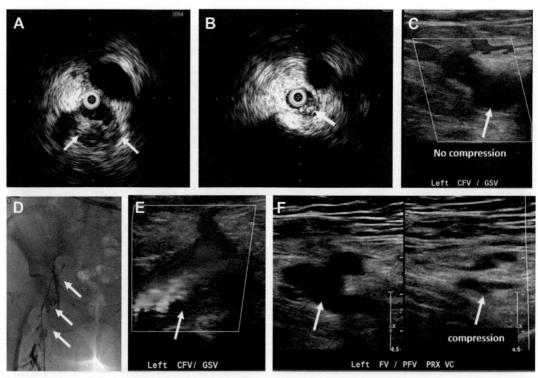

Fig. 11. Intravascular US (IVUS) in a 58-year-old male with left common iliac vein thrombosis. Patient presented for thrombectomy. (*A, B*) IVUS images obtained from the proximal and mid segments of the common iliac vein (CIV) demonstrate a filling defect and narrowing in the CFV compatible with thrombus (*arrows in A, B*). (*C*) Corresponding Doppler US of the left lower extremity reveals near occlusive thrombus in the left CIV (*arrow in C*) that propagated from the left femoral and popliteal veins (not shown). (*D*) Selective venogram showed a filling defect in the left femoral vein (FV) and common femoral vein (CFV) extending to the CIV (*arrows in D*). (*E, F*) Post thrombectomy gray scale (*E*), color Doppler (*F*) US images demonstrate patency and compressibility of the CIV and FV (*arrows*).

the necessity to surgically or medically manage carotid plaques.[54,55]

Lastly, IVUS is an application currently utilized for the guidance of various interventional procedures and assessment of vascular lumen and wall. IVUS aids in selected cases of balloon angioplasty and stent placement with complex vascular anatomy and unclear findings at angiography. It facilitates accurate measurements of the vessel dimensions and reveals the extent of the intravascular disease, and it allows accurate measurement of the vessel lumen and assessment of the atherosclerotic plaque for the selection of proper angioplasty balloon size as well as confirming full expansion and attachment of the stent or stent graft to the arterial wall. Additionally, IVUS provides guidance for percutaneous fenestration of a dissection flap, facilitates placement of vena cava filter, and aids in peripheral endovascular interventions (**Figs. 10 and 11**).[56,57]

SUMMARY

The advanced and innovative vascular US technologies discussed in this article make US a relevant and useful tool for vascular imaging and a modality of choice in complicated vascular cases. US portability, accessibility, and cost-effectiveness make this modality even more attractive over other imaging options. Significant advances in technology and availability of powerful and highly flow-sensitive new applications add value to traditional vascular US by boosting its potential to be the preferred imaging modality for evaluation of central abdominal and peripheral vasculature. These techniques can be used in conjunction with and offer a complementary role to Doppler US. With the added benefit of dynamic, real-time imaging along with increased visualization and characterization of small vessels and slow flow, US can rival other modalities, such as CT and MRI, especially in those situations where a patient may be unable to receive iodinated or gadolinium contrast.

Given the relatively new nature of these innovative vascular US applications, further research and experience are necessary to understand their full utility and potential. These techniques are readily accessible, however, on most new US machines, which makes them easy to trial in different clinical scenarios. With the exception of CEUS, which requires an intravenous line, the rest of the techniques are noninvasive and have a relatively short learning curve. Image optimization, identification of artifacts, and understanding the limitations of each technique are imperative to their utilization and to capitalize on their ability to make accurate diagnoses in challenging vascular cases.

DISCLOSURE

The authors have nothing to disclose.

REFERENCES

1. Revzin MV, Imanzadeh A, Menias C, et al. Optimizing Image Quality When Evaluating Blood Flow at Doppler US: A Tutorial. Radiographics 2019; 39(5):1501–23.
2. Kruskal JB, Newman PA, Sammons LG, et al. Optimizing Doppler and color flow US: application to hepatic sonography. Radiographics 2004;24(3): 657–75.
3. Di Siervi P, Bellizzi V, Pagano F, et al. The role of directional power Doppler in vascular characterization of renal masses. Arch Ital Urol Androl 2005; 77(1):69–72.
4. Di Siervi P, Pagano F, Bellizzi V, et al. The role of directional power Doppler in early detection of the onset of neoangiogenesis in a case of small hyperechoic renal lesion. Arch Ital Urol Androl 2009;81(4): 228–32.
5. Wilson SR, Greenbaum LD, Goldberg BB. Contrast-enhanced ultrasound: what is the evidence and what are the obstacles? AJR Am J Roentgenol 2009;193(1):55–60.
6. Harvey CJ, Blomley MJ, Eckersley RJ, et al. Developments in ultrasound contrast media. Eur Radiol 2001;11(4):675–89.
7. Huang DY, Yusuf GT, Daneshi M, et al. Contrast-enhanced ultrasound (CEUS) in abdominal intervention. Abdom Radiol (N Y) 2018;43(4):960–76.
8. Tang C, Fang K, Guo Y, et al. Safety of Sulfur Hexafluoride Microbubbles in Sonography of Abdominal and Superficial Organs: Retrospective Analysis of 30,222 Cases. J Ultrasound Med 2017;36(3):531–8.
9. Piscaglia F, Bolondi L. Italian Society for Ultrasound in M, Biology Study Group on Ultrasound Contrast A. The safety of Sonovue in abdominal applications: retrospective analysis of 23188 investigations. Ultrasound Med Biol 2006;32(9):1369–75.
10. Weinstein S, Jordan E, Goldstein R, et al. How to set up a contrast-enhanced ultrasound service. Abdom Radiol (N Y) 2018;43(4):808–18.
11. Albuquerque FC Jr, Tonnessen BH, Noll RE Jr, et al. Paradigm shifts in the treatment of abdominal aortic aneurysm: trends in 721 patients between 1996 and 2008. J Vasc Surg 2010;51(6):1348–52 [discussion: 1352–3].
12. Ten Bosch JA, Rouwet EV, Peters CT, et al. Contrast-enhanced ultrasound versus computed tomographic angiography for surveillance of endovascular abdominal aortic aneurysm repair. J Vasc Interv Radiol 2010;21(5):638–43.

13. Manning BJ, O'Neill SM, Haider SN, et al. Duplex ultrasound in aneurysm surveillance following endovascular aneurysm repair: a comparison with computed tomography aortography. J Vasc Surg 2009;49(1):60–5.

14. Andeweg CS, Mulder IM, Felt-Bersma RJ, et al. Guidelines of diagnostics and treatment of acute left-sided colonic diverticulitis. Dig Surg 2013; 30(4–6):278–92.

15. Elkouri S, Panneton JM, Andrews JC, et al. Computed tomography and ultrasound in follow-up of patients after endovascular repair of abdominal aortic aneurysm. Ann Vasc Surg 2004;18(3):271–9.

16. Abraha I, Luchetta ML, De Florio R, et al. Ultrasonography for endoleak detection after endoluminal abdominal aortic aneurysm repair. Cochrane Database Syst Rev 2017;(6):CD010296.

17. Abbas A, Hansrani V, Sedgwick N, et al. 3D contrast enhanced ultrasound for detecting endoleak following endovascular aneurysm repair (EVAR). Eur J Vasc Endovasc Surg 2014;47(5):487–92.

18. Ghouri YA, Mian I, Rowe JH. Review of hepatocellular carcinoma: Epidemiology, etiology, and carcinogenesis. J Carcinog 2017;16:1.

19. Raza SA, Jang HJ, Kim TK. Differentiating malignant from benign thrombosis in hepatocellular carcinoma: contrast-enhanced ultrasound. Abdom Imaging 2014;39(1):153–61.

20. Sereni CP, Rodgers SK, Kirby CL, et al. Portal vein thrombus and infiltrative HCC: a pictoral review. Abdom Radiol (N Y) 2017;42(1):159–70.

21. Tarantino L, Francica G, Sordelli I, et al. Diagnosis of benign and malignant portal vein thrombosis in cirrhotic patients with hepatocellular carcinoma: color Doppler US, contrast-enhanced US, and fine-needle biopsy. Abdom Imaging 2006;31(5): 537–44.

22. Fontanilla T, Noblejas A, Cortes C, et al. Contrast-enhanced ultrasound of liver lesions related to arterial thrombosis in adult liver transplantation. J Clin Ultrasound 2013;41(8):493–500.

23. Lu Q, Zhong XF, Huang ZX, et al. Role of contrast-enhanced ultrasound in decision support for diagnosis and treatment of hepatic artery thrombosis after liver transplantation. Eur J Radiol 2012;81(3): e338–43.

24. Sidhu PS, Ellis SM, Karani JB, et al. Hepatic artery stenosis following liver transplantation: significance of the tardus parvus waveform and the role of microbubble contrast media in the detection of a focal stenosis. Clin Radiol 2002;57(9):789–99.

25. Zheng RQ, Mao R, Ren J, et al. Contrast-enhanced ultrasound for the evaluation of hepatic artery stenosis after liver transplantation: potential role in changing the clinical algorithm. Liver Transpl 2010;16(6): 729–35.

26. Kim JS, Kim KW, Lee J, et al. Diagnostic Performance for Hepatic Artery Occlusion After Liver Transplantation: Computed Tomography Angiography Versus Contrast-Enhanced Ultrasound. Liver Transpl 2019;25(11):1651–60.

27. Sugi MD, Joshi G, Maddu KK, et al. Imaging of Renal Transplant Complications throughout the Life of the Allograft: Comprehensive Multimodality Review. Radiographics 2019;39(5):1327–55.

28. Kazmierski B, Deurdulian C, Tchelepi H, et al. Applications of contrast-enhanced ultrasound in the kidney. Abdom Radiol (N Y) 2018;43(4):880–98.

29. Wachsberg RH. B-flow imaging of the hepatic vasculature: correlation with color Doppler sonography. AJR Am J Roentgenol 2007;188(6):W522–33.

30. Wachsberg RH. B-flow, a non-Doppler technology for flow mapping: early experience in the abdomen. Ultrasound Q 2003;19(3):114–22.

31. Umemura A, Yamada K. B-mode flow imaging of the carotid artery. Stroke 2001;32(9):2055–7.

32. Tola M, Yurdakul M, Cumhur T. B-flow imaging in low cervical internal carotid artery dissection. J Ultrasound Med 2005;24(11):1497–502.

33. D'Abate F, Ramachandran V, Young MA, et al. B-Flow Imaging in Lower Limb Peripheral Arterial Disease and Bypass Graft Ultrasonography. Ultrasound Med Biol 2016;42(9):2345–51.

34. Morgan TA, Jha P, Poder L, et al. Advanced ultrasound applications in the assessment of renal transplants: contrast-enhanced ultrasound, elastography, and B-flow. Abdom Radiol (N Y) 2018;43(10): 2604–14.

35. Jiang ZZ, Huang YH, Shen HL, et al. Clinical Applications of Superb Microvascular Imaging in the Liver, Breast, Thyroid, Skeletal Muscle, and Carotid Plaques. J Ultrasound Med 2019;38(11):2811–20.

36. Shah PK. Biomarkers of plaque instability. Curr Cardiol Rep 2014;16(12):547.

37. Andrews JPM, Fayad ZA, Dweck MR. New methods to image unstable atherosclerotic plaques. Atherosclerosis 2018;272:118–28.

38. Oura K, Kato T, Ohba H, et al. Evaluation of Intraplaque Neovascularization Using Superb Microvascular Imaging and Contrast-Enhanced Ultrasonography. J Stroke Cerebrovasc Dis 2018; 27(9):2348–53.

39. Cantisani V, David E, Ferrari D, et al. Color Doppler ultrasound with superb microvascular imaging compared to contrast-enhanced ultrasound and computed tomography angiography to identify and classify endoleaks in patients undergoing EVAR. Ann Vasc Surg 2017;40:136–45.

40. Tokodai K, Miyagi S, Nakanishi C, et al. The utility of superb microvascular imaging for monitoring low-velocity venous flow following pancreas transplantation: report of a case. J Med Ultrason (2001) 2018; 45(1):171–4.

41. Kolkman RG, Brands PJ, Steenbergen W, et al. Real-time in vivo photoacoustic and ultrasound imaging. J Biomed Opt 2008;13(5):050510.

42. Jansen K, van Soest G, van der Steen AF. Intravascular photoacoustic imaging: a new tool for vulnerable plaque identification. Ultrasound Med Biol 2014;40(6):1037–48.

43. Jansen K, van der Steen AF, van Beusekom HM, et al. Intravascular photoacoustic imaging of human coronary atherosclerosis. Opt Lett 2011;36(5):597–9.

44. Karpiouk AB, Aglyamov SR, Mallidi S, et al. Combined ultrasound and photoacoustic imaging to detect and stage deep vein thrombosis: phantom and ex vivo studies. J Biomed Opt 2008;13(5):054061.

45. Sarvazyan A, Hall TJ, Urban MW, et al. An overview of elastography - an emerging branch of medical imaging. Curr Med Imaging Rev 2011;7(4):255–82.

46. Couade M, Pernot M, Prada C, et al. Quantitative assessment of arterial wall biomechanical properties using shear wave imaging. Ultrasound Med Biol 2010;36(10):1662–76.

47. Ramnarine KV, Garrard JW, Kanber B, et al. Shear wave elastography imaging of carotid plaques: feasible, reproducible and of clinical potential. Cardiovasc Ultrasound 2014;12:49.

48. Ramnarine KV, Garrard JW, Ummur P, et al. Letter to the editor: shear wave elastography may be superior to grayscale median for the identification of carotid plaque vulnerability: a comparison with histology–authors response. Ultraschall Med 2016;37(1):103–4.

49. Hoang P, Wallace A, Sugi M, et al. Elastography techniques in the evaluation of deep vein thrombosis. Cardiovasc Diagn Ther 2017;7(Suppl 3):S238–45.

50. Steel R, Ramnarine KV, Davidson F, et al. Angle-independent estimation of maximum velocity through stenoses using vector Doppler ultrasound. Ultrasound Med Biol 2003;29(4):575–84.

51. Avdal J, Lovstakken L, Torp H, et al. Combined 2-D vector velocity imaging and tracking doppler for improved vascular blood velocity quantification. IEEE Trans Ultrason Ferroelectr Freq Control 2017;64(12):1795–804.

52. Ekroll IK, Dahl T, Torp H, et al. Combined vector velocity and spectral Doppler imaging for improved imaging of complex blood flow in the carotid arteries. Ultrasound Med Biol 2014;40(7):1629–40.

53. Hansen KL, Udesen J, Oddershede N, et al. In vivo comparison of three ultrasound vector velocity techniques to MR phase contrast angiography. Ultrasonics 2009;49(8):659–67.

54. Kalashyan H, Saqqur M, Shuaib A, et al. Comprehensive and rapid assessment of carotid plaques in acute stroke using a new single sweep method for three-dimensional carotid ultrasound. Echocardiography 2013;30(4):414–8.

55. Kalashyan H, Shuaib A, Gibson PH, et al. Single sweep three-dimensional carotid ultrasound: reproducibility in plaque and artery volume measurements. Atherosclerosis 2014;232(2):397–402.

56. Manninen HI, Rasanen H. Intravascular ultrasound in interventional radiology. Eur Radiol 2000;10(11):1754–62.

57. Spiliopoulos S, Kitrou P, Katsanos K, et al. FD-OCT and IVUS intravascular imaging modalities in peripheral vasculature. Expert Rev Med Devices 2017;14(2):127–34.

Updates in Vascular Computed Tomography

Prabhakar Rajiah, MBBS, MD, FRCR, FSCMR

KEYWORDS

- CT • Vascular • Dual energy • CT angiography • Multienergy CT

KEY POINTS

- Computed tomography (CT) is a highly accurate technique in the evaluation of vascular disease.
- Recent advances in technology enable acquisition of images at high spatial resolution with low artifacts, radiation dose, and contrast.
- Using dual energy CT and photon counting CT, material composition can be characterized.

INTRODUCTION

Computed tomography angiography (CTA) has evolved into a vital noninvasive imaging technique in the evaluation of vascular diseases. CTA relies on optimal contrast opacification of the vasculature of interest following the injection of an appropriate volume of iodinated contrast medium at high flow rates. The advantages of computed tomography (CT) include its near-universal availability, rapid turnaround time, and high accuracy in the evaluation of vascular disease because of its isotropic submillimeter spatial resolution, multiplanar reconstruction capabilities, wide field of view, and excellent temporal resolution.[1] The use of ionizing radiation and iodinated contrast media are the concerns associated with the use of CT.[2] There is no conclusive evidence to link the low-dose radiation of CT with carcinogenesis; however, the linear no-threshold model, which implies that no radiation dose is safe and the risk progressively increases with the radiation dose, has gained credibility. Hence, it is imperative use the lowest possible radiation dose without compromising on image quality.[3] Iodinated contrast material was thought to be associated with the development of contrast-induced nephropathy in patients with risk factors and amplification of the DNA radiation damage by CT.[4,5] Recent evidence has shown the absence of any association between the intravenous CT contrast material and acute kidney injury, even in the presence of predisposing comorbidities,[6–8] questioning the need for prophylactic measures[9] such as volume expansion and decreasing dose of contrast.[10]

Recent advances in CTA have focused on improving the image quality, increasing the acquisition speed, eliminating artifacts, providing tissue/material characterization, and reducing the dose of radiation and iodinated contrast. This article reviews the current state of the art in vascular CT.

SCAN TECHNOLOGY

Multidetector CT scanners are the now the norm in vascular imaging, with current scanners ranging from 4 to 320 detector rows. The wide-array or volume CT scanners have a large z-coverage of up to 16 cm. The entire heart can be imaged in 1 R-R interval, which minimizes motion artifacts from cardiac arrhythmias. The entire body can be scanned in a few seconds, as a result of which motion artifacts can be minimized. Because contrast is required for only a short period of time, the total contrast volume injection is also reduced. Radiation doses are also lower with these scanners. With the use of electrocardiogram (ECG) gating, motion-free images of the coronary arteries can also be obtained in the same study. One study on a 320-volume CT scanner used prospective ECG triggering without medications (acquisition at 40%–50% R-R interval for HR ≥70 beats/min

Department of Radiology, Mayo Clinic, 200 1st Street SW, Rochester, MN 55904, USA
E-mail address: radpr73@gmail.com

Radiol Clin N Am 58 (2020) 671–691
https://doi.org/10.1016/j.rcl.2020.02.011

[bpm] and at 70%–80% R-R interval for HR <70 bpm) to obtain motion-free images of the aortic root, aortic valve, and the coronary arteries, with lower radiation doses.[11]

Ultrafast high-pitch helical mode (flash mode) is one of the several acquisition modes available with the latest generation of dual-source scanners. All these modes can be used either with or without ECG gating. Both the x-ray tubes can be operated at the same energy, which can achieve temporal resolution of up to 66 milliseconds with ECG gating, allowing generation of motion-free images of the aortic root and coronary arteries. Alternatively, the x-ray tubes can be operated at different energy levels (discussed later), providing dual-energy information. With the high-pitch helical mode, patients can be scanned at pitches of up to 3.4 without artifacts because of filling of data gaps by the data from the other x-ray tube. Because of the ultrafast acquisition, the entire aorta can be scanned in just 2 seconds[12,13] (Fig. 1). The absence of motion artifacts caused by such rapid scanning is beneficial in patients who cannot comply with breath-hold instructions, particularly in the emergency room and inpatient settings.[14] The rapid scanning obviates sedation/anesthesia in the pediatric population.[15] Multiple vascular beds, such as the aorta and coronary arteries or heart, head, and neck, can be scanned rapidly in 1 acquisition, saving radiation and contrast doses.[16,17]

The image quality of these scans is higher than that of conventional CTA[18] with less motion artifact and similar vascular attenuation.[19] Flash mode can be performed either without ECG gating or with prospective ECG triggering. The quality of both these modes has been shown to be comparable.[13,20,21] Motion-free images of the aortic root can be obtained even without ECG gating.[13,18] The addition of ECG gating did not substantially reduce motion artifacts in children.[22] Motion-free images of adjacent structures such as heart and pulmonary arteries can also be obtained using the flash mode, although the contrast bolus timing may be an issue with such a rapid acquisition. Motion-free images of the coronary arteries can also be obtained in the same study if the heart rate and variability are low (HR<63 bpm; variability<1.2 bpm) (12) (Fig. 2).

Radiation doses are lower with the flash mode because of decreased overlapping projection data.[12,23] Radiation doses are lower than conventional CTA by 50% to 72% for imaging the entire aorta.[23–25] Contrast dose is also lower with this mode, because arterial contrast is required only for the small duration of scanning.[26] High-pitch helical mode along with 70-kVp tube voltage and

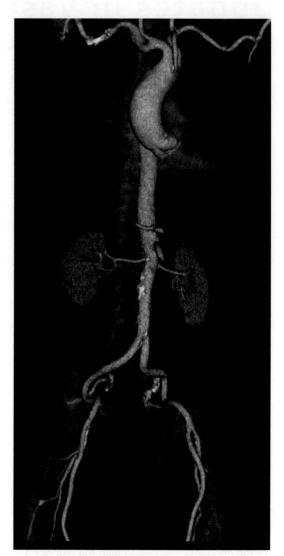

Fig. 1. Three-dimensional (3D) volume-rendered reconstruction of the aorta from an ungated high-pitch helical (flash mode) CTA scan acquired in a dual-source CT scanner. The scan was completed in less than 2 seconds.

iterative reconstruction can achieve radiation dose savings of 81% and contrast-dose savings of 33% with the same image quality of a 120-kVp scan.[27,28] Good-quality images of the renal arteries have been acquired using high-pitch helical mode with 51% contrast dose and 38% radiation dose reduction.[29] Transcatheter aortic valve replacement (TAVR) CTA of the chest, abdomen, and pelvis has been performed by using only 20 mL of contrast.[30,31]

Higher image noise is a challenge of high-pitch helical mode because of the presence of fewer redundant projection values to average.[32] Even with higher noise, the subjective image quality is

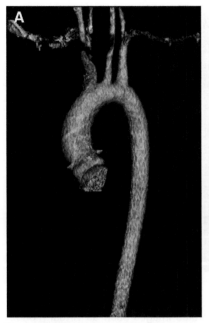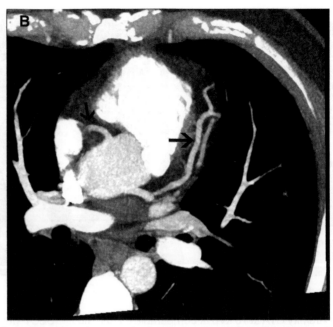

Fig. 2. (*A*) 3D volume-rendered reconstruction of the thoracic aorta obtained using the high-pitch helical mode of a dual-source CT scanner without ECG gating. (*B*) Maximum intensity projection (MIP) reconstruction in the same patient show excellent visualization of the coronary arteries (*arrows*).

comparable with a standard-pitch mode if good contrast opacification is achieved.[33] One study showed poorer image quality for abdominal than thoracic aorta,[25] whereas other studies have shown good quality even for abdominal aorta.[34,35] Noise is a significant challenge in morbidly obese individuals and with low-voltage techniques because of tube saturation.[36] Noise can be reduced by using iterative reconstruction techniques. ECG-gated flash acquisition requires a slow (<70 bpm) and steady heart rate and does not provide functional information because data are gathered from a single cardiac phase with the prospective ECG technique. In some instances, the contrast bolus may be out-run because of the rapid acquisition. Interpolation artifacts may be seen in the earlier generations of dual-source scanners with smaller x-ray detectors.[33] Lower spatial resolution, helical artifacts, and degraded section sensitivity profiles were also challenges associated with the earlier-generation scanners.[29]

LOW-TUBE-VOLTAGE CT

Vascular CT is typically performed at tube voltage of 120 to 140 kVp. Scanning at lower tube voltages (<120 kVp) has the advantage of lower radiation dose because of lower photon flux. However, the lower photon flux increases the image noise,

necessitating compensatory increase in tube currents up to 1500 mAs. Hence, this technique is generally limited to children and those with lean body habitus, and is typically avoided in obese individuals. Iterative reconstruction algorithms can also be used to maintain the image quality by decreasing the noise. Another advantage of low-kVp scanning is the higher signal of contrast caused by higher photoelectric attenuation of iodine as the x-ray energy approximates the k-edge of iodine, which is 33.2 keV. The mean energy of x-ray photons with peak voltage of 80 kVp is 43.7 keV and with peak voltage of 73 kVp is 33.2 keV.

Radiation and contrast-dose savings with maintained image quality have been shown in several CTA studies using tube voltage as low as 70 kVp (**Fig. 3**). A study on 256-slice CT with 100 kVp and 30 mL of iodinated contrast achieved 70% reduction in radiation dose with diagnostic performance comparable with a standard CT.[37] Aortoiliac CTA can be performed at 90 kVp with 60% lower contrast and similar vascular enhancement as a 120-kVp study.[38] At 80 kVp, radiation dose savings of 65% and contrast-dose savings of 30% can be obtained.[39–41] The 80-kVp scans of dual-energy CT also have improved vascular attenuation, diagnostic performance, and salvage of suboptimal studies compared with the mixed images, albeit at a higher noise.[42,43] Lower-

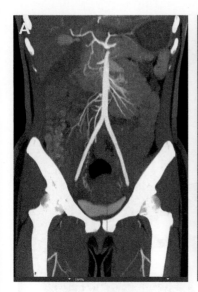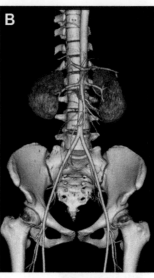

Fig. 3. Coronal reconstruction (*A*) and volume-rendered 3D reconstruction (*B*) of aortoiliac CTA in a 15-year-old boy performed at 70 kVp.

extremity CTA at 70 kVp at comparable diagnostic performance can be obtained with less than half the radiation dose and lower contrast volume of 1.2 mL/kg.[44]Lower-extremity CTA using 70-kVp, high-pitch acquisition and iterative reconstruction can achieve 81% radiation dose reduction and 33% contrast volume reduction.[27] Another dual-source CTA study also used 70 kVp and 80 mAs with 30 mL of contrast following timing bolus to generate good-quality images in peripheral arterial disease.[45] Automatic selection of tube potential and contrast volume based on weight can achieve contrast-dose savings of 20% without compromising image quality.[46] Another similar study that used automated attenuation-based tube voltage selection (70–150 kVp) and individualized low-volume contrast media protocols showed good quality for CTA of the aorta irrespective of the tube voltage.[47]

DUAL-ENERGY CT

Dual-energy CT (DECT) uses the differential attenuation properties of tissues/materials at different energy levels to separate them beyond that possible with a conventional CT. By calculating the attenuation of a voxel at 2 different energies and the prior knowledge of the attenuation coefficients of 2 or 3 dominant materials, the contribution of different tissues to each voxel can be estimated (2-material or 3-material decomposition). Dual-source and rapid kilovoltage-peak switching are the commonly used x-ray source-based technologies, whereas dual layer is the commercially available detector-based DECT technology.[48] In addition to conventional images,

DECT generates images such as virtual monoenergetic imaging (VMI), iodine maps, virtual noncontrast (VNC), and effective atomic number–based images.[48]

VMI mimics CT images obtained with a monoenergetic x-ray beam. In dual-energy CT, VMI can be generated from 40 to 200 keV (kiloelectron volts) by a process of linear combination of basis pair images at different ratios. VMI at 70 keV has the same attenuation as a conventional 120-kVp image, but with lower noise and artifacts.[49] VMI at low energy levels (<70 keV) shows higher signal of iodinated contrast because of higher photoelectric effect closer to the k-edge of iodine.[50] This property is advantageous in reducing the load of iodinated contrast (**Fig. 4**), salvaging suboptimal enhanced studies, generating CTA-quality images from a routine CT scan (**Fig. 5**), improving visualization of side branches, and improving lesion conspicuity. The optimal VMI energy for boosting contrast can range from 40 to 60 keV, depending on the vessel and vendor, with some scanners having higher noise at low energy levels, whereas others have consistently lower noise.[51] For example, 1 study with dual-layer CT found 50 keV to be the optimal energy level for aortic CTA with higher attenuation (by 91%), contrast/noise ratio (CNR) (by 85%), and signal/noise ratio (108%) than conventional 120-kVp level, salvaging all suboptimal enhanced studies.[50] Low-energy VMI has been used in several low-contrast-dose studies in different vascular beds,[52–60] with contrast material doses as low as 25 mL[56], iodine concentration as low as 15 g and contrast material reductions of up to 70% with maintained image quality and CNR.[57] Improved visualization of small

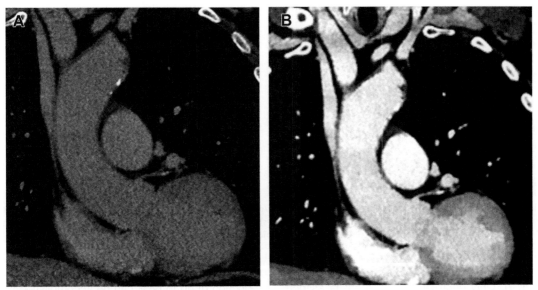

Fig. 4. (*A*) Conventional 120 kVp coronal CTA shows poor opacification of the thoracic aorta, which severely limits the vascular assessment. (*B*) Corresponding 40-keV VMI shows marked improvement in vascular signal, allowing assessment of the thoracic aorta.

branch vessels such as bronchial, intercostal, and vertebral arteries has been shown with low-energy VMI.[61] The detection of leaks in perigraft space of inclusion grafts and endoleaks has been shown to be improved with the use of low-energy VMI,[42,62–64] even in routine non-CTA scans.

Higher-energy VMI (>70 keV) can be used to decrease several artifacts, such as beam hardening, metallic artifact, and calcium blooming[65–68] (**Fig. 6**). VMI ≥ 90 keV has significantly lower hypo-attenuating and hyperattenuating beam hardening artifacts from high-density contrast material in

axillary and subclavian veins.[69] The best results for diagnostic assessment were provided at 130 keV with overcorrection of artifacts observed at higher keV values.[69]

Iodine maps are obtained by a 3-material decomposition of iodine, soft tissue, and Iodine maps can be displayed either in gray scale or color overlay over VNC images. It provides an objective measurement of contrast enhancement (in milligrams per milliliter), unrelated to Hounsfield units (HU). Iodine maps can be used to distinguish high-attenuation lesions in contrast

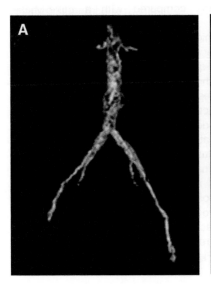

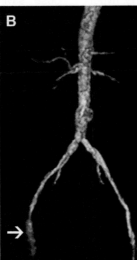

Fig. 5. (*A*) 3D volume-rendered image of the arterial vasculature from a conventional CT scan with poor arterial contrast opacification shows apparent truncation of the upper abdominal aorta, major mesenteric vessels, and the distal right iliac vasculature. (*B*) 3D volume-rendered image of the same arterial vasculature from a 40-keV VMI allows complete visualization of the upper abdominal aorta, major mesenteric vessels, and the distal right iliac vasculature (*arrow*).

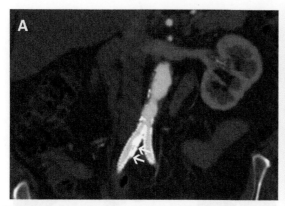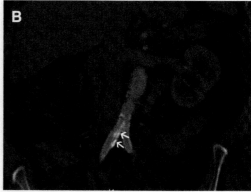

Fig. 6. (*A*) Coronal reconstruction of CT image at 120 kVp in a patient with bilateral kissing iliac artery stents shows blooming artifacts from the stent material (*arrows*). (*B*) Coronal reconstruction CT of VMI at 100 keV in the same patient shows significantly decreased calcium blooming artifact from the stents (*arrows*).

CT as contrast, hemorrhage, or calcification[60] (Fig. 7). Only contrast enhancement is associated with higher iodine uptake. Iodine maps can also help in characterizing masses, particularly thrombus, which does not show significant iodine uptake. One study on a rapid kilovoltage-peak switching scanner showed 1.74 mg/mL as the cutoff for distinguishing thrombus from a contrast admixture artifact in left atrial appendage,[70] but this number varies with the scanner and organ. Iodine maps are used for evaluating parenchymal perfusion, particularly in the heart and lungs. In the heart, iodine maps can be used for detecting myocardial ischemia with higher sensitivity and specificity than conventional CTA.[66] Iodine maps or derivatives, such as pulmonary blood volume maps, can be used to improve the diagnosis and provide prognostic information in acute pulmonary embolism, chronic pulmonary embolism, and chronic thromboembolic pulmonary hypertension.[71–74] Color iodine map overlays from venous-phase imaging increase the detection of subtle endoleaks with 100% accuracy,[63] while saving 28% radiation dose compared with single-energy biphasic studies (Fig. 8). Iodine maps also have lower artifacts from high-atomic-number metals, such as platinum embolization coils.[60]

Virtual noncontrast (VNC) images are derived from the same 3-material decomposition process as the iodine map, but with subtraction of pixels containing iodine. Because the VNC images have similar attenuation and noise [75], they can replace the true non contrast (TNC) images of a multiphasic vascular CT protocol, achieving 50% radiation-dose savings.[62,76,77] Image quality is not compromised, although some of the calcium can also be removed because it is not one of the 3 basis materials.[75,78] Further radiation dose reduction of up to 68% can be accomplished by acquiring only the delayed venous-phase images and generating virtual arterial-phase reconstructions, either from 40-keV low-energy VMI or from the low energy acquisition (80 kVp) in a dual-source scanner (Fig. 9). This technique has noninferior image quality and high diagnostic performance in the detection of endoleak (96%–100% sensitivity, specificity, accuracy) compared with true arterial-phase images.[62,76,79] VNC either on its own or along with iodine map can be used to characterize high-attenuation lesions encountered in contrast CT. Hemorrhage is seen in VNC but not in the iodine map, whereas extravasated contrast is seen in the iodine map but not in VNC (see Fig. 7). Similarly, VNC and iodine map can be used to detect and localize gastrointestinal bleeding with high diagnostic performance (area under the curve, 0.94) and 30% radiation dose savings compared with a triple-phase protocol.[80]

CTA has high accuracy in the evaluation of peripheral arterial disease.[81,82] This evaluation requires good-quality maximum intensity projections (MIPs) and three-dimensional (3D) reconstructions without bones. The conventional threshold-based bone subtraction techniques are time consuming and may erode vessels adjacent to bones, resulting in overestimation of luminal stenosis or mimicking of an occlusion. DECT can generate bone-subtracted images using 3-material decomposition of calcium, iodine, and blood[61] or 2-material decomposition of calcium and iodine.[83] The voxels with bone are assigned a low attenuation value (ie, −1024 HU) as a result of which bone-free MIP and 3D volume rendering (VR) images can be easily generated (Fig. 10). DECT bone subtraction takes substantially less time and is more robust than

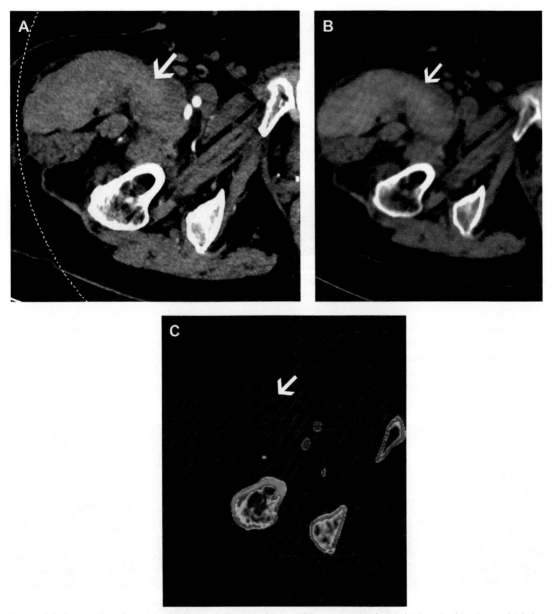

Fig. 7. (*A*) Conventional contrast-enhanced CT scan shows a large mass in the right inguinal region, which has high-attenuation areas (*arrow*), with concern for active extravasation versus hematoma. (*B*) Virtual noncontrast image at the same level shows that the high attenuation is present in the noncontrast CT (*arrow*), indicating that this is not an active contrast extravasation. (*C*) Iodine map shows that there is no iodine uptake in the lesion (*arrow*). These findings indicate that the mass is caused by a hematoma and not by contrast extravasation.

conventional techniques.[84,85] DECT MIPs are superior to single-energy bone-subtracted MIPs (sensitivity, 97.2% vs 77.1%; specificity, 94.1% vs 70.7%; accuracy, 94.7% vs 72.0%),[86] with less frequent erosion of vessels adjacent to the bone.[83] The performance is better in the aortoiliac and femoropopliteal regions as well as bypass grafts, but moderate at the knee and poor in the calf and pedal arteries, especially in critical limb ischemia.[87,88] With severely calcified vessels, DECT MIPs performed better than single-energy MIPs (91% to 96% vs 57% to 74%).[86] Incomplete bone subtraction may be seen in areas outside the central field of view (FOV) of the scanner, which can be manually subtracted. Some calcified plaques can also be removed as bone.[83,86] The resolution can be improved by isocenter positioning and regional batches.[61]

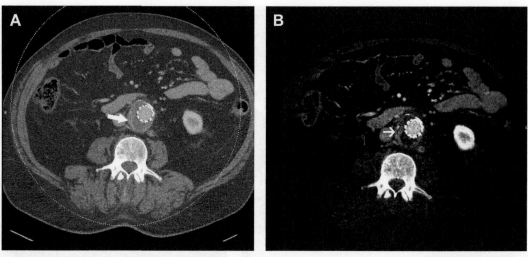

Fig. 8. (*A*) Axial CT scan in a patient with endovascular repair for abdominal aortic aneurysm shows subtle high-attenuation areas within the excluded aneurysmal sac, indicating endoleak (*arrow*). (*B*) Iodine map at the same level shows improved visualization of the endoleak (*arrow*).

In conventional CTA, calcified plaque cannot be removed and hence the MIPs are not accurate in grading the stenosis. Often an additional curved multiplanar reformation image has to be generated to accurately quantify luminal stenosis.[61] With DECT, calcified plaques can be removed using morphologic criteria to separate plaque and bone (**Fig. 11**), from which a CTA luminogram MIP can be generated, which saves additional postprocessing (**Fig. 12**). Similar to bone-

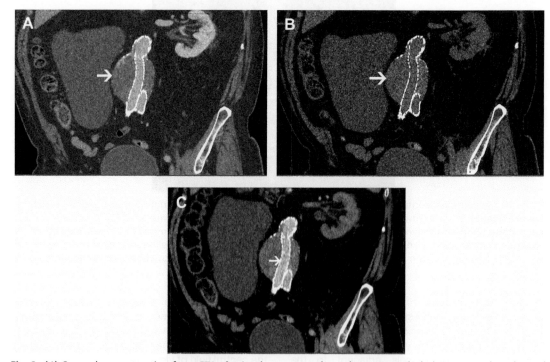

Fig. 9. (*A*) Coronal reconstruction from CTA obtained at venous phase shows an excluded aneurysmal sac (*arrow*) and endovascular aneurysm repair (EVAR). (*B*) Virtual noncontrast image reconstructed at the same level shows that there is no high attenuation within the aneurysmal sac (*arrow*). (*C*) VMI at 40 keV shows much higher attenuation (*arrow*) than the venous-phase image, equivalent to an arterial-phase image (virtual arterial reconstruction). Acquiring only the venous phase provides significant radiation dose savings.

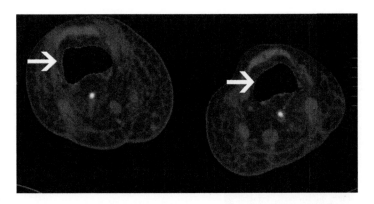

Fig. 10. Axial CT image with dual-energy bone subtraction, with the voxels containing bone assigned a low attenuation value of −1024 HU (*arrows*).

subtracted DECT images, calcified plaque subtraction is better for the pelvic and thigh arteries, especially for heavily calcified plaques in the larger vessels (>5 mm).[85] Over-removal of plaque may result in overestimation of luminal stenosis. The diagnostic performance of bone subtraction plus plaque removal was shown to be slightly lower than DECT bone subtraction alone (sensitivity, 84%; specificity, 56%; accuracy, 75%),[86,87] with better results at the aortoiliac level. Hence the findings should always be correlated with axial source images.[87] Recently a modified 3-material decomposition algorithm with calcium as the primary material has been developed with complete and selective calcium subtraction.[89] These datasets have higher CNR and higher accuracy (96.5% vs 93.1%) with comparable image quality.[89] This technique can potentially decrease inconclusive and false-positive CTA results in heavily calcified vessels.

DECT has been shown to be faster and superior to conventional bone subtraction in thorax, which often requires multiple clip planes in addition to threshold or region growing techniques.[61] Small branch vessels, such as intercostal arteries, are not eroded with DECT bone subtraction. The entire thorax may not fit into the smaller x-ray tube FOV, but, with the latest generation of scanners, this is not an issue anymore.[61] Advanced algorithms can be used to separate intravascular iodinated material from simultaneously administered high-atomic-number contrast media such as oral tantalum, tungsten, or rhenium contrast, with the tantalum appearing in iodine-only images and the rhenium in water-equivalent images.[90] DECT is still not widely available, involves additional cost, and may need new protocols for most of the scanners. Postprocessing may take additional time but can be automated and performed at the scanner.[48] With the dual-source scanners, there is a size limitation, because one of the x-ray detectors is smaller. There are higher beam hardening/streak artifacts on material-specific images in rapid kilovoltage-peak switching.[91]

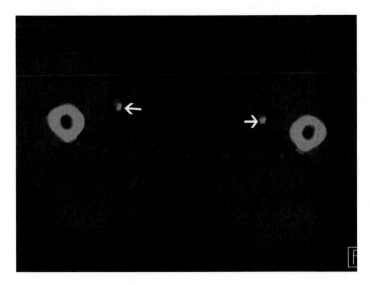

Fig. 11. Color-coded images of the plaques with the hard calcified plaque color coded as red (*arrows*) and the lumen with iodinated contrast color coded as blue.

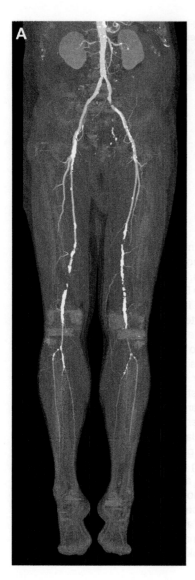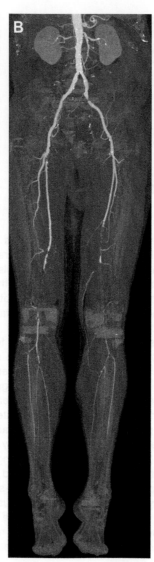

Fig. 12. (*A*) Dual-energy bone-subtracted MIPs show the presence of extensive calcifications in the superficial femoral arteries bilaterally, which precludes assessment of the luminal stenosis. (*B*) Dual-energy bone subtraction with additional removal of calcified plaque shows a luminogram that has significant narrowing of bilateral superficial arteries.

PHOTON-COUNTING COMPUTED TOMOGRAPHY

Photon-counting CT is an emerging technology with a semiconductor detector that converts the incident x-ray photons directly into positive and negative charge clouds. These clouds are pulled in opposite directions to generate an electrical pulse, whose height is proportional to the energy of the x-ray photon. The x-ray spectrum can be divided into several specific energy bins, albeit with some overlap.[92] Energy weighting is a technique in which more weight is assigned to 1 specific energy bin to highlight a specific tissue. Material decomposition can be achieved from energy-selective images and generation of basis image maps from 2 or 3 energy bins. Because of

energy weighting, the accuracy of detection of contrast agents can be increased.[92] K-edge imaging allows the measurement of the concentration of specific elements. Simultaneous multicontrast agent imaging is possible because of different k-edges allowing differentiation of multiple contrast agents, such as iodine or gadolinium with nanoparticles[93] There is also potential for novel contrast agents with high atomic numbers such as gold, platinum, xenon, bismuth, lutetium, tungsten, silver, and ytterbium because of higher spectral separation. Molecular CT imaging with targeted contrast agents is also possible.[92]

In addition, the CNR is higher in photon detector CT because of lower electronic noise and higher weighting of low-energy bins. This technique has the potential to reduce the radiation and contrast doses.[94,95] Photon detector CT scans also have high spatial resolution up to 0.07×0.07 mm^3 because of smaller detector elements and magnification factor.[92] The high spatial resolution is useful in the evaluation of small vascular structures and their disorders, such as vasculitis. The high spatial resolution along with material decomposition also has the potential to reduce calcium blooming and provide an accurate estimation of the severity of luminal stenosis, thus increasing the specificity of CT. This potential is particularly relevant in patients with critical limb ischemia for evaluation of calcified arteries below the level of knee. Other artifacts, such as beam hardening and metal, can also be reduced by using high-energy bins.[94] Photon-counting CT is still an experimental technology and is not commercially available, with only a few prototype scanners installed at select institutions.[92]

ULTRAHIGH SPATIAL RESOLUTION

High spatial resolution is beneficial in evaluating small vessels and elucidating fine details. High spatial resolution can also minimize or eliminate artifacts such as blooming from high-density structures such as calcium and metallic stents. The smallest clinically available detector element size, and hence the spatial resolution, is 0.5 mm, which is limited in evaluating small vessels (<3 mm) and vessels with calcium/metallic stents.[96] Prototype ultrahigh-resolution (UHR) scanners are now available with up to 0.25 × 0.25-mm detector element size, 1792 detector channels, and small x-ray focus size of 0.4 × 0.5 mm, which allows a reconstruction matrix of 2048 × 2048 or 1024 × 1024 and slice thickness of 0.25 mm.[96]

UHR CT will be useful in critical limb ischemia for the visualization of infrapopliteal and pedal arteries. UHR CT provides more detailed visualization of the distal vasculature, including digital arteries, pedal arch, and collateral vessels, than conventional CT. This information is important for interventional procedures below the knee, such as transmetatarsal retrograde puncture, which may be difficult to achieve even with invasive angiography. In a phantom study, UHR CT achieved twice the spatial resolution of conventional CT (29 line pairs per centimeter at 2% modulation transfer function vs 14 line pairs per centimeter for conventional CT), and yielded improved accuracy for evaluation of in-stent restenosis in a phantom study of renal artery stents.[97] UHR CT also decreases blooming

artifacts from calcium and stent, which improves the diagnostic accuracy of CTA compared with digital subtraction angiography (DSA).[96] With subtraction imaging of noncontrast from contrast images following orbital helical scanning, volume position matching, and zero clipping, calcium and stent can be removed.[96] UHR CT has also shown improved visualization of the entire course of the artery of Adamkiewicz from the aorta to the anterior spinal artery, which typically measures only 1 mm[98] (**Fig. 13**). Future developments may include evaluation of tissue perfusion.[92] The use of thinner sections may lead to higher radiation dose without the use of other techniques such as iterative reconstruction. Higher processing power, larger storage, and faster network traffic are required to manage the additional images generated because of thin slices.[92]

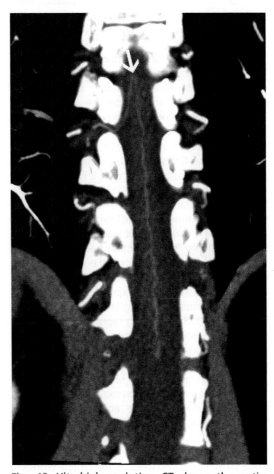

Fig. 13. Ultrahigh-resolution CT shows the entire course and characteristic hairpin bend of the artery of Adamkiewicz (*arrow*), which originates at the level of the right T8.

DYNAMIC COMPUTED TOMOGRAPHY ANGIOGRAPHY

Dynamic CTA (also called four-dimensional [4D] CTA, time-resolved CTA) refers to multiple CTA acquisitions at the same slice location. Wide-array or volume scanners can cover up to 16 cm of anatomy with a temporal resolution of 2 seconds for each dynamic acquisition. The anatomic coverage can be further increased by using the Fowler position.[99] The dual-source scanner has a shuttle mode, in which the table moves bidirectional in 2.5 seconds, providing a temporal resolution of 5 seconds for dynamic CTA with z-coverage of 27 to 48 cm (depending on the scan generation).[100,101] Following injection of contrast and then saline at 4 to 5 mL/s, a timing bolus or bolus tracking is used to initiate acquisition. On a 320-detector scanner, a timing bolus was used and scanning initiated 2 seconds before the preset delay time, for 16 intermittent phases. On dual-source CT, bolus tracking was used and 12 low-dose dynamic phases were acquired.[102] Low tube voltage (80 kVp) and tube current (120 mAs per rotation) are used to minimize radiation doses.[102]

Dynamic CTA is useful in the evaluation of endoleaks, aortic dissections, peripheral run-offs, arteriovenous malformations/fistulas, and surgical/procedural leak. Endoleaks can be seen in up to 40% of patients following endovascular aneurysm repair (EVAR).[103,104] Accurate classification of the endoleak determines the type and urgency of management. Conventional triphasic (noncontrast, arterial, venous) static CTA is usually adequate, but classification is limited when there is leakage of a large amount of blood or low-flow endoleaks that emerge in the late arterial phase.[105] Dynamic CTA can help with accurate classification, specifically the distinction between type I/III and II, evaluation of the source of endoleak, determination of flow direction, and identification of cause in patients with expanding aneurysmal sac. Other dynamic imaging techniques have limitations, with DSA requiring high radiation doses, contrast-enhanced ultrasonography (CEUS) and magnetic resonance (MR) imaging unable to evaluate stent graft position/fractures, CEUS being operator dependent, and MR imaging missing type I/III endoleaks.[99] Dynamic CTA shows that peak enhancement of the aorta and endoleak were achieved at 12 and 22 seconds following bolus threshold, respectively, with optimal detection of endoleak achieved at 27 seconds following bolus threshold.[106] As a result, the typical biphasic static CT, which acquires images 7 and 100 seconds after threshold, misses some endoleaks. Type I/III endoleaks enhance earlier along with the aortic lumen (0.28 seconds), whereas type II endoleaks enhance later (9.17 seconds)[100] (Fig. 14). The delay between peak aortic and endoleak enhancement was higher for type II than type I/III endoleaks (5.3 vs 2.0 seconds).[99] The HU index (HUendoleak/HUaorta) of type I/III endoleaks was also higher than the HU index of type II.[99] With DSA as the reference standard, dynamic CTA had 100% accuracy in the detection of endoleaks, compared with 55% accuracy for static CT scans,[106] with lower radiation and contrast doses.[105] The higher detection of endoleaks with dynamic CT could account for the type V endoleaks observed in static CTA. Addition of a static late venous phase (300 seconds) can detect low-flow endoleaks.[106] The 4D CTA technique does not replace conventional CTA, but provides complementary information in specific cases.

Dynamic CTA provides additional diagnostic information in patients with aortic dissection, such as delay in the enhancement between the true and false lumens, degree of oscillation of the flap, collapse of the true lumen, perfusion delay of arteries originating in the false lumen, quantification of asymmetrical renal perfusion, and dynamic occlusion of the aortic branches.[101] A dual-source study with 48-cm coverage, craniocaudal scanning, 6-second temporal resolution, 14-second scan delay after contrast injection, and 6 phases of scanning for 36 seconds demonstrated change of management in 21% of patients.[101] The radiation dose was 25% lower than the triphasic CT (CT dose index [CTDI] of 32.4 mGy vs 42 mGy).[101] The glomerular filtration rate can also be quantified using dynamic CTA.[107] Dynamic CTA may not replace triphasic CTA because it cannot cover the entire aorta in all patients and also does not have ECG gating, which is essential for the ascending aorta.

The diagnostic accuracy of static CTA in the evaluation of peripheral arterial disease is lower for the smaller leg vessels below the knee, especially those that are heavily calcified.[108] Delayed contrast enhancement of calf vessels caused by asymmetrical proximal stenosis and venous contamination caused by short arteriovenous transit time in ulcers/gangrene are additional challenges on top of lower contrast concentration further away from the heart.[102] Dynamic CTA with scan range of 48 cm in 8 phases of 3.5 seconds per phase at 100 kVp, 120 mAs, and 50 mL of contrast at 5 mL/s had higher arterial contrast, higher diagnostic confidence, and higher diagnostic performance (sensitivity and specificity) for the diagnosis of high-grade stenosis and occlusion in patients with critical limb ischemia than static CTA (specificity 97.1% vs 92.2%).[102] Similar

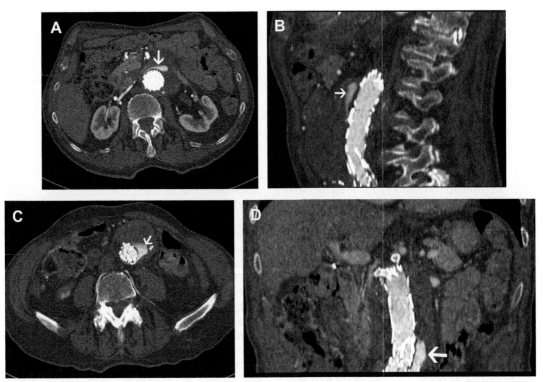

Fig. 14. (A) Axial CT reconstruction in the early arterial phase (20 seconds) of a dynamic CTA acquisition in a patient with EVAR shows an endoleak (*arrow*) originating at the level of the renal artery. (B) Sagittal CT reconstruction of the same phase as (A) shows the endoleak adjacent to the renal arterial origin (*arrow*). (C) Axial CT scan from a later dynamic acquisition (36 seconds) shows another endoleak that is originating from the level of the iliac limb (*arrow*). (D) Coronal CT reconstruction of the same phase as (C) shows the endoleak originating adjacent to the iliac limb (*arrow*).

results were obtained from a 256-slice GE CT scanner using 18 repeated axial acquisitions over calves with 2-second interphase delay with increased image quality and diagnostic confidence for the assessment of presence and degree of stenosis in below-the-knee arteries.[109] Lower leg muscle enhancement directly measured from dynamic CTA at 70 keV with 30 mL of contrasts has lower early enhancement and peak enhancement in ischemia.[110]

Dynamic CTA at 70 kVp has been shown to provide the diagnostic information required for therapy planning in children with venous malformation, such as flow dynamics, localization, volume, presence of thrombophlebitis, and lesion extension.[111] This information is advantageous compared with MR imaging, which requires sedation/anesthesia, and ultrasonography, which is operator dependent and cannot show the entire extent of the vascular anomaly essential for planning.[111] Radiation dose is a challenge in dynamic CTA but is minimized using low-dose protocols. The radiation dose of dynamic CTA is comparable with static triphasic CTA because of the smaller

anatomic coverage,[102] but it is 10% more than typical abdominal CTA[106] and lower than DSA.[102] Other challenges include the transfer and storage of multiple images, reconstruction and display technique, and communication to physicians.

ADVANCED RECONSTRUCTION ALGORITHMS

Nonlinear iterative reconstruction (IR) algorithms are now commonly used in vascular imaging. Unlike the simple linear filtered back-projection (FBP) technique, IR algorithms model an expected dataset that is then compared with the actual, acquired dataset. Noise is then detected and removed by an iterative process that uses the difference between the anticipated and actual image. IR algorithms can be either statistical, hybrid, or model based, operating either in the projection domain, image domain, or both. Statistical techniques assign a lower value to data with high noise, whereas model-based algorithms (partial or total) use system models that stimulate x-ray interaction with the object.[112] Statistical algorithms can either improve the image quality with radiation doses similar to FBP or maintain the image quality at lower radiation doses, but they cannot do both at the same time, whereas model-based algorithms can improve the image quality even at lower radiation doses. IR algorithms can improve the CNR in low-contrast-dose studies. Model-based algorithms also have lower image artifacts and higher spatial resolution.[112]

Several studies with different vendor algorithms on various vascular systems have shown the benefits of IR. One study showed that the image quality of an 80-kVp CT venography study was superior with model-based IR technique compared with hybrid iterative technique and FBP.[113] Using hybrid IR algorithm (Philips), abdominopelvic CTA was performed at 80 kVp and half-contrast volume (48 mL) for a 43% radiation-dose and 50% contrast-dose reduction with higher CNR.[114] With a model-based IR algorithm (Philips), good-quality TAVR CTA were obtained with an 80-kVp scan and low contrast volume (60 vs 80 mL) with significantly lower radiation dose.[115] Using the same algorithm, post-thoracic endovascular aortic repair (TEVAR) CTA was performed in obese patients at 80 kVp and low contrast volume (0.4 mL/kg) for 78% radiation-dose and 60% contrast-dose reduction with equivalent attenuation and image-quality score, lower noise, and higher or equivalent CNR compared with conventional images.[116] Similar results were shown in CTA aortography on 320-detector CT with IR that used 80 kVp and 40 mL of contrast medium for 48% reduction of radiation dose, without a significant difference in CNR.[117] Aortic CTA on third-generation dual-source CT with automated tube voltage selection, integrated circuit detector, and advanced IR showed higher image quality, lower noise, and higher CNR with substantial reduction of radiation dose and contrast dose compared with a routine 120-kVp scan with IR.[118] The tube voltage was reduced less than 120 kVp in 84% of CTA studies, with mean reduction of 21.1% for an average of 95 kVp, allowing radiation dose decrease by 44%. Interestingly, the radiation dose is lower by 19% even for cases selected for 120 kVp because of the use of integrated circuit detectors.[118] Contrast was used 37.5% less than second-generation dual-source CT studies.[118] A phantom study showed that model-based IR further improved the small vessel detectability of UHR CT, with lower noise and detection of submillimeter arteries up to 0.36 mm for model-based iterative reconstruction (MBIR) and 0.5 mm for FBP.[119] IR can also reduce artifacts, including those seen in the shoulder.[120] The challenges of IR include the long reconstruction times[121]; however, these have improved recently. At higher levels of IR algorithms, the images look artificial and plasticky, which some readers find disconcerting.

CINEMATIC RENDERING

Cinematic rendering (CR) is a novel postprocessing technique for the 3D visualization of CTA image data. Each voxel of a 3D volume is assigned a color and transparency based on its tissue composition using presets of ramp or trapezoidal functions. Unlike the VR technique that uses a simple unidirectional light model, CR uses a more complex global lighting model and Monte Carlo path tracing that computes the direction of the light photons and their interaction with tissues, including reflection off body surface, attenuation, penetration, refraction, and scattering in different directions.[122,123] Shadowing effects are also added, assuming that the light source can be obscured by objects within the visualized volume. This technique provides photorealistic images with high surface detail, realistic shadowing, higher depth, and higher shape perception (**Fig. 15**). Texture maps related to the brightness of surfaces within a virtual scene can also be generated.

CR has been shown to be of value in complex congenital heart diseases, providing detailed anatomic information with higher spatial impression and depth perception of the atrial appendages, pulmonary veins, peripheral pulmonary arteries, anterior interventricular sulcus, and aortic arch branches than conventional VR techniques.[124] CR allows a more accurate and faster comprehension of the surgical anatomy than conventional CT imaging, independent of the experience level of the surgeon.[125] CT has been shown to be useful in the evaluation of vascular abnormalities such as dissection,[126] mycotic aneurysm,[127] ductus aneurysm,[128] and vascular complications of pancreatitis such as pseudoaneurysm and portomesenteric thrombosis.[129] A black-blood CR technique that uses a preset with nonoverlapping soft tissue trapezoids (one with narrow plateau, centered at low attenuation, and another with broader plateau, centered at higher attenuation) can improve the intraluminal visualization, particularly within the heart.[130] CR requires higher computational power than VR. A recent study has shown that CR has lower accuracy and predictive values than conventional imaging or VR in the evaluation of vascular invasion in deep soft tissue sarcomas of extremities.[131]

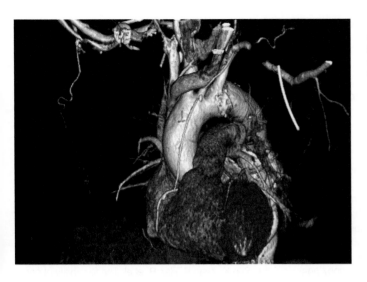

Fig. 15. Cinematic rendering of the aorta in a patient who had extensive surgical repair of the ascending aorta and arch. Cinematic rendering provides more photorealistic images with higher surface detail, realistic shadowing, and higher depth perception.

DEEP LEARNING TECHNIQUES

Deep learning is a subset of machine learning in which the computer progressively learns without any human input.[132] Deep learning relies on artificial neuronal networks. These networks have variable architectures with differences in numbers, layers, and connections.[132] Several applications of deep learning have been described in cardiovascular imaging,[132,133] broadly for the detection of disorders (classification), segmentation, quantification, and image enhancement. Deep convolutional neuronal network (DCNN) with a DetectNet detection network has been used for accurate automatic detection and segmentation of postoperative thrombus within an abdominal aortic aneurysm.[134] DCNN has also been shown to be highly accurate (slice level, 98.7%; patient level, 96.5%; site-level detection, 91.5%) in the automatic detection of aortic dissection.[135] The authors used a Mask R-CNN (regions with convolutional neuronal networks) to detect and segment the aorta from CTA, an area-wise screening method to remove unsatisfactory segmentation, Canny edge detector for extraction of edges and two residual neural networks (ResNets) to detection of aortic dissection. Deep learning based on 3D U-Net (a fully convolutional network [FCN]) combined intersection over union tracing algorithm has been used in the automatic segmentation, centerline analysis, vessel straightening, and measurement of true and false lumens with high correlation with standard technique and at much shorter time (3.16 ± 0.47 minutes vs 2 ± 0.4 hours).[136] Machine learning has been used to predict the expansion risk of abdominal aortic aneurysm using the major axis of the aneurysm and the aneurysm area.[137] Deep learning algorithms such as convolutional neuronal network (CNN) and general adversarial networks (GAN) can be used to decrease the noise, and can operate at the raw dose data from sensors by training of anatomy at standard and low-radiation doses.[138] At the image level, generator CNN has been used to transform low-dose CT images into routine-dose CT images using voxel-wise loss minimization.[139] Another group trained the CNN (with 18 convolution layers, each followed by a parametric rectified linear unit) to learn the noise distribution in low-dose images and obtain a customized noise model. Following this, the network generates low-noise images from low-dose aortic CTA images obtained at 80 kVp, with 40 mL of contrast, which allows 79% radiation dose and 50% contrast-dose savings.[140] Unlike IR algorithms, this deep learning technique is vendor neutral and is faster, with preserved image quality, improved details (not plasticky), and lower artifacts.[140] A deep learning technique using Improved GoogLeNet removed streak artifacts in a sparse-view CT reconstruction caused by missing projections by a technique of residual learning.[141]

SUMMARY

Vascular CTA is a highly accurate technique in the evaluation of vascular disease. Recent advances in technology enable acquisition of high-quality images at high spatial resolution with low artifacts, radiation dose, and contrast. Using dual-energy and photon counting CT, material composition can be characterized.

DISCLOSURE

The author has no financial disclosure or conflict of interest.

REFERENCES

1. Met R, Bipat S, Legemate DA, et al. Diagnostic performance of computed tomography angiography in peripheral arterial disease: a systematic review and meta-analysis. JAMA 2009;301(4):415–24.
2. Einstein AJ, Henzlova MJ, Rajagopalan S. Estimating risk of cancer associated with radiation exposure from 64-slice computed tomography coronary angiography. J Am Med Assoc 2007;298:317–23.
3. Rajiah P, Abbara S. Radiation exposure from medical imaging must not be taken out of context. Trends Cadiovasc Med 2016;26:66–7.
4. Piechowlak EI, Peter JFW, Kleb B, et al. Intravenous iodinated contrast agents amplify DNA radiation damage at CT. Radiology 2015;275:692–7.
5. Grudzenski S, Kuefner MA, Heckmann MB, et al. Contrast-medium enhanced radiation damage caused by CT examinations. Radiology 2009;253:706–14.
6. McDonald RJ, McDonald JS, Carter RE, et al. Intravenous contrast material exposure is not an independent risk factor for dialysis or mortality. Radiology 2014;273(3):714–25.
7. Davenport MS, Khalatbari S, Dillman JR, et al. Contrast material-induced nephrotoxicity and intravenous low-osmolality iodinated contrast material. Radiology 2013;267(1):94–105.
8. Hinson JS, Ehmann MR, Fine DM, et al. Risk of acute kidney injury after intravenous contrast media administration. Ann Emerg Med 2017;69(5):577–86.
9. Nijssen EC, Nelemans PJ, Rennenberg RJ, et al. Prophylactic intravenous hydration to protect renal function from intravascular iodinated contrast material (AMACING): long-term results of a prospective, randomized, controlled trial. EClinicalMedicine 2018;4-5:109–16.
10. Davenport MS, perazella MA, Yee J, et al. Use of intravenous iodinated contrast media in patients with kidney disease: Consensus statements from the American College of Radiology and the National Kidney Foundation. Radiology 2020;294:660–8.
11. Li Y, Fan Z, Xu L, et al. Prospective ECG-gated 320-row CT angiography of the whole aorta and coronary arteries. Eur Radiol 2012;22:2432–40.
12. Goetti R, Baumuller S, Feuchtner G, et al. High-pitch dual-source CT angiography of the thoracic aorta: Is simultaneous coronary artery assessment possible? AJR Am J Roentgenol 2010;194(4):938–44.
13. Beeres M, Wichman JL, Frellesen C, et al. ECG-gated versus non-ECG-gated High pitch dual source CT for whole body CT angiography (CTA). Acad Radiol 2016;23:163–7.
14. Nakagawa J, Tasaki O, Watanabe Y, et al. Reduction of thoracic aorta motion artifact with high-pitch 128-slice dual-source computed tomographic angiography: a historical control study. J Comput Assist Tomogr 2013;37:755–9.
15. Hedgire SS, Baliyan V, Ghoshhajra BB, et al. Recent advances in cardiac computed tomography dose reduction strategies: a review of scientific evidence and technical developments. J Med Imaging (Bellingham) 2017;4(3):0031211.
16. Sun K, Zhao R, Han R, et al. The feasibility of combined coronary and supraaortic angiography with single high-pitch acquisition dual source CT. Angiology 2015;3:2.
17. Wang Z, Chen Y, Wang Y, et al. Feasibility of low-dose contrast medium high pitch CT angiography for the combined evaluation of coronary, head and neck arteries. PLOS One 2014;9(6):e100025.
18. Beeres M, Schell B, Mastragelopoulos A, et al. High-pitch dual-source CT angiography of the whole aorta without ECG synchronization: Initial experience. Eur Radiol 2012;22:129–37.
19. Christensen JD, Seaman DM, Lungren MP, et al. Assessment of vascular contrast and wall motion of the aortic root and ascending aorta on MDCT angiography: dual-=source high-pitch vs non-gated single-source acquisition schemes. Eur Radiol 2014;24(5):990–7.
20. Karlo C, Leschka S, Goetti RP, et al. High-pitch dual-source CT angiography of the aortic valve-aortic root complex without ECG-synchronization. Eur Radiol 2011;21:205–12.
21. Wielandner A, Beitzke D, Schernthaner R, et al. Is ECG triggering for motion artefact reduction in dual-source CT angiography of the ascending aorta still required with high-pitch scanning? The role of ECG-gating in high-pitch dual-source CT of the ascending aorta. Br J Radiol 2016;89(1064):20160174.
22. Goo HW. Image quality and radiation dose of high-pitch dual-source spiral cardiothoracic computed tomography in young children with congenital heart disease: Comparison of non-ECG synchronization and prospective ECG triggering. Korean J Radiol 2018;19(6):L1031–41.
23. Liu Y, Xu J, Li J, et al. The ascending aortic image quality and the whole aortic radiation dose of high-pitch dual-source CT angiography. J Cardiothorac Surg 2013;228(8):228.

24. Apfaltrer P, Hanna EL, Schoepf UJ, et al. Radiation dose and image quality at high-pitch CT angiography of the aorta: intraindividual and interindividual comparisons with conventional CT angiography. AJR Am J Roentgenol 2012;199: 1402–9.

25. Manna C, Silva M, Cobelli R, et al. High-pitch dual-source CT angiography without ECT-gating for imaging the whole aorta: intraindividual comparison with standard pitch single-source technique without ECT-gating. Diagn Interv Radiol 2017; 23(4):293–9.

26. Rajiah P, Ciancebello L, Novak R, et al. Ultra-low dose contrast CT pulmonary angiography in oncology patients using a high pitch helical dual source technology. Diagn Interv Radiol 2019; 25(3):195–203.

27. Qi L, Meinel FG, Zhou CS, et al. Image quality and radiation dose of lower extremity CT angiography using 70 kVp, high pitch acquisition and sonogram-affirmed iterative reconstruction. PLOS One 2014;9(6):e99112.

28. Zhang LJ, Li X, Schoepf UJ, et al. Non-electrocardiogram-triggered 70-kVp high-pitch computed tomography angiography of the whole aorta with iterative reconstruction: Initial results. J Comput Assist Tomogr 2016;40(1):109–17.

29. Pang L, Zhao Y, Dong H, et al. High-pitch dual-source computed tomography renal angiography: Comparison with conventional low-pitch computed tomography angiography image quality, contrast medium volume, and radiation dose. J Comput Assist Tomogr 2015;39(5):737–40.

30. Azzalini L, Abbara S, Ghoshhajra BB. Ultra-low contrast computed tomographic angiography with 20-ml total dose for transcatheter aortic valve implantation planning. J Comput Assist Tomogr 2014;38:105 9.

31. Pulerwitz TC, Khalique OK, Nazif TN, et al. Very low intravenous contrast volume protocol for computed tomography angiography providing comprehensive cardiac and vascular assessment prior to transcatheter aortic valve replacement in patients with chronic kidney disease. J Cardiovasc Comput Tomogr 2014;10:316–21.

32. Primark AN, McCollough CH, Bruesewitz MR, et al. Relationship between noise, dose, and pitch in cardiac multi-detector row CT. Radiographics 2006;26: 1785–94.

33. Tacelli N, Femyi-Jardin M, Flohr T, et al. Dual-source chest CT angiography with high temporal resolution and high pitch modes: evaluation of image quality in 140 patients. Eur Radiol 2010;20: 1188–96.

34. Russo V, Garattoni M, Buia F, et al. 128-slice CT angiography of the aorta without ECG-gating: efficacy of faster gantry rotation time and iterative reconstruction in terms of image quality and radiation dose. Eur Radiol 2016;26:359–69.

35. Sahani D, Saini S, D'Souza RV, et al. Comparison between low (3:1) and high (6:1) pitch for routine abdominal/pelvic imaging with multislice computed tomography. J Comput Assist Tomogr 2003;27:105–9.

36. Flohr TG, Leng S, Yu L, et al. Dual-source spiral CT with pitch up to 3.2 and 75 ms temporal resolution: image reconstruction and assessment of image quality. Med Phys 2009;36:5641–53.

37. Ippolito D, Talei Franzesi C, Fior D, et al. Low kV settings CT angiography with low dose contrast medium volume protocol in the assessment of thoracic and abdominal aortic disease: a feasibility study. Br J Radiol 2015;88:20140140.

38. Nakayama Y, Awai K, Funama Y, et al. Lower tube voltage reduces contrast material and radiation doses on 16-MDCt aortography. AJR Am J Roentgenol 2006;187:W490–7.

39. Sigal-Cinqualbre AB, Hennequin R, Abada HT, et al. Low-kilovoltage multi-detector row chest CT in adults: feasibility and effect on image quality and iodine dose. Radiology 2004;231:169–74.

40. Utsunomiya D, Oda S, Funama Y, et al. Comparison of standard and low tube voltage MDCT angiography in patients with peripheral arterial disease. Eur Radiol 2010;20(11):2758–65.

41. Lezzi R, Santono M, Marnao R, et al. Low-dose multidetector CT angiography in the evaluation of infrarenal aorta and peripheral arterial occlusive disease. Radiology 2012;263(1):287–98.

42. Vlahos I, Godoy MC, Naidich DP. Dual-energy computed tomography imaging of the aorta. J Thorac Imaging 2010;25:289–300.

43. Godoy MC, Naidich DP, Marchiori E, et al. Single acquisition dual-energy multidetector computed tomography: analysis of vascular enhancement and post processing technique for evaluating the thoracic aorta. J Comput Assist Tomogr 2010;34:670–7.

44. Duan Y, Wang X, Yang X, et al. Diagnostic efficiency of low-dose CT angiography compared with conventional angiography in peripheral arterial occlusions. AJR Am J Roentgenol 2016;(6): W906–14.

45. Horehledova B, Mihl C, Milanese G, et al. CT angiography in the lower extremity peripheral artery disease. Feasibility of an ultra-low volume contrast media protocol. Cardiovasc Intervent Radiol 2018; 41(11):1751–64.

46. Vasconcelos R, Vrtiska T, Foley TA, et al. Reducing iodine contrast volume in CT angiography of the abdominal aorta using integrated tube potential selection and weight-based method without compromising image quality. AJR Am J Roentgenol 2017; 208(3):552–63.

47. Higashigaito K, Schmid T, Puippe G, et al. CT angiography of the aorta: prospective evaluation of

individualized low-volume contrast media protocols. Radiology 2016;280(3):960–8.

48. Rassouli N, Etesami M, Dhanntwari A, et al. Detector-based spectral CT with novel dual-layer technology: principles and applications. Insights Imaging 2017;8(6):589–98.

49. Rassouli N, Chalian H, Rajiah P, et al. Assessment of 70-keV virtual monoenergetic spectral images in abdominal CT imaging: a comparison study to conventional polychromatic 120-kVp images. Abdom Radiol 2017;42(1):2579–86.

50. Chalian H, Kalisz K, Rassouli N, et al. Utility of virtual monoenergetic images derived from a dual-layer detector-based spectral CT in the assessment of aortic anatomy and pathology: a retrospective case control study. Clin Imaging 2018;52: 292–301.

51. Kalisz K, Rassouli N, Dhanantwari A, et al. Noise characteristics of virtual monoenergetic images from a novel detector-based spectral CT scanner. Eur J Radiol 2018;98:118–25.

52. Yuan R, Shuman WP, Earls JP, et al. Reduced iodine load at Ct pulmonary angiography with dual-energy monochromatic imaging: comparison with standard CT pulmonary angiography- a prospective randomized trial. Radiology 2012;262(1): 290–7.

53. Raju R, Thompson AG, lee K, et al. Reduced iodine load with CT coronary angiography using dual-energy imaging: a prospective randomized trial compared with standard coronary CT angiography. J Cardiovasc Comput Tomogr 2014;8(4):282–8.

54. Dubourg B, Caudron J, Lestrat JP, et al. Single-source dual-energy CT angiography with reduced iodine load in patients referred for aortoiliofemoral evaluation before transcatheter aortic valve implantation: impact on image quality and radiation dose. Eur Radiol 2014;24(11):2659–68.

55. Almuairi A, Sun Z, Poovathumakadavi A, et al. Dual energy CT angiography of peripheral arterial disease: feasibility of using lower contrast medium volume. PLoS One 2015;10(9):e0139275.

56. Cavallo AU, Patterson AJ, Thomas R, et al. Low dose contrast CT for transcatheter aortic valve replacement assessment: results from the prospective SPECTACULAR study (spectral CT assessment prior to TAVR). J Cardiovasc Comput Tomogr 2020;14(1):68–74.

57. Shuman WP, O'Malley RB, Busey JM, et al. Prospective comparison of dual-energy CT aortography using 70 % reduced iodine dose versus single-energy CT aortography using standard iodine dose in the same patient. Abdom Radiol (NY) 2017;42:759–65.

58. Agrawal MD, Oliveira GR, Kalva SP, et al. Prospective comparison of reduced iodine dose virtual monochromatic imaging dataset from Dual-

energy CT angiography with standard iodine dose single energy CT angiography for abdominal aortic aneurysm. AJR Am J Roentgenol 2016;207: W125–32.

59. Xin L, Yang X, Huang N, et al. The initial experience of the upper abdominal CT angiography using low concentration contrast medium on dual energy spectral CT. Abdom Imaging 2015;40:2894–9.

60. Patino M, Prochowski A, Agarwal MD. Material separation using dual-energy CT: Current and emerging applications. Radiographics 2016;36: 1087–105.

61. Vlahos I, Chung R, Nair A, et al. Dual-energy CT: vascular applications. AJR Am J Roentgenol 2012;199:S87–97.

62. Stolzmann P, Frauenfelder T, Pfammatter T, et al. Endoleaks after endovascular abdominal aortic aneurysm repair: detection with dual-energy dual-source CT. Radiology 2008;249:682–91.

63. Ascenti G, Mazziotti S, lamberto S, et al. Dual-energy CT for detection of endoleaks after endovascular abdominal aortic aneurysm repair: usefulness of colored iodine overlay. AJR Am J Roentgenol 2011;196(6):1408–14.

64. Maturen KE, Kaza RK, Liu PS, et al. "Sweet spot" for endoleak detection: optimizing contrast to noise using low keV reconstructions from fast-switch kVp dual-energy CT. J Comput Assist Tomogr 2012;36: 83–7.

65. Yu L, Leng S, McCollough CH. Dual-energy CT-based monochromatic imaging. AJR Am J Roentgenol 2012;199(5 Suppl):S9–15.

66. Kalisz K, Halliburton S, Abbara S, et al. Update on cardiovascular applications of multienergy CT. Radiographics 2017;37(7):1955–74.

67. Bamberg F, Dierks A, Nikolou K, et al. Metal artifact reduction by dual energy computed tomography using monoenergetic extrapolation. Eur Radiol 2011;21:1424–9.

68. Secchi F, De Cecco CN, Speraman JV, et al. Monoenergetic extrapolation of cardiac dual energy CT for artifact reduction. Acta Radiol 2015;56(4): 413–8.

69. Laukamp KR, Gupta A, Grobe Hokamp N, et al. Role of spectral-detector CT in reduction of artifacts from contrast media in axillary and subclavian veins: single institution study in 50 patients. Acta Radiol 2019;18. 284185119868904.

70. Hur J, Kim YJ, Lee H-J, et al. Cardioembolic stroke: Dual-energy cardiac CT for differentiation of left atrial appendage thrombus and circulatory stasis. Radiology 2012;263(3):688–95.

71. Lu GM, Wu SY, Yeh BM, et al. Dual-energy computed tomography in pulmonary embolism. Br J Radiol 2010;83(992):707–18.

72. Ohno Y, Koyama H, Lee HY, et al. Contrast-enhanced CT- and MRI-based perfusion

assessment for pulmonary diseases: basics and clinical applications. Diagn Interv Radiol 2016; 22(5):407–21.

73. Kang MJ, Park CM, Lee CH, et al. Dual-energy CT: clinical applications in various pulmonary diseases. Radiographics 2010;30(3):685–98.

74. Rajiah P, Tanable Y, Partovi S, et al. State of the art: utility of multi-energy CT in the evaluation of pulmonary vasculature. Int J Cardiovasc Imaging 2019; 35(8):1509–24.

75. Numburi UD, Schoenhagen P, Flamm SD, et al. Feasibility of dual-energy Ct of the arterial phase: imaging after endovascular aortic repair. AJR Am J Roentgenol 2010;195:486–93.

76. Chandarana H, Godoy MCB, Vlahos I, et al. Abdominal aorta: evaluation with dual-source dual-energy multidetector CT after endovascular repair of aneurysms. Initial observations. Radiology 2008;249:692–700.

77. De Cecco CN, Darnell A, Macfas N, et al. Second generation dual-energy computed tomography of the abdomen: radiation dose comparison with 64- and 128-row single-energy acquisition. J Comput Assist Tomogr 2013;37:543–6.

78. Sommer WH, Graser A, Becker CR, et al. Image quality of virtual noncontrast images derived from dual-energy CT angiography after endovascular aneurysm repair. J Vasc Interv Radiol 2010;21: 315–21.

79. Maturen KE, Kleaveland PA, Kaza RK, et al. Aortic endograft surveillance: use of fast-switch kVp dual-energy computed tomography with virtual noncontrast imaging. J Comput Assist Tomogr 2011;35: 742–6.

80. Sun H, Hou XY, Xue HD, et al. Dual-source dual-energy CT angiography with virtual non-enhanced images and iodine map for active gastrointestinal bleeding: image quality, radiation dose and diagnostic performance. Eur J Radiol 2015;84:884–91.

81. Kock MC, Adrianensen ME, Pattynama PM, et al. DSA versus multi-detector row CT angiography in peripheral arterial disease: randomized controlled trial. Radiology 2005;237:727–37.

82. Albrecht T, Foert E, Holtkamp R, et al. 16-MDCT angiography of aortoiliac and lower extremity arteries: comparison with digital subtraction angiography. AJR Am J Roentgenol 2007;189:702–71.

83. Meyer BC, Werncke T, Hopfenmuller W, et al. Dual energy CT of peripheral arteries: Effect of automatic bone and plaque removal on image quality and grading of stenosis. Eur J Radiol 2008;68(3): 414–22.

84. Yamamato S, Mcwilliams J, Arellano C, et al. Dual-energy CT angiography of pelvic and lower extremity arteries: dual-energy bone subtraction versus manual bone subtraction. Clin Radiol 2009;64: 1088–96.

85. Sommer WH, Johnson TR, Becker CT, et al. The value of dual-energy bone removal in maximum intensity projections of lower extremity computed tomography angiography. Invest Radiol 2009;44: 285–92.

86. Brockmann C, Jochum S, Sadick M, et al. Dual-energy CT angiography in peripheral arterial occlusive disease. Cardiovasc Intervent Radiol 2009; 32:630–7.

87. Kau T, Eicher W, Reiterer C, et al. Dual-energy CT angiography in peripheral arterial occlusive disease-accuracy of maximum intensity projections in clinical routine and subgroup analysis. Eur Radiol 2011;21 98:1677–86.

88. Thomas C, Korn A, Keterlsen D, et al. Automatic lumen segmentation in calcified plaques: dual energy CT versus standard reconstructions in comparison with digital subtraction angiography. AJR Am J Roentgenol 2010;194:1590–5.

89. De Santis D, De Cecco CN, Schoepf UJ, et al. Modified calcium subtraction in dual-energy CT angiography of the lower extremity runoff: impact on diagnostic accuracy for stenosis detection. Eur Radiol 2019;4783–93.

90. Soesbe TC, Lewis MA, Nasr K, et al. Separating High-Z oral contrast from intravascular iodine contrast in an animal model using dual-layer spectral CT. Acad Radiol 2019;26(9):1237–44.

91. Kordbacheh H, Baliyan V, Singh P, et al. Rapid kVp switching dual-energy CT in the assessment of urolithiasis in patients with large body habitus: preliminary observations on image quality and stone characterization. Abdom Radiol 2019;44:1019–26.

92. Willemink MJ, Noel PB. The evolution of image reconstruction for CT- from filtered back projection to artificial intelligence. Eur Radiol 2019;29:2185–95.

93. Cormode DP, Si-Mohamed S, Bar-Ness D, et al. Multicolor spectral photon-counting computed tomography: in vivo dual contrast imaging with high count rate scanner. Sci Rep 2017;(7):4784.

94. Giersch J, Niederlohner D, Anton G. The influence of energy weighting on x-ray imaging quality. Nucl Instrum Methods Phys Res A 2004;531(1–2):68–74.

95. Pourmortexa A, Symons R, Reich DS, et al. Photon-counting CT of the brain: in vivo human results and image quality assessment. AJNR Am J Neuroradiol 2017;38(12):2257–63.

96. Tanaka R, Yoshioka K, Takagi H, et al. Novel developments in non-invasive imaging of peripheral arterial disease with CT: experience with state-of-the-art, ultra-high resolution CT and subtraction imaging. Clin Radiol 2019;74(1):51–8.

97. Onishi H, Tori M, Ota T, et al. Phantom study of instent restenosis at high spatial resolution CT. Radiology 2018;289(1):255–60.

98. Yoshioka K, Tanaka R, Takagi H, et al. Ultra-high resolution CT angiography of the artery of

Adamkiewicz: a feasibility study. Neuroradiology 2018;60(1):109–15.

99. Koike Y, Ishida K, Hase S, et al. Dynamic volumetric CT angiography for the detection and classification of endoleaks: application of cine imaging using a 320-row CT scanner with 16-cm detectors. J Vasc Interv Radiol 2014;25:1172–80.

100. Sommer WH, Becker CR, Haack M, et al. Time-resolved CT angiography for the detection and classification of endoleaks. Radiology 2012; 263(3):917–26.

101. Meinel FG, Nilolaou K, Widenhagen R, et al. Time-resolved CT angiography in aortic dissection. Eur J Radiol 2012;81(11):3254–61.

102. Sommer WH, Bamberg F, Johnson TR, et al. Diagnostic accuracy of dynamic computed tomographic angiographic of the lower leg in patients with critical limb ischemia. Invest Radiol 2012; 47(6):325–31.

103. Jones JE, Atkins MD, Brewster DC, et al. Persistent type 2 endoleak after endovascular repair of abdominal aortic aneurysm is associated with adverse late outcomes. J Vasc Surg 2007;46:1–8.

104. Bent CL, Jaskolka JD, Lindsay TF, et al. The use of dynamic volumetric CT angiography (DV-CTA) for the characterization of endoleaks following fenestrated endovascular aortic aneurysm repair (f-EVAR). J Vasc Surg 2010;51:203–6.

105. Hou K, Zhu T, Zhang W, et al. Dynamic volumetric computed tomography angiography is a preferred method for unclassified endoleaks by conventional computed tomography angiography after endovascular aortic repair. J Am Heart Assoc 2019; 8(8):e012011.

106. Lehmkuhl L, Andres C, Lucke C, et al. Dynamic CT angiography after abdominal aortic endovascular aneurysm repair: Influence of enhancement patterns and optimal bolus timing on endoleak detection. Radiology 2013;268(3):890–9.

107. Helck A, Sommer WH, Klotz E, et al. Determination of glomerular filtration rate using dynamic CT-angiography: simultaneous acquisition of morphological and functional information. Invest Radiol 2010;45:387–92.

108. Outwendijk R, Kock MC, van Dijk LC, et al. Vessel wall calcifications at multi-detector row CT angiography in patients with peripheral arterial disease: effect on clinical utility and clinical predictors. Radiology 2006;241:603–8.

109. Buls N, de Brucker Y, Aerden D, et al. Improving the diagnosis of peripheral arterial disease in below-the-knee arteries by adding time-resolved CT scan series to conventional run-off angiography. First experience with a 256-slice CT scanner. Eur J Radiol 2019;110:136–41.

110. Zhou X, Zhang D, Zhang H, et al. Quantitative analysis of lower leg muscle enhancement measured from computed tomographic angiography for diagnosis of peripheral arterial disease. J Comput Assist Tomogr 2020;44(1):20–5.

111. Henzler T, Vogler N, Lange B, et al. Low dose time-resolved CT-angiography in pediatric patients with venous malformations using 3rd generation dual-source CT: initial experience. Eur J Radiol Open 2016;3:216–22.

112. Halliburton SS, Tanabe Y, Partovi S, et al. The role of advanced reconstruction algorithms in cardiac CT. Cardiovasc Diagn Ther 2017;7(5):527–38.

113. Iyama Y, Nakaura T, Iyama A, et al. Usefulness of a low tube voltage knowledge-based iterative model reconstruction algorithm for computed tomography venography. J Comput Assist Tomogr 2017;41(55): 811–6.

114. Knipp D, Lane BF, Mitchell JW, et al. Computed tomographic angiography of abdomen and pelvis in azotemic patients using 80 kVp technique and reduce dose iodinated contrast. J Comput Assist Tomogr 2017;41:141–7.

115. Ippolito D, Riva L, Talei F, et al. Computed tomography angiography combined with knowledge-based iterative reconstruction algorithm for transcatheter aortic valve implantation planning: Image quality and radiation dose exposure with low-kv and low-contrast protocol. J Comput Assist Tomogr 2020;44(1):13–9.

116. Hou P, Feng X, Liu J, et al. Low tube voltage and iterative model reconstruction in follow-up CT angiography after thoracic endovascular aortic repair: Ultra-low radiation exposure and contrast medium dose. Acad Radiol 2018;25(4):494–501.

117. Chen H, Zhang Y, Zhang W, et al. Low-dose CT in convolutional neural network. Biomed Opt Express 2017;8(2):679–94.

118. Mangold S, De Cecco CN, Wichmann JL, et al. Effect of automated tube voltage selection, integrated circuit detector and advanced iterative reconstruction on radiation dose and image quality of 3rd generation dual-source aortic CT angiography: an intra-individual comparison. Eur J Radiol 2016;85:972–8.

119. Morisaka H, Shimizu Y, Adachi T, et al. Effect of Ultra high-resolution computed tomography and model-based iterative reconstruction on detectability of simulated submillimeter artery. J Comput Assist Tomogr 2020;44(1):32–6.

120. Rajiah P, Schoenhagen P, Mehta D, et al. Low-dose, wide-detector array thoracic aortic CT angiography using an iterative reconstruction technique results in improved image quality with lower noise and fewer artifacts. J Cardiovasc Comput Tomogr 2012;6(3):205–13.

121. Cho YJ, Schoepf UJ, Silverman JR, et al. Iterative image reconstruction techniques: cardiothoracic computed tomography applications. J Thorac Imaging 2014;29:198–208.

122. Johnson PT, Schneider R, Lugo-Fagundo C, et al. MDCT angiography with 3D rendering: a novel cinematic rendering algorithm for enhanced anatomic detail. AJR Am J Roentgenol 2017; 209(2):309–12.

123. Rowe SP, Chu LC, Recht HS, et al. Black-blood cinematic rendering: a new method for cardiac CT intraluminal visualization. J Cardiovasc Comput Tomogr 2019. [Epub ahead of print].

124. Roschi F, Purbojo A, Ruffer a, et al. Initial experience with cinematic rendering for the visualization of extracardiac anatomy in complex congenital heart defects. Interact Cardiovasc Thorac Surg 2019;28(6):916–21.

125. Elshafei M, Binder J, Baecker J, et al. Comparison of cinematic rendering and computed tomography for speed and comprehension of surgical anatomy. JAMA Surg 2019;154(98):738–44.

126. Colli AC, Tua L, Punzo B, et al. Cinematic rendering: an alternative to classical volume rendering for acute aortic dissection. Ann Thorac Surg 2019;108(2):e121.

127. Rowe SP, Chu LC, Zimmerman SL, et al. 3D CT cinematic rendering of mycotic aneurysms. Emerg Radiol 2016;25(6):723–8.

128. Rowe SP, Johnson PT, Fishman EK. MDCT of ductus diverticulum: 3D cinematic rendering to enhance understanding of anatomic configuration and avoid misinterpretation as traumatic aortic injury. Emerg Radiol 2018;25(2):209–13.

129. Rowe SP, Chu LC, Fishman EK. Initial experience with 3D CT cinematic rendering of acute pancreatitis and associated complications. Abdom Radiol 2019. [Epub ahead of print].

130. Rowe SP, Johnson PT, Fishman EK. Cinematic rendering of cardiac CT volumetric data: Principles and initial observations. J Cardiovasc Comput Tomogr 2018;12:56–9.

131. Li K, Yan R, Ma H, et al. Value of cinematic rendering from volumetric computed tomography data in evaluating the relationship between deep soft tissue sarcomas of the extremities and adjacent major vessels: a preliminary study. J Comput Assist Tomogr 2019;43(3):386–91.

132. Litjens G, Ciompi F, Woleterink JM, et al. State-of-the-art deep learning in cardiovascular imaging analysis. JACC Cardiovasc Imaging 2019;12(8): 1549–65.

133. Retson T, Besser A, Sall S, et al. Machine learning and deep neural networks in thoracic and cardiovascular imaging. J Thorac Imaging 2019;34(3): 192–201.

134. López-Linares K, Aranjuelo N, Kabongo L, et al. Fully automatic detection and segmentation of abdominal aortic thrombus in post-operative cta images using deep convolutional neural networks. Med Image Anal 2018;46:202–14.

135. Xu X, He Z, Niu K, et al. An automatic detection scheme of acute Stanford Type A Aortic dissection based on DCNNs in CTA images. ICMSSP 2019; Proceedings of the 2019 4th International Conference on Multimedia systems and signal processing. Guangzhou, China, May 2019. p. 16–20.

136. Yu, T, Lu, B, Yong, W, et al, A 3D deep convolutional neural network for automatic segmentation and measurement of Type B aortic dissection. Radiological Society of North America 2019 Scientific Assembly and Annual Meeting. Chicago IL, December 1 - December 6, 2019. Available at: archive.rsna.org/2019/19006706.html Accessed January 3, 2020

137. Hirata K, Nakaura T, Nakagawa M, et al. Machine learning to predict the rapid growth of small abdominal aortic aneurysm. J Comput Assist Tomogr 2020;44(1):37–42.

138. Chen C-M, Chu S-Y, Hsu M-Y, et al. Low-tube voltage (80 kvp) CT aortography using 320-row volume CT with adaptive iterative reconstruction: lower contrast medium and radiation dose. Eur Radiol 2013;24:460–8.

139. Wolterink JM, Leiner T, Viergever MA, et al. Generative adversarial networks for noise reduction in low-dose ct. IEEE Trans Med Imaging 2017; 36(12):2536–45.

140. Wang Y, Yu M, Wang M, et al. Application of artificial intelligence-based image optimization for computed tomography angiography of the aorta with low tube voltage and reduced contrasts medium volume. J Thorac Imaging 2019;34:393–9.

141. Xie S, Zheng X, Chen Y, et al. Artifact removal using improved GoogLeNet for spare-view CT reconstruction. Sci Rep 2018;8(91):6700.

Magnetic Resonance Lymphangiography

Govind B. Chavhan, MD, DABR[a],*, Christopher Z. Lam, MD[a], Mary-Louise C. Greer, MD[a], Michael Temple, MD[a,b], Joao Amaral, MD[a,b], Lars Grosse-Wortmann, MD[a,c]

KEYWORDS

- MR Lymphangiography • Chylothorax • Chyloperitoneum • Plastic bronchitis
- Lymphatic anomalies • Lymphedema

KEY POINTS

- Dynamic contrast-enhanced magnetic resonance lymphangiography is a novel technique to image central conducting lymphatics performed by injecting gadolinium-based contrast agent into groin lymph nodes.
- It includes both T2-weighted imaging and postintranodal injection T1-weighted imaging.
- Current applications include assessment of plastic bronchitis in patients with Fontan surgery, chylothorax, chyloperitoneum, and intestinal lymphangiectasia.

INTRODUCTION

The lymphatic system is an important component of the circulatory system with essential physiologic functions including nutrition, fluid balance, immunity, and clearing of waste products.[1] It returns excess interstitial fluid and protein to the systemic circulation. Along with lymphoid tissues such as lymph nodes and spleen, it plays an important role in the immunity and clearance of cellular debris including bacteria and proteins. The lymphatic system is also a transporter of long-chain lipids absorbed from the intestine and proteins synthesized in the liver.

Lymph constitutes the excess of tissue fluid, which is derived from blood plasma and removed from the interstitial tissue via the lymphatic system. Lymph contains nutrients, hormones, fatty acids, toxins, and cellular waste products. The most commonly manifested clinical features of lymphatic system disorders are lymphedema, ascites, and pleural effusion, which result from accumulation of tissue fluids due to impaired lymphatic drainage. However, in recent years, the lymphatic system has been implicated in various diseases including inflammatory bowel disease, cancer, and cardiovascular disorders.[2]

Most of the lymphatic system consists of a network of small vessels; hence it is difficult to image it and especially to introduce contrast media into these small lymphatic ducts. However, in the last few years, the lymphatic imaging has been advanced by combining soft tissue contrast and resolution offered by MR imaging, supplemented by the injection of contrast media via a lymph node.[3–5] These recent advances in imaging methods, along with the development of newer lymphatic interventional techniques have prompted progress in the imaging and treatment of lymphatic pathologies.[6–8] These advances have focused on the visualization of the central conducting lymphatics (CCLs) such as the cisterna chyli and thoracic duct by dynamic

[a] Department of Diagnostic Imaging, The Hospital for Sick Children and Medical Imaging, University of Toronto, 555 University Avenue, Toronto, Ontario M5G 1X8, Canada; [b] Division of Image Guided Therapy (IGT), Department of Diagnostic Imaging, The Hospital for Sick Children, Toronto, Ontario, Canada; [c] Division of Cardiology, Department of Paediatrics, The Hospital for Sick Children, University of Toronto, 555 University Avenue, Toronto, Ontario M5G 1X8, Canada
* Corresponding author.
E-mail address: govind.chavhan@sickkids.ca
Twitter: @govindchavhan (G.B.C.)

Radiol Clin N Am 58 (2020) 693–706
https://doi.org/10.1016/j.rcl.2020.02.002
0033-8389/20/© 2020 Elsevier Inc. All rights reserved.

contrast-enhanced magnetic resonance lymph-angiography (DCMRL) as well as in the imaging of the extremity's lymphatic system.

In this review, the authors discuss the anatomy of the lymphatic system and various methods of imaging of the lymphatic system and focus on the DCMRL technique along with its current and potential clinical applications.

ANATOMY OF THE LYMPHATIC SYSTEM

The lymphatic system consists of a network of small terminal lymphatic ducts and larger lymphatic ducts, with lymph nodes interspersed throughout the lymphatic pathways.[9] Terminal lymphatics are small lymphatic vessels originating in tissues of the body. The lymph collected by terminal ducts from tissues is drained into larger lymphatic ducts that in turn drain into the veins. The lymphatic ducts contain valves, similar to veins, for unidirectional lymph flow from tissues and organs into the systemic venous system. Lymph enters lymph nodes via afferent lymphatic vessels and leaves via efferent lymphatic ducts. Lymph nodes regulate the composition of lymph and mount an immune response if pathogens are detected.

The lymphatic vessels from the right side of the head and neck; right upper extremity; and right side of the chest, lung, and heart drain into the right lymphatic duct. The right lymphatic duct is short (approximately 1.25 cm) and opens directly into the venous system at the junction of the right subclavian and right internal jugular veins.[9] The lymph from the rest of the body including lower extremities; abdomen including liver and intestine; left upper extremity; left side of the chest, head, and neck is drained by the thoracic duct (Fig. 1).The thoracic duct is a long channel, measuring approximately 38 to 45 cm in adults. It typically enters the venous system at the left venous angle formed by the junction of the left subclavian and left internal jugular veins. It starts as a triangular or saccular dilation over the first or second lumbar vertebral body, the cisterna chyli, and runs on the right side of the aorta over the spine. It crosses over to the left side at approximately the fifth thoracic vertebral body in the superior mediastinum and ultimately runs on the left side of the spine. The anatomy of the thoracic duct is variable. Similarly, the cisterna chyli can have variable shape including an inverted Y or V and a string of pearls.[10] The cisterna chyli measures approximately 5 to 20 mm in width and 5 to 7 cm in craniocaudal dimension in adults, and its caliber may change with contraction of the lymphatic pathways.[10] The thoracic duct transports approximately 1.5 to 2.5 L of lymph/chyle daily.[11]

The lymphatic vessels can be divided into 3 types depending on their origin: soft tissue, liver, and intestinal lymphatic ducts.[12] The intestinal lymphatic system absorbs the long-chain lipids from the intestine, reflected by higher concentration of lipids and proteins (60% of the blood level) in the intestinal lymph (also known as chyle). The liver lymphatic system delivers the proteins that are synthesized by the liver into the blood stream, and in fact, liver lymph contains the highest concentration of proteins of all lymph (80%–90% of the blood level), compared with a lower concentration of proteins in the peripheral lymph (17%–30% of the blood level).[13,14] Understanding of the biochemical differences of different types of lymph can help in the diagnosis of the origin of the lymphatic leaks by biochemical analysis of composition of the chylous fluid.

METHODS OF IMAGING THE LYMPHATIC SYSTEM

Over the years, imaging of the lymphatic system has evolved from direct lymphangiography through cannulation of peripheral lymphatic ducts on the dorsum of feet and hands and interstitial injection of contrast media into interdigital web spaces to injection of contrast media directly into lymph nodes.[1] Modalities of lymphatic imaging include lymphoscintigraphy, fluoroscopic lymphangiography, and, more recently, MR imaging.

Lymphoscintigraphy

Lymphoscintigraphy is performed by injection of radioactive tracers intracutaneously or subcutaneously into the feet or hands. The tracers are rapidly absorbed into terminal lymphatic ducts. Lymphoscintigraphy provides dynamic information but lacks spatial resolution and anatomic details.

Fluoroscopic Peripheral Lymphangiography

Direct lymphangiography is performed through cannulation of peripheral lymphatic ducts on the dorsum of feet or hands, interstitial injection into interdigital web spaces, or cannulation of lymph nodes in the groins and injection of iodized oil-based contrast media (Lipiodol; Guerbet LLC, Bloomington, IN, USA).

Injections directly into peripheral ducts or into the interstitium can be technically challenging and time consuming especially in small children. Furthermore, this peripheral technique may not be adequate to visualize CCL including retroperitoneal

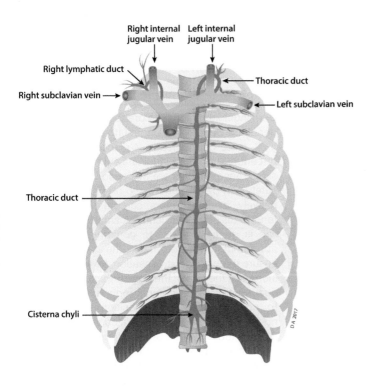

Right internal jugular vein
Left internal jugular vein
Right lymphatic duct
Thoracic duct
Right subclavian vein
Left subclavian vein
Thoracic duct
Cisterna chyli

Fig. 1. Normal anatomy of the lymphatic system. (*From* Chavhan GB, Amaral JG, Temple M, Itkin M. MR Lymphangiography in Children: Technique and Potential Applications. *Radiographics.* 2017;37(6):1775-1790; with permission.)

lymphatic channels, the cisterna chyli, and the thoracic duct.

Injection of contrast media into the groin lymph nodes for selective visualization of CCL has been used for many decades.[15] Ultrasound-guided intranodal injection of oil-based contrast media with imaging of CCL under fluoroscopy has been refined in children and successfully used for subsequent lymphatic interventions in recent years.[5,16] This technique provides excellent spatial resolution, but it is limited by exposure to ionizing radiation, longer examination time than DCMRL, somewhat limited dynamic information due to slow movement of viscous contrast media, and limited information about the relationship of lymphatic ducts with surrounding structures.[4] Importantly, oil-based contrast media poses a potential risk of paradoxic embolization in children with right to left shunts from congenital heart disease or large pulmonary arteriovenous malformations. Cerebral lipiodol embolism has been reported in a child with congenital heart disease and plastic bronchitis (PB) after lymphatic embolization due to direct connection between a lymphatic channel and a pulmonary venous branch.[17]

The limitations of intranodal injection fluoroscopic lymphangiography using lipiodol were overcome by injection of gadolinium-based contrast media (GBCM) into groin lymph nodes

in swine models, in conjunction with MR imaging[3] and subsequently used for planning selective lymphatic embolization in children with PB.[4,8,18] This technique is called DCMRL, which is described later and is the focus of this article.

Peripheral Magnetic Resonance Lymphangiography

Lymphatic ducts in the lower and upper extremities can be imaged by MR imaging using T2-weighted images[19-21] or with injection of GBCM into the dermal plane in the feet and hands on T1-weighted images.[22-24] These peripheral MR lymphangiography methods have been used to effectively plan treatments such as lymphovenous bypass in cases of lymphedema.[20-22,24] T2-weighted MR lymphangiography has several limitations including difficulty to visualize smaller lymphatic ducts because of insufficient signal from small amounts of fluid within them and difficulty to differentiate lymphatic ducts from other overlapping fluid-containing structures and veins. Also, it is a static imaging technique that lacks dynamic information, which is important when it comes to demonstrating lymphatic reflux or leakage. Similar to fluoroscopic peripheral lymphangiography, peripheral DCMRL could be technically challenging and time consuming and has not been reported in children yet.

Newer Lymphatic Imaging Approaches

The liver is one of the major producers of lymph fluid. Normally, lymphatic flow is from the liver to the CCL. Hence, the liver lymphatics are not opacified by groin intranodal contrast injection. Until recently, there was no imaging method to visualize liver lymphatics. However, Biko and his colleagues have reported an MR imaging method to image liver lymphatics using T1-weighted MR images and angiographic sequences after injecting GBCM into lymphatics in the liver.[25] In this initial experience, they demonstrated lymphatic flow from liver toward bowel and leakage of contrast into the duodenum in patients with protein losing enteropathy, and leakage into the peritoneal cavity as well as retrograde mesenteric lymphatic perfusion in patients with chylous ascites.

TECHNIQUE OF DYNAMIC INTRANODAL MAGNETIC RESONANCE LYMPHANGIOGRAPHY

After confirming appropriateness of indication, MR compatibility, and normal renal function, ultrasound of the groins is performed to identify good size lymph nodes for cannulation, done in advance of scheduling the DCMRL. This is especially important for infants who may not have sufficiently large lymph nodes for cannulation. Small children undergo the entire procedure under general anesthesia, whereas adolescents and adult patients can undergo the lymph node cannulation under local anesthetic. The following steps are followed in sequence.

Positioning

The patient is placed supine on a detachable MR imaging table, outside the scanning room, with posterior elements of the torso coil underneath the patient before induction of anesthesia or the start of cannulation. Anterior elements of the coil are placed when the patient is taken into the scanner, after the lymph node cannulation.

Lymph Node Cannulation

Both inguinal regions are prepped and draped under sterile conditions. Under ultrasound guidance, a 22- to 25-gauge needle is placed in the medulla or central part of an inguinal lymph node on each side. These needles are MR conditional, and their safety can be predetermined on phantoms. Alternatively, angiocatheters can be used but they tend to dislodge frequently. A small volume of saline is gently injected to confirm the needle is appropriately located within the medulla and to ensure there is no extravasation. Injection of saline increases the size of the node (Fig. 2). Some investigators have used contrast-enhanced ultrasound to confirm the needle position in the lymph nodes.[26] The needle is then connected to long 21-inch tubing with a 3-way stopcock on the end and taped in place (Fig. 3). The needle position is again confirmed with saline injection under ultrasound visualization. If the needle is not well positioned or extravasation of normal saline is noted, then the needle is repositioned or another lymph node is cannulated. Syringes with contrast media (dilute gadolinium) and saline flush are connected to the 3-way stopcock (see Fig. 3). The patient is then transferred to the MR imaging scanner.

Contrast Media

Any routinely used GBCM can be used for DCMRL. The dose used for DCRML is the same standard dose of 0.1 mmol/kg used for routine intravenous injection. A double dose of 0.2 mmol/kg can be used occasionally in larger patients. The guidelines and precautions used for

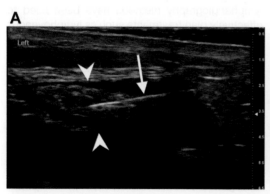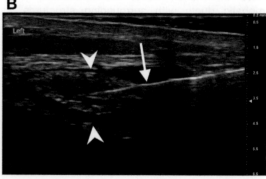

Fig. 2. Groin lymph node cannulation for MR lymphangiography in an 8-month-old baby. Longitudinal ultrasound image of the left groin (A, B) shows a lymph node (*arrowheads*) with a needle (*arrow*) within the central echogenic medulla. The lymph node size increases with injection of saline (B).

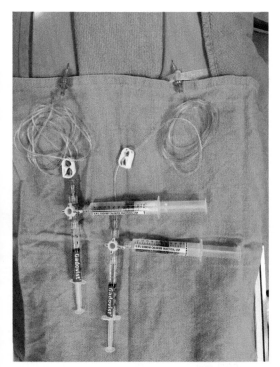

Fig. 3. Photograph simulating setup of bilateral groin needles in a phantom. The needles are connected to a long 21-inch tubing with a 3-way stopcock on each end, which in turn are connected to syringes with contrast media (Gadovist) and saline flush.

intravenous injection of GBCM, including assessment of renal function, need to be followed for DCMRL. The total amount of GBCM can be diluted with normal saline 1:1 for older children and adults and 1:2 or 1:3 for younger children to reduce T2 effects of concentrated gadolinium causing darkening from paramagnetic effects of undiluted gadolinium.[4] This practice also increases the volume available for injection, which can be useful in smaller children. Some centers do not dilute the contrast material. The total volume is divided and half of the amount is injected on each side. The entire tubing is primed with contrast containing solution. A syringe with normal saline is also attached to the 3-way stopcock on each side to flush the system and push the contrast remaining in the tube. Contrast media is administered by slow-hand injection and not by pressure injector.

MR Imaging Examination

DCMRL can be performed on 1.5 T or 3 T scanners.[4,8,18] However, 3 T scanners can potentially provide better visualization of thin lymphatic ducts due to better signal and smaller voxel size achieved at 3 T scanners.[27] Mid-neck to the lesser trochanter is the typical coverage for DCMRL. Some investigators use a plastic tray over the abdomen and pelvis to lift the weight of the anterior coil off the patient, to protect the sterile field and minimize dislodgement of the tubing and cannulae.[4]

The 2 main components of MR lymphangiography include T2-weighted imaging and postcontrast dynamic T1-weighted imaging (DCMRL), both acquired with fat suppression. The sequence parameters are listed in **Table 1.** As discussed earlier under Peripheral Lymphangiography, T2-weighted lymphatic imaging has several limitations including lack of dynamic information about lymph flow. However, it should be part of the MR lymphangiography for several complementary advantages. T2-weighted images help to localize areas of lymphedema, which may remain undetected by DCMRL. They also provide anatomic information of the cisterna chyli and thoracic duct that can be complementary to DCMRL in cases where the contrast does not propagate into the thoracic duct due to distal obstruction or lymph leak. Furthermore, static, noncontrast T2-weighted MR lymphangiography can be useful in procedural planning for DCMRL and potential intervention. There are no data on frequency of visualization of cisterna chyli and thoracic duct on heavily T2-weighted images. However, on routine T2-weighted images, they are visualized only in approximately 15% of the patients.[10] In our experience with optimized heavily T2-weighted imaging, this demonstrates lymphatic ducts with significantly higher frequency.

Dynamic imaging of passage of contrast from the injection (first passage of contrast) through the lymphatic ducts is performed using T1-weighted 3D gradient echo sequences such as T1-weighted high-resolution isotropic volume examination, volumetric interpolated breath-hold examination, and liver acquisition with volume acquisition in the coronal plane that can be acquired within 15 to 30 seconds. The usual flip angle of 10° for this sequence is increased to 25° to improve the contrast between opacified lymphatics and soft tissues. A precontrast mask is acquired that is used for subtraction. The images are acquired every minute from the start of intranodal injection of contrast until it reaches the venous angle between left subclavian and left internal jugular veins. More frequent imaging (every 30 seconds) can be performed if there is suspected chylolymphatic reflux, defined as passage of contrast from CCL into lymphatic ducts away from the expected direction of flow. Images in axial plane can be acquired in between coronal runs as required to assess the ducts. Washout of contrast

Table 1
MR lymphangiography sequences

Seq #	Sequence	Plane	TR/TE (ms)	Flip Angle (Degrees)	Matrix/SL	ETL	Pixel Band-Width (Hz)	Approximate Time
1	Single-shot T2 fatsat	Coronal	2248/160	90	264 × 230/3 mm	96	399	3 min
2	Single-shot T2 fatsat	Axial	1376/160	90	268 × 237/3 mm	98	404	4 min
3	3D T2 FSE	Coronal	3168/740	180	288 × 256/2 mm	129	167	4 min
4	T1W 3D GRE (VIBE/THRIVE/LAVA)	Coronal	3.5/1.7	25	308 × 362/2.6 mm	1	574	20–30 s
GBCM 0.1 mmol/kg, 1:1–1:3 dilution; half dose on each side of groin lymph node hand injected slowly								
5	T1W 3D GRE (VIBE/THRIVE/LAVA) every minute till contrast seen at the venous angle	Coronal	3.5/1.7	25	308 × 362/2.6 mm	1	574	20–30 s
6	T1W 3D GRE (VIBE/THRIVE/LAVA) as required	Axial	3.1/1.5	25	180 × 180/3 mm	1	720	20–30 s

Abbreviations: ETL, echo train length; FSE, fast spin echo; GRE, gradient echo; LAVA, liver acquisition with volume acquisition; NSA, number of signal averages; SL, slice thickness; THRIVE, T1-weighted high-resolution isotropic volume examination; VIBE, volumetric interpolated breath-hold examination.

from normal lymphatic ducts typically occurs within 15 to 30 minutes.[4] The dynamic images are reformatted using maximum intensity projection. Some centers use time-resolved MR angiography for the dynamic imaging.

Postprocedure

The patient is monitored for several hours for any local complications such as skin damage/burn adjacent to lymph nodes, skin discharge, and hematoma or systemic complications, including anesthetic effects.

IMAGE ANALYSIS

MR lymphangiography techniques have been applied first in patients with lymphatic disorders, limiting the knowledge of the normal lymphatic anatomy. As mentioned, there is high anatomic variability in the lymphatic system, including the shape and size of the cisterna chyli, which can appear as a single straight tube, straight thick tube, sausage-shaped tube, tortuous tube, or a focal plexus[10] (Fig. 4). In some patients, no distinct cisterna chyli may be identifiable (see Fig. 4). The

thoracic duct can have a variable diameter along its course and may show significant tortuosity as a normal variant. The lymphatic ducts are also slightly tortuous, and they can have an interrupted appearance at intervals caused by constrictions at the location of the valves.[9] This knotted or beaded appearance of lymphatic ducts can help to differentiate them from other channels such as small veins.

First passage of contrast (Fig. 5): the contrast material usually appears in the retroperitoneal lymphatics at the aortic bifurcation and along iliac ducts approximately within 2 minutes of the start of intranodal injection. A normal cisterna chyli is typically opacified within 3 to 6 minutes. The contrast then moves rapidly superiorly from the cisterna chyli through the thoracic duct, reaching the venous angle approximately in the next 2 to 3 minutes.[4] There is almost complete washout of contrast material from the normal CCL in 15 to 20 minutes with contrast excretion seen in the renal collecting system and urinary bladder.[4]

Lymphatic abnormalities: lymphangiectasia represents dilatation and increased tortuosity of lymphatic ducts. Presence of several lymphatic

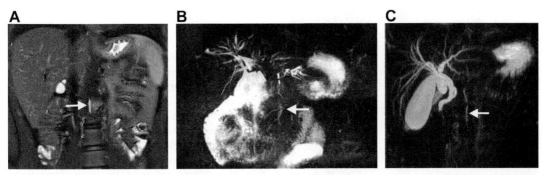

Fig. 4. Variable morphology of cisterna chyli. (*A*) Coronal T2-weighted image of the abdomen in a 17-year-old boy with nonspecific abdominal pain shows a usual slightly bulbous cisterna chyli (*arrow*). (*B*) Coronal T2-weighted MRCP image in a 10-year-old child with history of choledochal cyst resection demonstrates an irregular cisterna chyli (*arrow*) joined by lumbar trunks. (*C*) Coronal T2-weighted MRCP image in another 15-year-old child with choledocholithiasis demonstrates a thin tubular cisterna chyli (*arrow*).

channels in the same region with flow in a similar direction is considered collateralization.[4] Lymphangiectasia and collateralization indicate some drainage abnormality in the lymphatic system. Thoracic duct dilatation, lymphangiectasia, and collateralization can be seen with proximal obstruction or congestion of the lymphatic system due to elevated central venous pressure (**Fig. 6**).

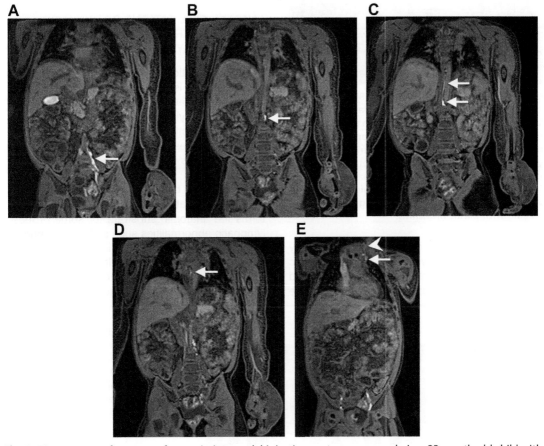

Fig. 5. First passage of contrast after groin intranodal injection up to venous angle in a 23-month-old child with protein losing enteropathy and areas of lymphedema over upper extremities. It demonstrates normal central conducting lymphatics. Coronal 3D T1-weighted images at 4 minutes (*A*), 5 minutes (*B*), 6 minutes (*C*), 7 minutes (*D*), and 8 minutes (*E*) after injection of contrast demonstrate progressive passage of the contrast (*arrows*) up to the venous angle (*arrowhead*).

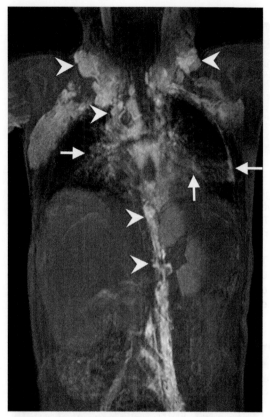

Fig. 6. MR lymphangiography in an 8-year-old child with history of Fontan surgery and plastic bronchitis. A coronal 3D T1-weighted image with thin maximum intensity projection (MIP) reconstruction at 22 minutes after injection of contrast demonstrates extensive lymphangiectasia (*arrowheads*) in retroperitoneum, mediastinum, supraclavicular, and axillary regions. Chylolymphatic reflux is seen into cervical and axillary lymph nodes, left lung, and pleural region (*arrows*) in keeping with plastic bronchitis.

Lymphangiectasia seen on MR lymphangiography has been correlated with decreased lymphatic drainage on lymphoscintigraphy, pointing toward mechanical or functional obstruction as the culprit.[28] Normal passage of the lymph is from peripheral to central conducting ducts and ultimately to the venous system via the thoracic duct. If contrast flows from the CCL into lymphatic ducts away from the expected direction of flow, it is called chylolymphatic reflux or retrograde lymphatic flow. Other abnormalities of the lymphatic system include segmental obstruction or leakage from the lymphatic channels and thoracic duct. Pleural and pericardial leakage can be seen as an area of progressive accumulation of contrast followed by slow dispersion.[4] However, nonvisualization of pleural and pericardial leakage on CDMRL does not completely exclude it. Lymphedema is typically seen as ill-defined areas of heterogeneous and granular increased signal abnormality in the soft tissues on T2-weighted images (Fig. 7). It is predominantly seen in subcutaneous tissues that are also hypertrophied. It represents abnormal lymphatic drainage and stagnation of the affected area.

CLINICAL APPLICATIONS OF DYNAMIC CONTRAST-ENHANCED MAGNETIC RESONANCE LYMPHANGIOGRAPHY

Clinical applications of DCMRL are still emerging because this is a relatively new technique. Currently, indications of DCMRL include assessment of PB, chylous pleural effusion and ascites, protein losing enteropathy, and lymphatic anomalies. Many of these conditions are interrelated and in many cases the pathophysiology is poorly understood.

As proposed by Drs Dori and Itkin,[18,29,30] pulmonary lymphatic perfusion syndrome (PLPS) forms the anatomic substrate for some of these lymphatic abnormalities such as PB and congenital chylothorax. In PLPS, a congenital abnormality has been postulated, resulting in retrograde lymphatic flow from the thoracic duct toward the mediastinum and lung parenchyma through the

A
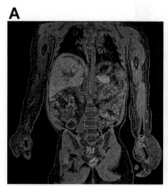

B
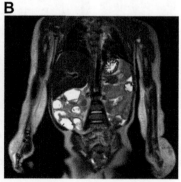

Fig. 7. Lymphedema in a 23-month-old child with protein losing enteropathy. (*A*) Coronal 3D T1-weighted and (*B*) coronal T2-weighted images demonstrate thickening and granularity of subcutaneous tissue of both upper extremities in keeping with lymphedema.

aberrant lymphatic vessels, in comparison with normal lymphatic flow from lung parenchyma toward the thoracic duct. PLPS can present at any age, from newborns as a neonatal chylothorax, to older children or adults as an idiopathic chylothorax or PB.[29] It is hypothesized that in-utero occlusion or stenosis of the downstream segment of the thoracic duct results in the development of aberrant lymphatic collaterals that are often clinically insignificant.[30] However, they may become symptomatic after silent trauma, a respiratory infection, or increased central venous pressure (CVP) as in Fontan patients, especially if the collaterals abut the serous and mucosal surfaces such as pleura, pericardium, and bronchi, leading to leakage from them. DCMRL demonstrates retrograde flow of the contrast toward the lung parenchyma. The superior segment of the thoracic duct is often stenosed or occluded in cases with PLPS,[30] although it can be challenging to demonstrate this with certainty.

Plastic Bronchitis

PB is a rare and potentially fatal condition involving airway obstruction caused by casts that can lead to significant asphyxia.[18] It is characterized by expectoration of branching bronchial casts that are formed by exudation of proteinaceous material and sometimes cells in the airways. PB can occur in patients after single-ventricle palliation, cystic fibrosis, sickle cell anemia, asthma, and lymphangiomatosis.[31,32] In patients with total cavopulmonary connection (TCPC), the prevalence of plastic bronchitis is approximately 4%.[33]

PLPS serves as the likely anatomic substrate for the condition. Elevated CVP in TCPC patients results in increased lymph production, mainly by the liver as well as increased impedance to lymphatic drainage.[8] This causes congestion in the central lymphatic system, and in the presence of PLPS, it can result in overflow of lymph into the lung parenchyma and/or into the airways, resulting in protein leakage into the airways.[8,18] This may be mediated by a potential inflammatory component, as evidenced by presence of fibrin and inflammatory cells in bronchial casts of Fontan patients with plastic bronchitis.[34] Histologically, dilatation of subpleural and interlobular lymphatics has been shown in patients with plastic bronchitis and intestinal lymphangiectasia in patients with protein losing enteropathy.[35] Abnormal tracer uptake in lungs of plastic bronchitis patients has been demonstrated on lymphoscintigraphy.[18] Children with single ventricle physiology have been shown to have lymphatic abnormalities in fetal life, indicating a possible congenital cause

or predisposition, which may be unveiled by the underlying cardiac anomaly.[36–38] Early lymphatic abnormalities, including dilated lymphatic collaterals in supraclavicular regions, mediastinum, and lungs, have been demonstrated even before TCPC and after superior cavopulmonary connection (SCPC).[36] In some of these patients, after SCPC, elevated innominate vein pressure leads to impedance to lymphatic flow, which, in combination with congenital anatomic susceptibility, leads to lymphatic collateralization in the lower neck and chest. Greater extent and distribution of these neck and chest lymphatic collaterals on T2-weighted images have been correlated with worse outcome after planned Fontan surgery including failure of Fontan and longer hospital stay.[36]

Diagnosis of PB has primarily been by direct visualization of endobronchial casts in the expectoration or on flexible bronchoscopy. DCMRL in patients with PB demonstrates abnormal lymphatic flow from the thoracic duct toward pulmonary parenchyma[8,18,39] (Fig. 8). Medical treatment attempts include sildenafil, steroids, mucolytics, heparin, and midodrine. In most cases, medical treatment improves symptoms but does not treat the underlying condition. Cardiac transplantation can lead to resolution of the disease presumably due to normalization of CVP and return of normal pulsatile pulmonary flow as compared with the passive venous flow of the Fontan circulation. Normalization of CVP by fenestration of the Fontan circuit resulting into resolution of plastic bronchitis symptoms has also been reported.[40] Recently, selective embolization of lymphatic channels in the lungs and thoracic duct stenting has been successfully used to treat the disease in children and adults with close to 90% success rate.[8,18,41] DCMRL therefore plays an important role in planning of the embolization treatment in these patients. Identification of all lymphatic pathways from the abdomen toward the chest on DCMRL is essential in interventional treatment planning. These communications can consist of a single thoracic duct or 2 thoracic ducts or can be through the retroperitoneal/mediastinal pathways.

Chylothorax and Chyloperitoneum

Chylothorax and chyloperitoneum can be congenital and isolated or associated with lymphatic dysplasia. They can occur secondary to trauma, surgery, severe infection such as tuberculosis or fungal infestations, as well as malignancy.[11,42] Chylothorax can also result from thrombosis of the SVC or subclavian veins, likely due to resistance to the flow of lymph from the thoracic duct into the veins.

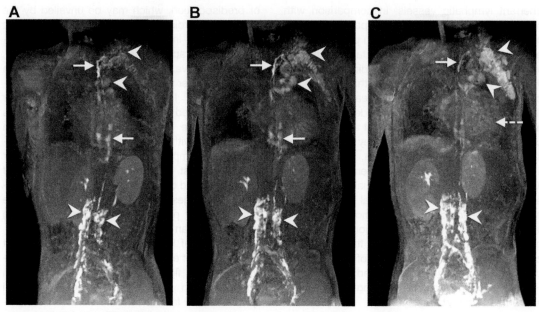

Fig. 8. Plastic bronchitis in a 4-year-old child with Fontan surgery. Coronal 3D T1-weighted images with thin maximum intensity projection (MIP) reconstruction at 8 minutes (*A*), 10 minutes (*B*), and 16 minutes (*C*) after injection of contrast demonstrate an abnormal ectatic lymphatic duct extending from retroperitoneum to the left side of superior mediastinum (*arrows*), lymphangiectasia in retroperitoneum (*arrowheads*) and mediastinum (*arrowheads*), and extensive and progressive chylolymphatic reflux into left supraclavicular and axillary lymph nodes. There is also chylolymphatic reflux into the lungs (*dashed arrows*).

Congenital chylothorax and chyloperitoneum can result from aplasia, hypoplasia, obstruction, valvular incompetence, or leakage from the thoracic duct. Its prevalence is greater in Noonan, Down, and Turner syndromes.[11] Children with Noonan syndrome and clinical evidence of lymphatic dysfunction frequently have central lymphatic abnormalities characterized by retrograde intercostal flow, pulmonary lymphatic perfusion, and thoracic duct abnormalities.[43]

Congenital lymphatic flow disorders often manifest in utero as hydrops, ascites, or pleural effusions. In most cases, isolated neonatal chylothorax is discovered on prenatal ultrasound.[44] Pulmonary lymphangiectasia can be associated with chylothorax and seen as nutmeg appearance of lungs on fetal MR imaging.[45,46] Isolated chylous ascites can also be detected on prenatal ultrasound. Postnatally, DCRML can provide an excellent imaging of the lymphatic abnormalities in these patients. In most patients with idiopathic chylothorax, there is an abnormal pulmonary lymphatic flow from the thoracic duct toward lung parenchyma (**Fig. 9**). Dilation of the thoracic duct is also often observed in these patients. In some cases of chylous ascites, frank extravasation of the contrast into the peritoneal cavity can be seen on DCMRL (**Fig. 10**). In other

cases of chylothorax and chyloperitoneum, MR lymphangiography will help to show preserved integrity of CCL.

Chylothorax and chyloperitoneum have been treated with drainage, dietary modifications, and medical therapy with secretion inhibitors such as octreotide or somatostatin. Refractory cases are treated with pleurodesis, pleuroperitoneal shunts, surgical ligation, or embolization of the thoracic duct.[11,42] Thoracoamniotic shunts can be placed in utero in cases with antenatally detected chylothorax to prevent underdevelopment of the lung.[47] After birth, embolization of retrograde pulmonary lymphatic flow with Lipiodol can result in complete resolution of the congenital chylothorax.[48] If the thoracic duct is found to be occluded at the level of the neck, a microsurgical thoracic duct to vein connection can be attempted.

Chylothorax in Pediatric Patients After Cardiac Surgery

Chylothorax after surgery for congenital cardiac disease is common in children, with an incidence of 2.8% to 3.9%.[49,50] It is associated with increased mortality and length of hospital stay, incurring a high cost for the care of these patients.[49] Traditionally, surgical trauma to the

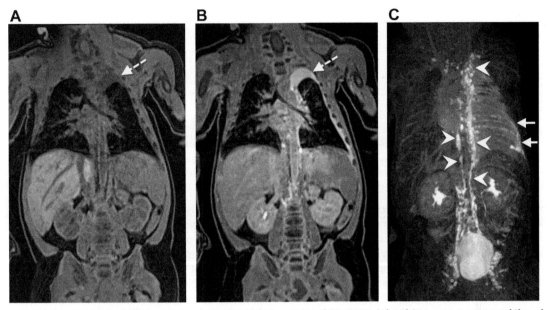

Fig. 9. Congenital left chylothorax in a 7-week-old baby. Coronal 3D T1-weighted images precontrast (*A*) and 18 minutes after injection of contrast (*B*) demonstrate left pleural effusion with opacification on postcontrast image suggesting lymphatic leak (*dashed arrows*). A thin MIP reconstruction image (*C*) shows abnormal tortuous CCL (*arrowheads*) without a single normal looking thoracic duct and chylolymphatic reflux into left pleural cavity (*arrows*).

thoracic duct or its branches has been assumed to be the cause of the chylothorax. However, a recent study using DCMRL to image these patients identified that the trauma of the thoracic lymphatic occurred only in a minority (8%) of the patients.[51] The majority (56%) in this study had PLPS, and the rest of the patients (36%) had central lymphatic flow disorder, which is characterized by abnormal central lymphatic flow, effusion in more than one compartment, and dermal backflow.[51] In this series, the imaging findings of those patients who had PLPS were similar to the imaging findings in patients with PB, and some patients in this series had both PB and chylothorax.

Protein Losing Enteropathy

Protein losing enteropathy (PLE) is characterized by rapid loss of serum proteins into the gut lumen. The resulting hypoproteinemia can lead to edema, ascites, pleural, and pericardial effusions due to an imbalance between oncotic and hydrostatic pressures. Diagnosis is usually made by virtue of

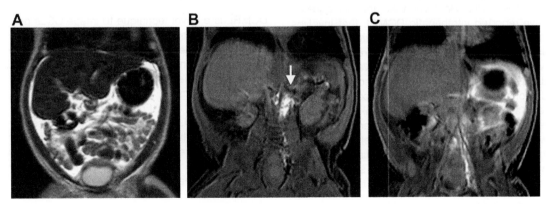

Fig. 10. Congenital chyloperitoneum in an 8-week-old baby from chyle leak. Coronal T2-weighted (*A*), and post nodal injection coronal 3D T1-weighted images at 3 minutes (*B*) and 15 minutes (*C*) after injection of contrast demonstrate contrast leakage from retroperitoneal lymphatic channel (*arrow on B*) with progressive opacification of ascites on left side of the abdomen.

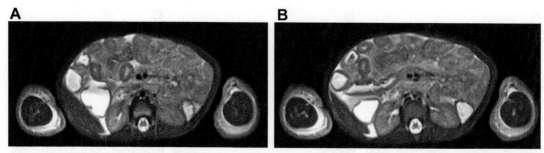

Fig. 11. Protein losing enteropathy (PLE) in a 23-month-old child. Axial T2-weighted images of the abdomen (*A, B*) demonstrate mild ascites, mesenteric edema, and diffuse bowel wall thickening in keeping with PLE. This child had normal CCL as demonstrated in **Fig. 5**.

clinical symptoms and increased fecal concentrations of alpha-1-antitrypsin. Occasionally, the site of protein leakage can be localized by scintigraphy.[52] PLE is either caused by lymphatic abnormalities or chronic mucosal injury as occurs in inflammatory bowel disease or neoplasm. Lymphatic abnormalities include primary intestinal lymphangiectasia and secondary lymphangiectasia from congestive heart failure.[52] PLE seen in patients with Fontan are likely the result of a combination of lymphatic congestion from elevated CVP and increased lymph production by the liver. Increased hepatic lymph production is also result of increased CVP. Mild bowel wall thickening, mesenteric edema, and ascites are typical imaging findings of PLE caused by intestinal lymphangiectasia (**Fig. 11**). DCMRL via intranodal injection in the groin cannot reliably directly visualize normal intraperitoneal, liver, and intestinal lymphatics. However, findings of lymphatic congestion in CCL in Fontan patients is typically apparent, in contrast to normal CCL in PLE from other causes, such as isolated congenital intestinal lymphangiectasia.[1] Until recently, there was no method to image liver lymphatics that are likely to play a significant role in the pathogenesis of PLE. However, Biko and colleagues[25] have reported intrahepatic DCMRL that involves injection of GBCA directly in the liver lymphatics and tracking the passage of contrast using T1-weighted MR images. Normally liver lymphatics drain into the CCL. Using this technique, they demonstrated chylolymphatic reflux into mesentery and bowel as well as frank intraluminal leakage of contrast into the duodenum in cases with PLE.[25] This technique is likely to play an important role in better understanding the pathogenesis of PLE and hopefully open some new avenues for therapeutic interventions in PLE.

Lymphatic Malformations

Lymphatic malformations are a group of poorly understood developmental lymphatic anomalies

that include common cystic lymphatic malformations, generalized lymphatic anomalies (GLA) including a proliferative disorder Kaposiform lymphangiomatosis, lymphatic malformations in Gorham-Stout disease, channel type lymphatic malformations, "acquired" progressive lymphatic anomalies, and a variety of primary lymphedema.[53,54] These conditions have overlapping features and are often difficult to differentiate. GLA or lymphangiomatosis is a rare disease consisting of multiple lymphatic malformations infiltrating different tissues with a wide spectrum, from single-organ involvement to generalized disease involving multiple systems. The predominant sites of involvement in GLA are lungs and pleura, resulting in interstitial lung disease and chylothorax.

MR lymphangiography in these conditions can show pleural effusions, significant dilation of the thoracic duct on T2-weighted imaging, and presence of PLPS if any. DCMRL can help to map CCL and find potentially treatable abnormalities such as collaterals, leakages, and obstruction.[4]

SUMMARY

DCMRL is a novel technique to image CCLs performed by injecting GBCA into groin lymph nodes and following the passage of contrast through the lymphatic system using T1-weighted MR images. To date, it has been successfully applied to image and guide treatment of the lymphatic abnormalities associated with Fontan procedure such as plastic bronchitis. It is also useful in the assessment of chylothorax and chyloperitoneum and their potential treatment planning. Its role in other areas such as intestinal lymphangiectasia and lymphatic anomalies is likely to increase.

DISCLOSURE

All authors have no funding to disclose related to this work.

REFERENCES

1. Chavhan GB, Amaral JG, Temple M, et al. MR lymphangiography in children: technique and potential applications. Radiographics 2017;37(6):1775–90.
2. Betterman KL, Harvey NL. The lymphatic vasculature: development and role in shaping immunity. Immunol Rev 2016;271(1):276–92.
3. Dori Y, Zviman MM, Itkin M. Dynamic contrast-enhanced MR lymphangiography: feasibility study in swine. Radiology 2014;273(2):410–6.
4. Krishnamurthy R, Hernandez A, Kavuk S, et al. Imaging the central conducting lymphatics: initial experience with dynamic MR lymphangiography. Radiology 2015;274(3):871–8.
5. Nadolski GJ, Itkin M. Feasibility of ultrasound-guided intranodal lymphangiogram for thoracic duct embolization. J Vasc Interv Radiol 2012;23(5):613–6.
6. Itkin M, Krishnamurthy G, Naim MY, et al. Percutaneous thoracic duct embolization as a treatment for intrathoracic chyle leaks in infants. Pediatrics 2011;128(1):e237–41.
7. Nadolski GJ, Itkin M. Thoracic duct embolization for nontraumatic chylous effusion: experience in 34 patients. Chest 2013;143(1):158–63.
8. Dori Y, Keller MS, Rychik J, et al. Successful treatment of plastic bronchitis by selective lymphatic embolization in a Fontan patient. Pediatrics 2014;134(2):e590–5.
9. Gray H. Chapter VIII. In: Lewis WH, editor. The lymphatic system in anatomy of human body. 20th edition; 2000. New York. Available at: Bartleby.com 2000. Accessed January 11, 2017.
10. Pinto PS, Sirlin CB, Andrade-Barreto OA, et al. Cisterna chyli at routine abdominal MR imaging: a normal anatomic structure in the retrocrural space. Radiographics 2004;24(3):809–17.
11. Tutor JD. Chylothorax in infants and children. Pediatrics 2014;133(4):722–33.
12. Hsu MC, Itkin M. Lymphatic anatomy. Tech Vasc Interv Radiol 2016;19(4):247–54.
13. Szabó G, Pósch E, Magyar Z. Interstitial fluid, lymph and oedema formation. Acta Physiol Acad Sci Hung 1980;56(4):367–78.
14. Witte CL, Witte MH, Dumont AE, et al. Protein content in lymph and edema fluid in congestive heart failure. Circulation 1969;40(5):623–30.
15. Hall RC, Krementz ET. Lymphangiography by lymph-node injection. JAMA 1967;202(13):1136–9.
16. Rajebi MR, Chaudry G, Padua HM, et al. Intranodal lymphangiography: feasibility and preliminary experience in children. J Vasc Interv Radiol 2011;22(9):1300–5.
17. Kirschen MP, Dori Y, Itkin M, et al. Cerebral lipiodol embolism after lymphatic embolization for plastic bronchitis. J Pediatr 2016;176:200–3.
18. Dori Y, Keller MS, Rome JJ, et al. Percutaneous lymphatic embolization of abnormal pulmonary lymphatic flow as treatment of plastic bronchitis in patients with congenital heart disease. Circulation 2016;133(12):1160–70.
19. Laor T, Hoffer FA, Burrows PE, et al. MR lymphangiography in infants, children, and young adults. AJR Am J Roentgenol 1998;171(4):1111–7.
20. Arrivé L, Derhy S, Dahan B, et al. Primary lower limb lymphoedema: classification with non-contrast MR lymphography. Eur Radiol 2018;28(1):291–300.
21. Crescenzi R, Donahue PMC, Hartley KG, et al. Lymphedema evaluation using noninvasive 3T MR lymphangiography. J Magn Reson Imaging 2017;46(5):1349–60.
22. Zeltzer AA, Brussaard C, Koning M, et al. MR lymphography in patients with upper limb lymphedema: The GPS for feasibility and surgical planning for lympho-venous bypass. J Surg Oncol 2018;118(3):407–15.
23. Pieper CC, Schild HH. Interstitial transpedal MR-lymphangiography of central lymphatics using a standard MR contrast agent: feasibility and initial results in patients with chylous effusions. Rofo 2018;190(10):938–45.
24. Mazzei MA, Gentili F, Mazzei FG, et al. High-resolution MR lymphangiography for planning lymphatico-venous anastomosis treatment: a single-centre experience. Radiol Med 2017;122(12):918–27.
25. Biko DM, Smith CL, Otero HJ, et al. Intrahepatic dynamic contrast MR lymphangiography: initial experience with a new technique for the assessment of liver lymphatics. Eur Radiol 2019;29(10):5190–6.
26. Nadolski GJ, Ponce-Dorrego MD, Darge K, et al. Validation of the position of injection needles with contrast-enhanced ultrasound for dynamic contract-enhanced MR lymphangiography. J Vasc Interv Radiol 2018;29(7):1028–30.
27. Chavhan GB, Babyn PS, Singh M, et al. MR imaging at 3.0 T in children: technical differences, safety issues, and initial experience. Radiographics 2009;29(5):1451–66.
28. Notohamiprodjo M, Weiss M, Baumeister RG, et al. MR lymphangiography at 3.0 T: correlation with lymphoscintigraphy. Radiology 2012;264(1):78–87.
29. Itkin M, McCormack FX. Nonmalignant adult thoracic lymphatic disorders. Clin Chest Med 2016;37(3):409–20.
30. Itkin M. Interventional treatment of pulmonary lymphatic anomalies. Tech Vasc Interv Radiol 2016;19(4):299–304.
31. Seear M, Hui H, Magee F, et al. Bronchial casts in children: a proposed classification based on nine cases and a review of the literature. Am J Respir Crit Care Med 1997;155(1):364–70.
32. Madsen P, Shah SA, Rubin BK. Plastic bronchitis: new insights and a classification scheme. Paediatr Respir Rev 2005;6(4):292–300.

33. Schumacher KR, Singh TP, Kuebler J, et al. Risk factors and outcome of Fontan-associated plastic bronchitis: a case-control study. J Am Heart Assoc 2014; 3(2):e000865.

34. Racz J, Mane G, Ford M, et al. Immunophenotyping and protein profiling of Fontan-associated plastic bronchitis airway casts. Ann Am Thorac Soc 2013; 10(2):98–107.

35. Languepin J, Scheinmann P, Mahut B, et al. Bronchial casts in children with cardiopathies: the role of pulmonary lymphatic abnormalities. Pediatr Pulmonol 1999;28(5):329–36.

36. Biko DM, DeWitt AG, Pinto EM, et al. MRI evaluation of lymphatic abnormalities in the neck and thorax after fontan surgery: relationship with outcome. Radiology 2019;291(3):774–80.

37. Saul D, Degenhardt K, Iyoob SD, et al. Hypoplastic left heart syndrome and the nutmeg lung pattern in utero: a cause and effect relationship or prognostic indicator? Pediatr Radiol 2016;46(4):483–9.

38. Lam CZ, Bhamare TA, Gazzaz T, et al. Diagnosis of secondary pulmonary lymphangiectasia in congenital heart disease: a novel role for chest ultrasound and prognostic implications. Pediatr Radiol 2017; 47(11):1441–51.

39. Dori Y, Keller MS, Fogel MA, et al. MRI of lymphatic abnormalities after functional single-ventricle palliation surgery. AJR Am J Roentgenol 2014;203(2): 426–31.

40. Wilson J, Russell J, Williams W, et al. Fenestration of the Fontan circuit as treatment for plastic bronchitis. Pediatr Cardiol 2005;26(5):717–9.

41. Itkin MG, McCormack FX, Dori Y. Diagnosis and treatment of lymphatic plastic bronchitis in adults using advanced lymphatic imaging and percutaneous embolization. Ann Am Thorac Soc 2016;13(10): 1689–96.

42. Lopez-Gutierrez JC, Tovar JA. Chylothorax and chylous ascites: management and pitfalls. Semin Pediatr Surg 2014;23(5):298–302.

43. Biko DM, Reisen B, Otero HJ, et al. Imaging of central lymphatic abnormalities in Noonan syndrome. Pediatr Radiol 2019;49(5):586–92.

44. Rocha G, Fernandes P, Rocha P, et al. Pleural effusions in the neonate. Acta Paediatr 2006;95(7): 791–8.

45. Biko DM, Johnstone JA, Dori Y, et al. Recognition of neonatal lymphatic flow disorder: fetal MR findings and postnatal MR lymphangiogram correlation. Acad Radiol 2018;25(11):1446–50.

46. Seed M, Bradley T, Bourgeois J, et al. Antenatal MR imaging of pulmonary lymphangiectasia secondary to hypoplastic left heart syndrome. Pediatr Radiol 2009;39(7):747–9.

47. Wilson RD, Baxter JK, Johnson MP, et al. Thoracoamniotic shunts: fetal treatment of pleural effusions and congenital cystic adenomatoid malformations. Fetal Diagn Ther 2004;19(5):413–20.

48. Gray M, Kovatis KZ, Stuart T, et al. Treatment of congenital pulmonary lymphangiectasia using ethiodized oil lymphangiography. J Perinatol 2014;34(9): 720–2.

49. Mery CM, Moffett BS, Khan MS, et al. Incidence and treatment of chylothorax after cardiac surgery in children: analysis of a large multi-institution database. J Thorac Cardiovasc Surg 2014;147(2): 678–86.e1 [discussion: 685–6].

50. Bauman ME, Moher C, Bruce AK, et al. Chylothorax in children with congenital heart disease: incidence of thrombosis. Thromb Res 2013;132(2):e83–5.

51. Savla JJ, Itkin M, Rossano JW, et al. Post-operative chylothorax in patients with congenital heart disease. J Am Coll Cardiol 2017;69(19):2410–22.

52. Braamskamp MJ, Dolman KM, Tabbers MM. Clinical practice.Protein-losing enteropathy in children. Eur J Pediatr 2010;169(10):1179–85.

53. Wassef M, Blei F, Adams D, et al. Vascular anomalies classification: recommendations from the International Society for the Study of Vascular Anomalies. Pediatrics 2015;136(1):e203–14.

54. ISSVA Classification of Vascular Anomalies ©2018 International Society for the Study of Vascular Anomalies. Available at: issva.org/classification. Accessed October 27, 2018.

Pulmonary Vascular Disease Evaluation with Magnetic Resonance Angiography

Bradley D. Allen, MD, MS[a],*, Mark L. Schiebler, MD[b],
Christopher J. François, MD[b]

KEYWORDS

- Magnetic resonance angiography • Pulmonary arteries • Pulmonary embolism
- Pulmonary hypertension

KEY POINTS

- Pulmonary magnetic resonance angiography (pMRA) is an effective nonionizing examination for the exclusion of pulmonary embolism.
- pMRA with cardiac magnetic resonance imaging provides quantitative information predictive of outcome in patients with pulmonary hypertension.
- Knowledge of common pMRA artifacts is crucial.
- Future uses of noncontrast magnetic resonance angiography and four-dimensional flow magnetic resonance imaging for pMRA remain to be explored.

INTRODUCTION

Historically, magnetic resonance angiography (MRA) has been used for the evaluation of the systemic circulation, including the thoracic and abdominal aorta and branches, the renal arteries, upper and lower extremity peripheral vasculature, and head and neck vasculature. This technique most commonly uses gadolinium-based contrast agents to opacify the vasculature of interest, and, because magnetic resonance (MR) imaging is not limited by concerns related to ionizing radiation, multiple images can be acquired over the course of contrast transit to provide time-resolved MRA (TR-MRA) or dynamic, contrast-enhanced MRA (CE-MRA). Noncontrast MRA techniques are also available, and, with improved MR imaging hardware and acceleration approaches, extremely high spatial and temporal resolution MRA images can be acquired.

With these improvements, there has been increasing use of MRA for the evaluation of pulmonary vascular diseases, including pulmonary embolism (PE) and pulmonary hypertension (PH). These commonly encountered diseases can result in significant morbidity and mortality if not correctly diagnosed, and medical imaging plays an important role in evaluating the underlying causes and complications of these and other pulmonary vascular diseases. Most commonly, pulmonary vascular assessment relies on computed tomography angiography (CTA) and can be supplemented by nuclear medicine ventilation-perfusion (VQ) scintigraphy. In PH, invasive measurement of right heart pressure and estimated pulmonary vascular resistance is also commonly performed. One of the key advantages of pulmonary MRA (pMRA) relative to these other techniques is the opportunity to evaluate pulmonary

a Department of Radiology, Northwestern University Feinberg School of Medicine, 737 North Michigan Avenue, Suite 1600, Chicago, IL 60611, USA; b Department of Radiology, University of Wisconsin, 600 Highland Avenue, Madison, WI 53792, USA
* Corresponding author.
E-mail address: bdallen@northwestern.edu

Radiol Clin N Am 58 (2020) 707–719
https://doi.org/10.1016/j.rcl.2020.02.006
0033-8389/20/© 2020 Elsevier Inc. All rights reserved.

radiologic.theclinics.com

Table 1
Suggested pulmonary magnetic resonance angiography protocol

	Series	Use	Notes
1	Three-plane single-shot fast spin echo	Localizer	—
2	Precontrast coronal T1-weighted 3D SGRE	Assess for appropriate anatomic coverage	Must have adequate AP coverage Wrap artifact from shoulders should be minimized
3	Pulmonary arterial-phase T1-weighted 3D SGRE	PA visualization Lung parenchymal perfusion assessment	Fluoro triggered Bolus timing and truncation artifacts can reduce diagnostic accuracy
4	Immediate postcontrast T1-weighted 3D SGRE	PA visualization	Can be helpful if series 3 is degraded
5	Low-flip-angle postcontrast T1-weighted 3D SGRE	Pulmonary and systemic vasculature visualization	Performed 1–2 min after injection Low flip angle allows increased signal in vessels even though contrast is diluted
6	T1-weighted 2D axial fat saturated	Assess nonvascular structures	—
Optional Series			
1	Axial maximal intensity projections of series 3	PA visualization	Can be helpful, particularly for novice readers
2	Time-resolved MRA	PA visualization Lung parenchymal perfusion assessment	Can allow for quantification of pulmonary hemodynamics
3	4D flow MR imaging	Velocity and flow visualization and quantification	Allows hemodynamic assessment of pulmonary vasculature in single acquisition Requires specialized postprocessing and viewing software
3	Cardiac cine imaging	Cardiac qualitative and quantitative function	Useful in pulmonary hypertension evaluation

Abbreviations: 2D, two-dimensional; 3D, three-dimensional; AP, anteroposterior; PA, pulmonary artery; SGRE, spoiled gradient echo.

vascular anatomy, hemodynamic physiology, lung parenchymal perfusion, and (optionally) right and left ventricular function with a single examination without exposure to ionizing radiation.

This article provides an overview of pMRA acquisition techniques and its performance and potential in commonly encountered pulmonary vascular diseases. It also provides an outlook for additional pMRA applications and advanced techniques that are actively being investigated.

PULMONARY MAGNETIC RESONANCE ANGIOGRAPHY TECHNIQUE

MRA evaluation of the pulmonary vasculature is best accomplished using CE-MRA, with imaging timing optimized for visualization of the pulmonary arteries (PAs). In general, gadolinium-based contrast agent is injected through a peripheral intravenous catheter, and timing for PA imaging can be performed using test timing bolus or fluoroscopic triggering. For high-quality imaging, a 0.1-mmol/kg dose of high-relaxivity contrast agent is recommended. Note that several gadolinium-based contrast agents have been approved for MRA, but not specifically for pMRA. The contrast can be diluted in normal saline for a total injected volume of 30 mL with injection rate of 1.5 mL/s, which helps improve artifacts related to contrast bolus timing (discussed later). Proper imaging timing is crucial for high-quality pMRA, and our protocol consists of manual fluoroscopic triggering with real-time two-dimensional (2D) images

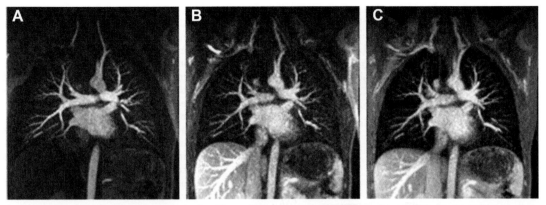

Fig. 1. Normal pulmonary angiogram maximal intensity projections in a 13-year-old girl with chest pain. The PA phase (*A*), immediate postinjection (*B*), and low-flip-angle 60-second delayed image (*C*) are displayed. There is excellent contrast bolus timing in PA phase with progressive visualization of the pulmonary veins and systemic vasculature during delayed imaging. In this young girl, pMRA was an effective modality for excluding PE with no exposure to ionizing radiation.

acquired in an axial or sagittal oblique orientation and scanning initiated when contrast is seen in the right ventricle.[1]

An effective pMRA protocol has previously been described by Nagle and colleagues[1] and is outlined in **Table 1**. A typical CE-MRA protocol consists of a rapid three-dimensional (3D) spoiled gradient-echo sequence acquired in the coronal orientation.[2] To limit respiratory motion artifact, which can significantly degrade image quality,

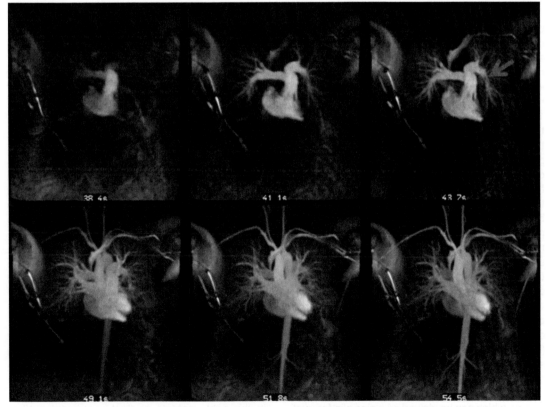

Fig. 2. Time-resolved pulmonary MRA in a 54-year-old woman with breast cancer. Sequential images (*top row, left to right and bottom row, left to right*) show filling of the pulmonary vasculature, enhancement of the pulmonary parenchyma, filling of the pulmonary veins, and opacification of the systemic vasculature. There is filling defect consistent with PE in the left interlobar PA (*blue arrow*).

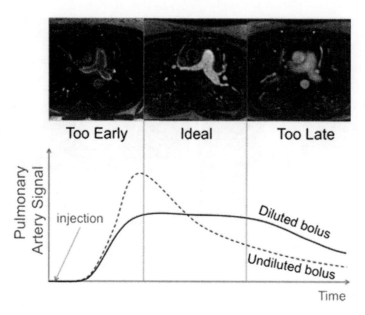

Fig. 3. The impact of contrast bolus timing and bolus length on pulmonary MRA image quality. In this example, all images were acquired using elliptic centric k-space sampling, meaning the low-spatial-frequency data were acquired first. The too-early image shows poor opacification of the central PAs with apparent edge enhancement. This appearance is related to sampling the low spatial frequencies (center of vessels) before contrast has arrived in the vessel, and high spatial frequencies (vessel walls) after contrast has arrived. The too-late image appears less sharp and in part is related to lack of contrast remaining in the vessel during high-spatial-frequency sampling as well as reduced signal-to-noise ratio (SNR) caused by overall less contrast in the vessel. The graph shows the impact of bolus dilution (*solid line*), which allows the contrast peak to be spread over a longer period of time, but at a slightly lower concentration. The result is a longer window for adequate arterial-phase imaging with the trade-off of slightly lower SNR. (*From* Nagle SK, Schiebler ML, Repplinger MD, et al. Contrast enhanced pulmonary magnetic resonance angiography for pulmonary embolism: Building a successful program. *Eur J Radiol.* 2016;85(3):553-563; with permission.)

breath holding is generally required but can be difficult for patients with cardiopulmonary diseases. Recent advances in image acceleration, namely 2D autocalibrated parallel imaging, now allows both shorter breath holds and higher spatial resolution.[3,4] Imaging can be performed at both 1.5 T and 3.0 T, with slightly higher spatial resolution available at 3.0 T without a significant reduction in signal-to-noise ratio.[5] Of note, it is our practice to perform sequential MR images immediately after and approximately 30 to 60 seconds following the initial PA phase images. These series tend to be helpful for problem solving if contrast bolus timing or other artifacts degrade the initial pMRA and also allow for evaluation of the pulmonary veins and systemic vasculature. When properly implemented, pMRA examinations take less than 10 minutes on the scanner and can be deployed in the emergency setting[1] (Fig. 1).

Time-resolved MRA can be included as a part of pMRA, which allows for imaging of the first pass of contrast through the pulmonary vasculature[6] (Fig. 2). This technique also uses 3D gradient-echo sequence and leverages acceleration approaches and optimized k-space sampling strategies to generate images with high spatial and temporal resolution, which can be viewed as a cine clip for qualitative assessment of pulmonary hemodynamics and also used to qualitatively or quantitatively assess lung parenchymal perfusion.[7–9]

ARTIFACTS ASSOCIATED WITH PULMONARY MAGNETIC RESONANCE ANGIOGRAPHY

In addition to respiratory motion artifact, poor PA opacification caused by suboptimal contrast bolus timing and truncation (Gibbs ringing) artifact can reduce both image quality and diagnostic accuracy.

Pulmonary Artery Opacification

On contrast-enhanced pMRA, the high signal in the PA is caused by the T1-shortening effect of gadolinium-based contrast agent in the PAs. As described earlier, timing of imaging relative to arrival of the contrast bolus is critical to allow adequate opacification of the pulmonary tree. Challenges associated with timing are among the primary benefits of pMRA relative to CTA, because MRA allows multiple acquisitions without concerns related to radiation exposure,[10] and delayed images may have improved PA opacification.

Two key parameters determine optimal contrast opacification: (1) image timing relative to bolus arrival, and (2) bolus length. For image timing relative to the contrast bolus, fluoroscopic triggering is used with imaging initiated when contrast is seen in the right ventricle or right ventricular outflow tract. Exact trigger timing may be site, scanner, and injector specific so feedback to the technologist regarding image quality related to triggering is

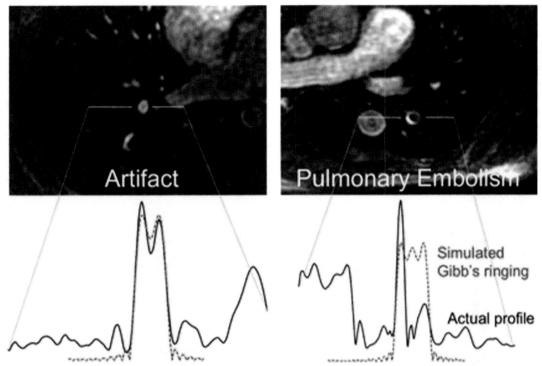

Fig. 4. Truncation (Gibbs ringing) artifact can mimic PE, although the true signal decrease in PE (*black curve, bottom left*) is generally much greater relative to signal decrease from truncation artifact (*red curves*). (*From* Nagle SK, Schiebler ML, Repplinger MD, et al. Contrast enhanced pulmonary magnetic resonance angiography for pulmonary embolism: Building a successful program. *Eur J Radiol.* 2016;85(3):553-563; ;with permission.)

important. Depending on k-space sampling strategies (standard cartesian vs elliptic centric), initiating the scan too early or too late can result in image blur or inappropriate edge enhancement (**Fig. 3**). The narrower the bolus, the more difficult it becomes to align the contrast bolus timing with the selected k-space sampling scheme.[1] Therefore, increasing the bolus duration by diluting the contrast with saline and injecting over a longer time period (~20 seconds) allows more flexibility with contrast bolus timing with minimal impact on the overall signal in the PAs.

Truncation Artifact

Truncation (Gibbs) artifact is a well-known artifact in MR imaging that can lead to image interpretation challenges in pMRA, particularly when evaluating for PE. In MR imaging, high-spatial-frequency structures such as vessel edges are approximated by progressively higher frequency wave functions, and at sharp boundaries, such as a small vessel edge, infinite k-space sampling is required. Given the practical need to truncate higher spatial frequencies in k-space

approximations of these edges, ripples of signal intensity can occur near sharp boundaries in reconstructed images.[11] In larger anatomic structures such as the aorta or main PA, there is usually little problem generating adequate spatial frequencies to approximate the vessel walls without truncation artifact affecting signal in the vessel center. However, in small vessels, usually with intraluminal diameters on the order of 3 to 5 voxels, signal loss from destructive interference of the truncation artifact ripples can occur.

However, these artifacts can closely approximate true filling defects related to PE.[12] Importantly, because the artifact is closely related to vessel size rather than contrast timing, it is likely to be present on all phases of images and therefore persistence of the filling defect on delayed series does not necessarily imply that the finding is a PE.[1] A study by Bannas and colleagues[12] showed that, by comparing the signal decrease in the central filling defect relative to surrounding blood, signal could be used to distinguish artifact from thrombus. A signal decrease of greater than 51% on pulmonary arterial-phase images or 47% on delayed-phase images resulted in a sensitivity of

100% and specificity of 90% for distinguishing PE from truncation artifact (Fig. 4).

One approach to mitigate these artifacts is to increase the spatial resolution of the acquisition, which shifts the truncation artifact to smaller vessels. However, this change leads to prolonged scan times, longer breath holds, and decreased signal-to-noise ratio.[12] As such, appropriately balancing scan parameters with the presence of this artifact is important for overall image quality optimization. There are occasions when exclusion of PE on pMRA is not possible because of the presence of Gibbs artifact and a CTA chest needs to be obtained.

SELECTED CLINICAL APPLICATIONS OF PULMONARY MAGNETIC RESONANCE ANGIOGRAPHY
Pulmonary Embolism

After myocardial infarction and stroke, PE is the third most common cause of acute cardiovascular disease.[13] Acute PE can be fatal in up to 30% of patients if not diagnosed and treated promptly, but a mortality rate of only 2% to 10% when appropriately managed.[14] The multicenter Prospective Investigation of Pulmonary Embolism Diagnosis (PIOPED) II study showed that computed tomography (CT) pulmonary

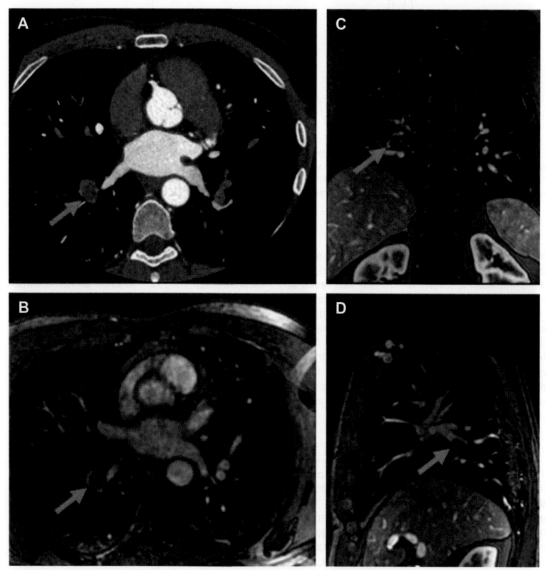

Fig. 5. A 56-year-old man with chest pain with cardiac risk factors. A questioned filling defect (*arrows*) was seen in the righter interlobar PA at coronary CTA (*A*). PE was confirmed on pulmonary MRA. (*B*) Axial reformat, (*C*) coronal, and (*D*) sagittal reformat.

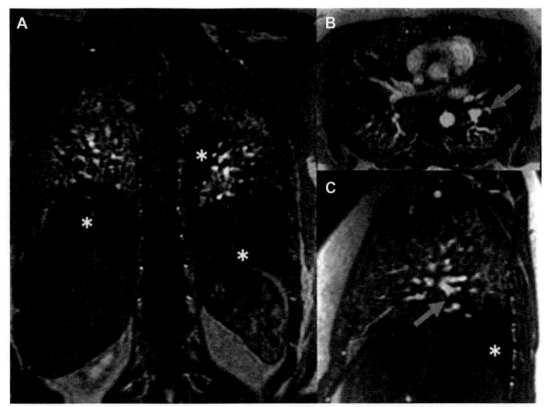

Fig. 6. A 30-year-old woman presenting to the emergency department with pleuritic chest pain and history of oral contraceptive use. Coronal image (A) and axial (B) and sagittal (C) multiplanar reformats show large, peripheral, wedge-shaped perfusion defects in the right and left lower lobes (asterisks). Bilateral pulmonary emboli are seen in the right interlobar PA (orange arrow) and a segmental left lower lobe PA (blue arrow).

angiography had high sensitivity and specificity for diagnosing PE and has since become the standard of care in PE evaluation.[15] CT is associated with medical exposure to ionizing radiation, which is associated with a small but nonzero risk of radiation-induced malignancies.[10,16] The risk of radiation-induced malignancy may be slightly higher in women and younger patients, particularly when performing chest CT, and therefore the risks and benefits of CT imaging must be weighed.[17] Moreover, allergies to iodinated contrast agents are common and patients may be ineligible for CTA or require allergy prep medications, which could delay diagnosis.

As mentioned earlier, pMRA is a radiation-free alternative to CTA for pulmonary angiography. The PIOPED III study was a prospective, multi-center trial evaluating the efficacy of contrast-enhanced pMRA for diagnosis of PE in 371 patients. Although this study showed modest sensitivity (78%) and high specificity (99%) for diagnosis of PE, the results were limited by a large percentage of technically inadequate images, which ranged from 11% to 52% of included

patients across the 7 sites involved in the study.[18] Note that most of the technically inadequate scans in this study were related to poor arterial enhancement or motion artifact. As discussed, arterial enhancement can be optimized, and more experienced centers were more successful than less experienced centers in limiting this artifact. It is also important to note that the MRA techniques used in PIOPED III were performed on older-generation hardware and did not consistently use parallel imaging, thus the scans were longer, which likely led to more motion-related artifacts as well as images with lower spatial resolution.

A study by Kalb and colleagues[19] explored the utility of time-resolved pMRA, delayed 3D gradient-echo CE-MRA, and steady-state free precession (SSFP) imaging for the diagnosis of PE. All sequences provided 99% to 100% specificity, whereas sensitivity was highest for the delayed CE-MRA sequence (73%). Combining all 3 sequences, the sensitivity for PE diagnosis reached 84% with a specificity of 100%. More recently, the authors published a retrospective study evaluating 190 patients who underwent pMRA for

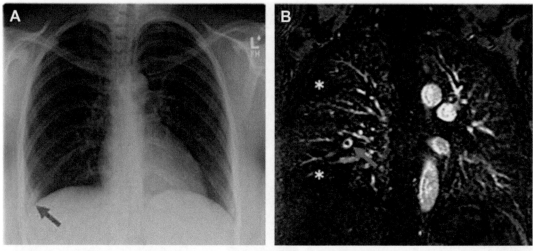

Fig. 7. A 24-year-old woman presenting to the emergency department with pleuritic right chest pain. A peripheral, wedge-shaped opacity in the right lower lung on chest radiograph is suspicious for pulmonary infarction (*blue arrow, A*). Pulmonary MRA confirms a right lower lobe PE (*orange arrow*) with associated parenchymal perfusion defects (*asterisks*).

evaluation of PE and found a negative predictive value of 97% at 3 months of follow-up, which is similar to published reports for CTA. Moreover, there was a technical success rate of 97%, again highlighting that experienced centers can consistently and effectively perform pMRA for PE.[20]

Image interpretation of pMRA for PE is essentially the same as CTA and requires evaluating the PAs for filling defects consistent with PE (**Fig. 5**). As described earlier, several artifacts that are unique to MRA (truncation MRA and contrast bolus timing issues) must be considered when reviewing MRA images. However, in our experience, the ability to observe perfusion defects in the lung parenchyma as well as to perform multiple delayed phases of imaging can add diagnostic confidence when performing MRA, and we have not found there to be a substantial difference in technical challenges between CTA and MRA in everyday clinical practice. One key potential advantage of pMRA relative to CTA is the opportunity to evaluate lung parenchymal perfusion (**Figs. 6 and 7**), although dual-energy CT iodine mapping may allow similar visualization and possibly quantification.[21] A second advantage is that the pMRA methods allow multiple contrast-enhanced series to be performed in a sequential manner, so that the reader is not reliant on 1 series of data. A third advantage is that there is more upper abdominal coverage so the gall bladder, pancreas, common bile duct, and some of the renal collecting systems are routinely visualized.

Pulmonary Hypertension

PH is a condition of increased pressure in the PAs and is defined by having a mean PA pressure (mPAP) greater than 25 mm Hg at right heart catheterization.[22] There are multiple underlying pathologic entities that can result in PH, and the disease can be subclassified based on the underlying cause as pulmonary arterial hypertension (type 1), PH secondary to left heart disease (type 2), PH secondary to lung disease or hypoxia(type 3), chronic thromboembolic PH (CTEPH; type 4), and miscellaneous other causes (type 5).[23] Overall, PH is increasingly recognized as a contributing cause of morbidity and mortality,[24,25] and, with newer treatments being explored to treat both the symptoms and underlying mechanisms driving all types of PH, imaging will continue to play a critical role in diagnosis and monitoring.

Pulmonary MRA combined with cardiac MR imaging (CMR) can provide a comprehensive assessment of the pulmonary vasculature, physiology, and cardiac function in patients with PH.[26] Thus, there is the potential for a single examination to be used for diagnosis and treatment follow-up. The main objective for initial MR imaging in patients with suspected PH is to identify potential underlying disorders associated with PH and establish a baseline of right heart function (**Fig. 8**). As such, time-resolved or multiphase pMRA can allow the visualization of shunt lesions such as partial anomalous pulmonary venous return and atrial septal defects. Moreover, pMRA

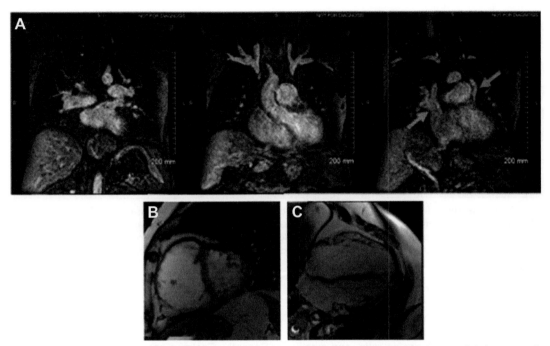

Fig. 8. Pulmonary MRA and cardiac MR imaging in a patient with PH. The pMRA examination (*A*) shows a right upper lobe partial anomalous pulmonary venous return (*orange arrow*), which was associated with a sinus venosus atrial septal defect (not pictured). Short-axis (*B*) and 4-chamber (*C*) cardiac MR imaging shows significant right ventricle and right atrium enlargement consistent with chronic left-to-right shunt. Incidental note was made of a persistent left superior vena cava (*blue arrow*).

evaluation for PE and pulmonary perfusion in the setting of CTEPH can also be assessed. Results from the Assessing the Spectrum of Pulmonary Hypertension Identified at a Referral Centre (ASPIRE) registry in the United Kingdom showed that qualitative MR pulmonary perfusion images had sensitivity of 97% and specificity of 92% for diagnosing CTEPH, which was at least as good as standard perfusion scintigraphy (sensitivity 96%, specificity 90%). Although not routinely performed, quantitative perfusion parameters such as pulmonary transit time have been shown to correlate with mPAP in pulmonary arterial hypertension[8,27,28] and have also been correlated with risk of mortality in this disease.[29] The CMR portion of the examination allows the assessment of cardiac mass, right and left heart volumes, and global and regional function such as bowing of the interventricular septum. Increasingly, newer techniques in myocardial feature tracking and strain analysis allow the assessment of left ventricular diastolic function. Both 2D and four-dimensional (4D) phase-contrast MR imaging can also be included to assess flow through the PAs and valvular heart disease as potential markers of the underlying cause of PH. Follow-up examinations can be performed to track changes in right and left heart function, pulmonary vasculature size, degree of thromboembolism, and pulmonary perfusion.

Other Pulmonary Magnetic Resonance Angiography Applications

An additional pMRA application is the evaluation of pediatric congenital heart disease, particularly congenital shunt lesions, tetralogy of Fallot, double-outlet right ventricle, pulmonary stenosis or atresia, and the status of repaired lesions. The potential for pMRA, when combined with phase-contrast MR imaging and CMR, to provide anatomic and functional information without radiation exposure makes it an ideal test for diagnosing and follow-up in patients with these and other congenital diseases (**Fig. 9**).

ONGOING RESEARCH AND FUTURE DIRECTIONS
Noncontrast Pulmonary Magnetic Resonance Angiography

Non–contrast-enhanced MRA (NCE-MRA) is an appealing alternative to CE-MRA because of concerns related to gadolinium-based contrast agents, including gadolinium deposition and,

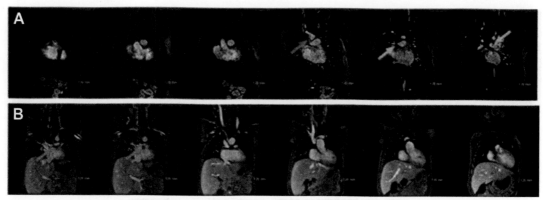

Fig. 9. Sequential slice of pulmonary MRA in 2 patients with congenital heart disease. (*A*) A 22-month-old girl with unrepaired double-outlet right ventricle, Blalock-Taussig shunt (*blue arrow*) and bilateral, right greater than left PA stenosis (*green arrows*). (*B*) A 21-month-old boy with repaired D-transposition of the great arteries and bidirection Glenn shunt with pMRA showing a widely patent Glenn shunt (*orange arrows*).

historically, nephrogenic systemic fibrosis. There have been few studies comparing NCE-MRA with CE-MRA or CTA in the PAs, partly because these techniques have often offered lower spatial resolution, poor signal-to-noise ratio, and significant motion artifacts, which limit their effectiveness in evaluating the PAs, particular for the detecting of PE. Several noncontrast approaches, including balanced SSFP (bSSFP) imaging, 3D fresh blood imaging using 3D fast spin echo, and arterial spin labeling, have been used in the evaluation of PE with varying degrees of success.[19,30] Recently, Edelman and colleagues[31] have developed both breath-hold and free-breathing NCE-MRA acquisition called quiescent interval single shot (QISS) and used a radial k-space sampling

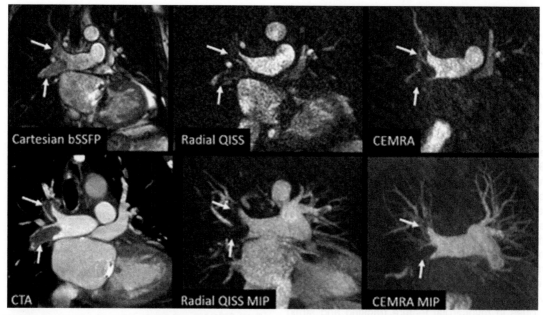

Fig. 10. A 68-year-old man with shortness of breath and suspected perivalvular leak after mitral valve repair with PE incidentally noted during cardiac MR imaging. A large occlusive thrombus (*arrows*) is seen in the right inter-lobar PA with a small thrombus seen in the right upper lobe PA. The noncontrast radial QISS acquisition (*middle column*) shows excellent agreement with contrast-enhanced pulmonary MRA (*third column*) and CTA images (*bottom left*) and the clots are significantly more conspicuous than bSSFP MR imaging (*top left*). MIP, maximum intensity projection. (*From* Edelman RR, Silvers RI, Thakrar KH, et al. Nonenhanced MR angiography of the pulmonary arteries using single-shot radial quiescent-interval slice-selective (QISS): a technical feasibility study. *Journal of Cardiovascular Magnetic Resonance.* 2017;19(1):48; with permission.)

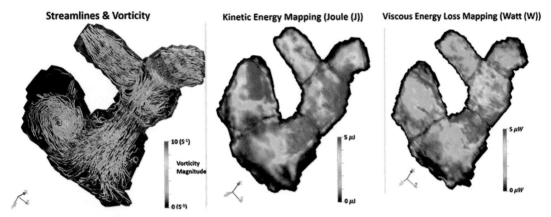

Fig. 11. Advanced hemodynamic characterization of the PAs and right heart chambers using 4D flow MR imaging. In this patient with PH, there is reduced right PA (RPA) and left PA (LPA) vorticity, kinetic energy, and viscous energy loss relative to normal controls, whereas these hemodynamic parameters are not significantly different from control subjects in the main PA (MPA), right ventricle (RV), and right atrium (RA). (*Courtesy of* Mohammed Elbaz, PhD.)

strategy that allows images with high spatial and temporal resolution that are robust to respiratory motion artifact (**Fig. 10**). In their initial feasibility study, these approaches both adequately identified all PA segments with acceptable imaging time (2 minutes with breath holds and 3.4 minutes with free-breathing approach). They also detected central pulmonary emboli in 1 patient with improved contrast-to-noise ratio relative to standard bSSFP images.[31]

Ferumoxytol-enhanced Pulmonary Magnetic Resonance Angiography

Ferumoxytol is an ultrasmall superparamagnetic iron oxide that is an approved treatment of iron deficiency anemia but can also be used off label as an intravascular MR imaging contrast agent because of its T1 and T2 shortening effects.[32] There is increasing interest in using this agent in vascular imaging as an alternative to gadolinium, particularly in patients who are not eligible for gadolinium contrast, such as pregnant women or patients with renal failure.[33,34] Moreover, because of its intravascular half-life of 10 to 14 hours and in combination with rapid imaging techniques or respiratory navigator techniques, ferumoxytol may allow free-breathing MRA assessment of the pulmonary vasculature, which can potentially reduce the diagnostic impact of respiratory motion and contrast bolus timing artifacts. A recent animal study suggests ferumoxytol-enhanced pMRA using both conventional MRA and free-breathing ultrashort-echo-time MRA pulse sequences provides adequate depiction of pulmonary vasculature with image quality that is comparable with standard gadolinium-enhanced pMRA.[33]

However, further studies are required to assess performance for clinical detection of PE or other pulmonary vascular diseases.

Four-dimensional Flow Magnetic Resonance Imaging

Time-resolved, 3D phase-contrast (4D flow) MR imaging is an increasingly used tool for the noninvasive evaluation of vascular hemodynamics.[35] This technique measures the 3D blood flow velocity field in vessels of interest and allows qualitative and quantitative evaluation of blood flow, velocity, and other derived parameters, such as wall shear stress and pulse wave velocity.[36,37]

There has been great interest in applying this technique in the PAs, particularly in the setting of PH, because of how the disease affects more proximal PA pressures, which can manifest as changes in blood flow patterns, velocity, and other derived parameters such as vortical and retrograde flow, pulse wave velocity, and wall shear stress, which have all been used to correlate PH severity.[38] Intracardiac parameters measured with 4D flow, including tricuspid valve regurgitant fraction and increasing right ventricular kinetic energy, have also been correlated with relative disease severity.[39] Several studies have focused on qualitative changes in the main PA (MPA). The time period of MPA vortex flow correlated with mean PA pressures (mPAPs)[40] and an additional study found that vortex formation occurs at mPAPs greater than 16 mm Hg.[41] Other groups have shown that decreasing MPA wall shear stress correlates with increased pulmonary vascular resistance and mPAP.[38,42] More recently, Elbaz and colleagues[43] showed that 4D flow-derived vorticity, kinetic energy, and viscous energy loss are reduced in the right and left PAs in patients with PH and that the decrease in the left PA correlates with both right and left ventricular systolic function[44] (**Fig. 11**).

REFERENCES

1. Nagle SK, Schiebler ML, Repplinger MD, et al. Contrast enhanced pulmonary magnetic resonance angiography for pulmonary embolism: building a successful program. Eur J Radiol 2016; 85(3):553–63.

2. Benson DG, Schiebler ML, Repplinger MD, et al. Contrast-enhanced pulmonary MRA for the primary diagnosis of pulmonary embolism: current state of the art and future directions. Br J Radiol 2017; 90(1074):20160901.

3. Griswold MA, Jakob PM, Heidemann RM, et al. Generalized autocalibrating partially parallel acquisitions (GRAPPA). Magn Reson Med 2002;47(6): 1202–10.

4. Brau AC, Beatty PJ, Skare S, et al. Comparison of reconstruction accuracy and efficiency among autocalibrating data-driven parallel imaging methods. Magn Reson Med 2008;59(2):382–95.

5. Nael K, Fenchel M, Krishnam M, et al. 3.0 Tesla high spatial resolution contrast-enhanced magnetic resonance angiography (CE-MRA) of the pulmonary circulation: initial experience with a 32-channel phased array coil using a high relaxivity contrast agent. Invest Radiol 2007;42(6):392–8.

6. Carr JC, Laub G, Zheng J, et al. Time-resolved three-dimensional pulmonary MR angiography and perfusion imaging with ultrashort repetition time. Acad Radiol 2002;9(12):1407–18.

7. Attenberger UI, Ingrisch M, Dietrich O, et al. Time-resolved 3D pulmonary perfusion MRI: comparison of different k-space acquisition strategies at 1.5 and 3 T. Invest Radiol 2009;44(9):525–31.

8. Jeong HJ, Vakil P, Sheehan JJ, et al. Time-resolved magnetic resonance angiography: evaluation of intrapulmonary circulation parameters in pulmonary arterial hypertension. J Magn Reson Imaging 2011; 33(1):225–31.

9. Krishnam MS, Tomasian A, Lohan DG, et al. Low-dose, time-resolved, contrast-enhanced 3D MR angiography in cardiac and vascular diseases: correlation to high spatial resolution 3D contrast-enhanced MRA. Clin Radiol 2008;63(7):744–55.

10. Hong J-Y, Han K, Jung J-H, et al. Association of exposure to diagnostic low-dose ionizing radiation with risk of cancer among youths in South Korea. JAMA Netw Open 2019;2(9):e1910584.

11. Czervionke LF, Czervionke JM, Daniels DL, et al. Characteristic features of MR truncation artifacts. AJR Am J Roentgenol 1988;151(6):1219–28.

12. Bannas P, Schiebler ML, Motosugi U, et al. Pulmonary MRA: differentiation of pulmonary embolism from truncation artefact. Eur Radiol 2014;24(8): 1942–9.

13. Sadigh G, Kelly AM, Cronin P. Challenges, controversies, and hot topics in pulmonary embolism imaging. AJR Am J Roentgenol 2011;196(3):497–515.

14. Nikolaou K, Thieme S, Sommer W, et al. Diagnosing pulmonary embolism: new computed tomography applications. J Thorac Imaging 2010; 25(2):151–60.

15. Stein PD, Fowler SE, Goodman LR, et al. Multidetector computed tomography for acute pulmonary embolism. N Engl J Med 2006;354(22):2317–27.

16. Hall EJ, Brenner DJ. Cancer risks from diagnostic radiology: the impact of new epidemiological data. Br J Radiol 2012;85(1020):e1316–7.

17. Einstein AJ, Henzlova MJ, Rajagopalan S. Estimating risk of cancer associated with radiation exposure from 64-slice computed tomography coronary angiography. JAMA 2007;298(3):317–23.

18. Stein PD, Chenevert TL, Fowler SE, et al. Gadolinium-enhanced magnetic resonance angiography for pulmonary embolism: a multicenter prospective study (PIOPED III). Ann Intern Med 2010;152(7): 434–43. w142-433.

19. Kalb B, Sharma P, Tigges S, et al. MR imaging of pulmonary embolism: diagnostic accuracy of contrast-enhanced 3D MR pulmonary angiography, contrast-enhanced low–flip angle 3D GRE, and Non-enhanced free-induction FISP sequences. Radiology 2012;263(1):271–8.

20. Schiebler ML, Nagle SK, François CJ, et al. Effectiveness of MR angiography for the primary diagnosis of acute pulmonary embolism: clinical outcomes at 3 months and 1 year. J Magn Reson Imaging 2013;38(4):914–25.

21. Nakazawa T, Watanabe Y, Hori Y, et al. Lung perfused blood volume images with dual-energy computed tomography for chronic thromboembolic pulmonary hypertension: correlation to scintigraphy with single-photon emission computed tomography. J Comput Assist Tomogr 2011;35(5):590–5.

22. Galie N, Humbert M, Vachiery JL, et al. 2015 ESC/ERS guidelines for the diagnosis and treatment of pulmonary hypertension: the joint task force for the diagnosis and treatment of pulmonary hypertension of the European Society of Cardiology (ESC) and the European Respiratory Society (ERS): Endorsed by: Association for European Paediatric and Congenital Cardiology (AEPC), International Society for Heart and Lung Transplantation (ISHLT). Eur Heart J 2016;37(1):67–119.

23. Simonneau G, Robbins IM, Beghetti M, et al. Updated clinical classification of pulmonary hypertension. J Am Coll Cardiol 2009;54(1 Supplement): S43–54.

24. George MG, Schieb LJ, Ayala C, et al. Pulmonary hypertension surveillance: United States, 2001 to 2010. Chest 2014;146(2):476–95.

25. Hyduk A, Croft JB, Ayala C, et al. Pulmonary hypertension surveillance–United States, 1980-2002. MMWR Surveill Summ 2005;54(5):1–28.

26. Swift AJ, Wild JM, Nagle SK, et al. Quantitative magnetic resonance imaging of pulmonary hypertension: a practical approach to the current state of the art. J Thorac Imaging 2014;29(2):68–79.

27. Skrok J, Shehata ML, Mathai S, et al. Pulmonary arterial hypertension: MR imaging-derived first-pass bolus kinetic parameters are biomarkers for pulmonary hemodynamics, cardiac function, and ventricular remodeling. Radiology 2012;263(3):678–87.

28. Ley S, Mereles D, Risse F, et al. Quantitative 3D pulmonary MR-perfusion in patients with pulmonary arterial hypertension: correlation with invasive pressure measurements. Eur J Radiol 2007;61(2):251–5.

29. Swift AJ, Telfer A, Rajaram S, et al. Dynamic contrast-enhanced magnetic resonance imaging in patients with pulmonary arterial hypertension. Pulm Circ 2014;4(1):61–70.

30. Ohno Y, Yoshikawa T, Kishida Y, et al. Unenhanced and contrast-enhanced MR angiography and perfusion imaging for suspected pulmonary thromboembolism. Am J Roentgenol 2017;208(3):517–30.

31. Edelman RR, Silvers RI, Thakrar KH, et al. Nonenhanced MR angiography of the pulmonary arteries using single-shot radial quiescent-interval slice-selective (QISS): a technical feasibility study. J Cardiovasc Magn Reson 2017;19(1):48.

32. Knobloch G, Colgan T, Wiens CN, et al. Relaxivity of Ferumoxytol at 1.5 T and 3.0 T. Invest Radiol 2018;53(5):257–63.

33. Knobloch G, Colgan T, Schiebler ML, et al. Comparison of gadolinium-enhanced and ferumoxytol-enhanced conventional and UTE-MRA for the depiction of the pulmonary vasculature. Magn Reson Med 2019;82(5):1660–70.

34. Hope MD, Hope TA, Zhu C, et al. Vascular imaging with ferumoxytol as a contrast agent. Am J Roentgenol 2015;205(3):W366–73.

35. Dyverfeldt P, Bissell M, Barker AJ, et al. 4D flow cardiovascular magnetic resonance consensus statement. J Cardiovasc Magn Reson 2015;17(1):72.

36. van Ooij P, Potters WV, Nederveen AJ, et al. A methodology to detect abnormal relative wall shear stress on the full surface of the thoracic aorta using four-dimensional flow MRI. Magn Reson Med 2015;73(3):1216–27.

37. Markl M, Wallis W, Strecker C, et al. Analysis of pulse wave velocity in the thoracic aorta by flow-sensitive four-dimensional MRI: reproducibility and correlation with characteristics in patients with aortic atherosclerosis. J Magn Reson Imaging 2012;35(5):1162–8.

38. Barker AJ, Roldan-Alzate A, Entezari P, et al. Four-dimensional flow assessment of pulmonary artery flow and wall shear stress in adult pulmonary arterial hypertension: results from two institutions. Magn Reson Med 2015;73(5):1904–13.

39. Reiter U, Reiter G, Fuchsjager M. MR phase-contrast imaging in pulmonary hypertension. Br J Radiol 2016;89(1063):20150995.

40. Reiter G, Reiter U, Kovacs G, et al. Magnetic resonance-derived 3-dimensional blood flow patterns in the main pulmonary artery as a marker of pulmonary hypertension and a measure of elevated mean pulmonary arterial pressure. Circ Cardiovasc Imaging 2008;1(1):23–30.

41. Reiter G, Reiter U, Kovacs G, et al. Blood flow vortices along the main pulmonary artery measured with MR imaging for diagnosis of pulmonary hypertension. Radiology 2015;275(1):71–9.

42. Schäfer M, Kheyfets VO, Schroeder JD, et al. Main pulmonary arterial wall shear stress correlates with invasive hemodynamics and stiffness in pulmonary hypertension. Pulm Circ 2016;6(1):37–45.

43. Elbaz MSM, Reddy V, Gordon D, et al. Impact of pulmonary hypertension on viscous energy loss, kinetic energy and vorticity in the right heart: a pilot 4D Flow CMR study. Bellevue (WA): Society of Cardiovascular Magnetic Resonance; 2019.

44. Elbaz MSM, Reddy V, Abbasi M, et al. Left and right heart ventricular-vascular coupling in pulmonary venous hypertension. International Society of Magnetic Resonance in Medicine 27th Annual Meeting and Exhibition. Montreal, QC, Canada, May 11-16, 2019, 2019.

Imaging Thoracic Aortic Aneurysm

Kimberly G. Kallianos, MD[a], Nicholas S. Burris, MD[b],*

KEYWORDS

• Thoracic • Aorta • Ectasia • Aortopathy • Aneurysm

KEY POINTS

- Cross-sectional imaging (CTA and MRA) plays a central role in management of patients with thoracic aortic aneurysm.
- Maximal aortic diameter is the primary metric used to estimate risk and determine the need for surgical repair, although diameter measurement are subject to error related to image artifact and measurement technique.
- Optimal imaging surveillance requires selection of imaging modality (CTA vs MRA) based on patient-specific characteristics and indications, in addition to consistent measurement protocols based on double-oblique images to minimize measurement error.
- Most TAAs are classified as degenerative and associated with fusiform dilation of the ascending aorta, whereas root aneurysms are typically seen in aortic-related connective tissue disorders and descending thoracoabdominal aneurysms are strongly associated with atherosclerosis.

INTRODUCTION

Thoracic aortic aneurysm (TAA) is a chronic condition that manifests as progressive dilation of the thoracic aorta resulting from degradation of the normal smooth muscle cells and extracellular matrix proteins that provide integrity to the aortic wall. TAA is broadly classified into three categories based on cause: (1) degenerative, (2) genetically mediated, and (3) inflammatory (ie, aortitis). Degenerative aneurysms are the most common; are associated with advanced age; occur in the absence of a defined genetic aortopathy or familial clustering; and are associated with cardiovascular risk-factors, such as atherosclerosis and hypertension. Genetically mediated TAAs are those that occur in the setting of a known clinical syndrome (eg, Marfan, Ehlers-Danlos) or in the setting of a genetic mutation in molecular pathways known to be associated with TAA (eg, transforming growth factor-β signaling pathway).[1]

The prevalence of TAA has increased from 3.5 to 7.6 per 100,000 persons between 2002 and 2014.[2] In part, this is caused by increasing rates of incidental detection on unrelated imaging studies (eg, lung cancer screening, coronary computed tomography angiography [CTA]/calcium scoring). Incidental aortic dilation (>4.0 cm) is present in about 3% of patients greater than 55 years old.[3] Maximal aortic diameter is currently the primary metric used to guide surveillance strategy and timing of surgical intervention for patients with TAA. As aortic diameter increases so does the risk of developing life-threatening complications, the most common of which is aortic dissection (ie, delamination of the aortic wall) and less commonly rupture (ie, transmural tearing). In the absence of acute complications, TAAs grow slowly over years or even decades, with typical growth rates in the range of 1 to 3 mm/y. When the aorta size reaches its biomechanical "hinge

Funding: Dr N.S. Burris - Research Scholar Grant (RSCH 1801), Radiologic Society of North America.
[a] Department of Radiology and Biomedical Imaging, University of California, San Francisco, 505 Parnassus Avenue, M-391, San Francisco, CA 94143-0628, USA; [b] University of Michigan, Frankel Cardiovascular Center, Room 5588, 1500 East Medical Center Drive, Ann Arbor, MI 48109-5868, USA
* Corresponding author.
E-mail address: nburris@med.umich.edu

Radiol Clin N Am 58 (2020) 721–731
https://doi.org/10.1016/j.rcl.2020.02.009

point," usually about 6 cm in diameter, wall integrity rapidly declines, growth accelerates, and the incidence of complications rapidly increases. Current guidelines recommend surgical repair of the ascending aorta before the maximal diameter "hinge point" is reached, typically at a threshold of 5.5 cm.[4] The primary management objective for TAA is to identify aortic growth early and to surgically replace the aorta before it reaches a high-risk size.

Noninvasive imaging surveillance plays a central role in the management of TAA through its ability to determine maximal aneurysm diameter and monitor for growth and other complications. Transthoracic echocardiography is used to monitor TAA that is limited to the root and proximal ascending aorta; however, CTA and magnetic resonance angiography (MRA) are the most common imaging modalities for evaluation of TAA because they can evaluate the entire thoracic aorta without the limitations of acoustic windows. Current guidelines generally lack detailed recommendations for the frequency of imaging surveillance and there are variations in approaches between physicians and centers; however, it is generally agreed that in degenerative TAA where the degree of dilation is mild or moderate (4.0–5.0 cm), annual follow-up imaging is appropriate with spacing to biennial or triennial if aortic dimensions have shown long-term stability.[5,6] When aortic dimensions are clearly increasing or approaching surgical thresholds, imaging frequency is typically increased to biannual.

NORMAL AORTIC ANATOMY

The thoracic aorta is divided into the following regions: aortic root, ascending aorta, aortic arch, and descending aorta. The aortic root includes the annulus, aortic valve, and sinuses of Valsalva. The conventional aortic anatomy consists of three sinuses corresponding to the aortic valve cusps (right, left, and noncoronary). The three sinuses of Valsalva taper and form a "waist" at their junction with the tubular ascending segment (ie, the sinotubular junction [STJ]). The tubular ascending aorta extends from the STJ to the first arch vessel, and is so named given its lack of branches and resemblance to simple "tube." Beyond the tubular segment, the aorta arch gives rise to the arch vessels (innominate, left common carotid, and left subclavian) from the proximal aortic arch. The distal arch beyond the left subclavian artery to the region of the ligamentum arteriosum is called the aortic isthmus. This region is of clinical significance, because it is a common site of nonfatal traumatic aortic injury and coarctation. The

descending thoracic aorta extends to the diaphragmatic hiatus.[7] Guidelines suggest that aortic diameters be reported at specific aortic locations along the aortic length including the sinuses of Valsalva, STJ, midascending aorta, proximal and distal arch, middescending aorta, and at the diaphragmatic hiatus.[5] Either sinus-to-sinus or sinus-to-commissure measurements may be reported for the sinuses of Valsalva.

Normal sizes for the thoracic aorta have been defined from several reference populations. In general, aortic size increases with patient age, male gender, and body size.[8,9] However, measurement techniques can introduce variability into the reported size of the thoracic aorta. These include measuring the aorta using gated versus nongated imaging technique (and when gated, during systole vs diastole), from inner versus outer edge, and in the axial versus double-oblique planes. The next section explores best practices of measurement technique.[10]

The range of mean ascending aortic diameters (including gated and nongated examinations) in the literature by computed tomography (CT) ranges from 29.0 to 37.2 mm for females, and 30.8 to 39.1 mm for males, with the larger diameters reported for studies without electrocardiographic (ECG)-gating.[11] Although in general it is accepted that the maximal diameter of the ascending thoracic aorta should be lower than 40 mm in healthy individuals,[6] some series have shown that the normal range (within two standard deviations of the mean) for males and females can extend above this level. Considering the significant impact of patient size on normal aortic diameter, indexing aortic dimensions to adjust for patient body size (ie, height or body surface area) is appropriate for optimal definition of pathologic aortic dilation; however, clinical application of indexed aortic measurements in adults is limited because of the lack of comprehensive population nomograms to determine reference ranges.

IMAGING TECHNIQUE

When selecting an imaging technique, the strengths and weaknesses of various imaging modalities should be considered in relation to the clinical context. The American College of Radiology Appropriateness Criteria for TAA initial imaging rates CTA and MRA as "usually appropriate."[12] For preprocedure planning before thoracic endovascular repair (TEVAR), CTA chest, abdomen, and pelvis is rated at 9 "usually appropriate," whereas MRA and CTA chest alone are rated at 7 "usually appropriate." CTA is often preferable to MRA following TEVAR given the increased artifact as a result of metal stent (particularly those composed of stainless steel) and the increased ability of CTA to detect postoperative infection and endoleak. Pros and cons of CTA versus MRA are summarized in **Table 1**.

Measurement Techniques

Measurement techniques can introduce significant variability into the reported size of the thoracic aorta. Different measurement techniques used in clinical practice by different centers have been shown to result in a lower reproducivity for CT compared with echocardiography.[13] One method to reduce this variability is through the use of double-oblique or orthogonal measurements. Double-oblique measurement obtained orthogonal to the aortic centerline allows creation of a true short axis reformation of the aortic diameter and has been shown to allow more accurate measurement of aortic size compared with axial measurement (**Fig. 1**). Axial measurement may result in a significant overestimation of aortic size, up to 6 mm or 21% increase in size according to Hager and colleagues.[8] In one series, axial measurements were shown to overestimate aortic size at multiple locations (with the exception of the aortic arch) and resulted in the misclassification of 13% of patients into either aneurysmal or surgical candidate categories (**Fig. 2**).[14] It is also important to recognize that different measurement approaches at the aortic wall such as inner to inner, leading edge, or outer to outer can also introduce variation in aortic diameter.[15] Consensus as

to which of these methods is preferred has not been established for CT and MR imaging, although leading edge to leading edge is a frequent standard used with echocardiography. Within a center, consistent technique should be adopted to decrease measurement variability between serial scans.

IMAGING PROTOCOLS

The thoracic aorta is best evaluated with cross-sectional imaging, either CT or MR imaging. Although CTA and MRA imaging techniques are routinely used to evaluate the aortic size and structure, specific CT and MR imaging protocols are additive in evaluating thoracic aortic pathology.

Computed Tomography

The standard multidetector CT evaluation of TAA consists of contrast-enhanced CTA. Noncontrast CT may be obtained before CTA to assess for intramural hematoma (IMH) in the setting of concern for acute aortic syndrome or to assess for calcification or surgical material in a postoperative patient. It is important to distinguish aortic wall thickening resulting from atherosclerosis, which presents as circumferential aortic wall thickening that is stable over time, from acute IMH, which tends to be eccentric in location and hyperdense of non-contrast series (**Fig. 3**). Contrast-enhanced CTA of the aorta may be performed with bolus tracking or use of a timing bolus to ensure optimal enhancement of the thoracic aorta.

Table 1
Pros/cons of imaging modalities

Characteristic	Pros and Cons of CTA vs MRA	
	CTA	**MRA**
Radiation	Ionizing radiation (x-ray) + DNA damage	Nonionizing (radiofrequency) No DNA damage
Spatial resolution (typical)	0.5–1.5 mm^3	0.7–1.5 mm^3 (variable)
Number of acquisitions	Usually single	Usually multiple
Set-up and scan time	Short (5–10 min)	Long (45–60 min)
Acquisition complexity	Easy	More difficult
Patient participation	Minimal	Significant: multiple breath hold
Modality strength	Anatomy and postsurgical evaluation	Soft tissue characterization and hemodynamic/functional assessment
Contrast risk	Iodinated contrast: 1. Contrast-induced nephropathy • Rare 2. Severe allergy: ∼1:1000	Gadolinium contrast: 1. Nephrogenic systemic fibrosis • Extremely rare 2. Gadolinium deposition in brain (unclear clinical significance) 3. Severe allergy: ∼1:100,000

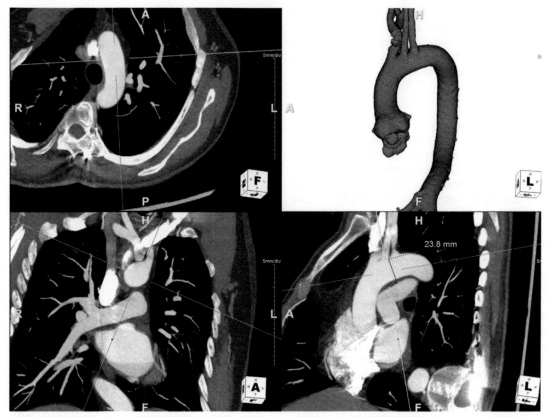

Fig. 1. Double oblique measurement technique of the aortic arch and three-dimensional reformation of the thoracic aorta in a patient with connective tissue disease undergoing routine surveillance.

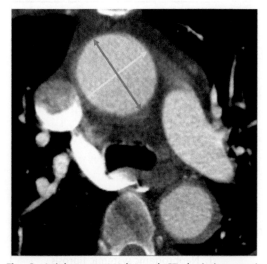

Fig. 2. Axial contrast-enhanced CT depicting aortic measurement perpendicular to the aortic axis (*yellow arrow*) versus overestimation of aortic size when measurement is obtained parallel to aortic axis (*blue arrow*).

Postcontrast delayed phase images may also be obtained in patients with endovascular repair of TAA or dissection (TEVAR) to assess for endoleak or in patients with inflammatory TAA/aortitis to evaluate for periadventitial enhancement indicative of active inflammation.

ECG-gating, either prospective or retrospective, may be employed, and if done, care should be made to compare aortic measurements at equivalent phases of the cardiac cycle on subsequent examinations. Benefits of ECG-gated analysis of the thoracic aorta include a reduction in motion artifact, which is particularly helpful when evaluating the aortic root/ascending aorta or in cases of suspected aortic dissection (**Fig. 4**). ECG-gated CTA also can allow concurrent assessment of the proximal coronary arteries. Roos and colleagues[16] demonstrated that prospective and retrospective ECG-gating reduced motion artifacts throughout the thoracic aorta, although the greatest improvement in image quality was noted at the level of the aortic valve.

In general, aortic size is slightly larger in systole compared with diastole.[17] Mao and colleagues[18] demonstrated that the ascending aorta measured

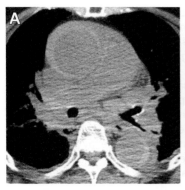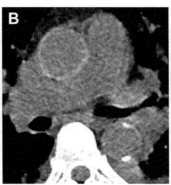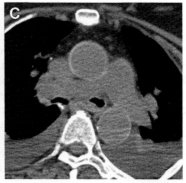

Fig. 3. (A) Axial noncontrast CT of the chest in a patient with acute intramural hematoma. (B) Axial noncontrast CT of the chest in a patient with aortic wall thickening as a result of atherosclerosis. (C) Follow-up CT of the second patient 6 months later demonstrates stable findings.

1.7 mm larger at end systole (35% of the R-R interval) compared with end diastole. de Heer and colleagues[17] also demonstrated larger diameters in systole for the aortic valve annulus, sinuses of Valsalva, and STJ, in the range of 0.4 to 1.0 mm. CTA before transcatheter aortic valve replacement has shown an 8% higher annulus area in systole, with greater variability among patients without significant annular calcification.[19,20] Diastolic images are most commonly used for aortic measurements to minimize motion artifact.

MR Imaging

A unique benefit of MR imaging is the ability to perform high-quality vascular imaging without the need for potentially nephrotoxic contrast agents and without ionizing radiation exposure. Disadvantages of MR imaging include the slightly lower spatial resolution compared with CT, reduced ability to evaluate burden of calcified atherosclerosis, artifacts in the setting of metallic stents or implants, and the potential for patient claustrophobia. A variety of sequences can be performed to evaluate the aortic wall and lumen (black blood spin echo or fast spin echo imaging), aortic valve morphology (steady state free precession cine),

and valve function (phase contrast imaging).[21] MR imaging of the aorta is most commonly performed using gadolinium-based contrast agents, although iron-based agents (eg, ferumoxytol) are being increasingly used given their high relaxivity and long intravascular half-life.[22] Gadolinium-enhanced MRA is typically performed in arterial phase, after bolus injection, although slow continuous infusion protocols have been described.[23] A significant advantage of MR imaging is the ability to perform noncontrast MRA using steady state free precession (ie, "white blood") techniques, with comparable measurement quality compared with contrast-enhanced techniques.[24] Three-dimensional (3D) noncontrast MRA techniques have also been shown to be feasible for evaluation of the aortic annulus before transcatheter aortic valve replacement, and employ both respiratory and cardiac gating.[25]

Multiplanar and Three-Dimensional Analysis

Beyond the benefits of multiplanar reformats for aortic measurements (discussed previously), an additional benefit of CTA and MRA is the ability to easily create 3D reconstructions of TAA. Volume-rendered 3D reconstructions are easily

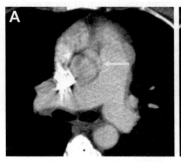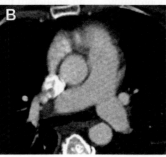

Fig. 4. (A) Nongated axial contrast-enhanced chest CT depicting motion-related artifact at the aortic root simulating aortic dissection (arrow). (B) Repeat CT with cardiac gating shows resolution of the artifact.

generated using a variety of clinical 3D image analysis software tools, and are useful in providing a visual overview of the extent of disease, especially during procedure planning. Additionally, the volumetric nature of CTA and MRA data is well suited for 3D printing, which allows rapid creation of anatomic models. 3D printed models allow clinicians, surgeons, and patients the opportunity to comprehend complex cardiovascular anatomy and pathology in a more tangible manner than achieved with computer-based 3D models and may assist in planning endovascular or open surgical repair.[26]

Safety and Quality

There has been increased focus on the risks associated with radiation exposure in medical imaging. This risk is particularly relevant for TAA patients who often undergo repeated imaging as a part of imaging surveillance, and may be subjected to a significant radiation doses over their lifetime. Zoli and colleagues[27] evaluated the cumulative radiation dose exposure of patients with TAA who underwent TEVAR and subsequent imaging follow-up, and identified that such patients would be exposed to 89 mSv over 1 year when adhering to an institutional surveillance protocol, with a lifetime radiation exposure of greater than 350 mSv. They concluded that this was associated with an increased lifetime risk of malignancy of 2.7%. Eliminating nonessential sequences, such as noncontrast and delayed-phase CTA, when not clinically indicated, can significantly reduce radiation doses. Retrospective ECG-gating is associated with a higher radiation dose compared with nongated examinations, often nearly two-fold greater.[16] Other scanner and protocol-related methods, such as tube current modulation, iterative reconstruction, and dual-energy CT, can substantially reduce patient radiation dose.[28]

Recent studies have questioned the causal relationship of iodinated contrast and acute kidney injury, as discussed in the American College of Radiology Manual on Contrast Media 10.3.[29] However, the possibility of contrast-induced nephropathy and postcontrast kidney injury remain a consideration in the selection of aortic imaging modality. Vascular imaging techniques that reduce or eliminate the use of iodine based intravenous contrast (eg, MR imaging) may be preferable, particularly in patients with preexisting renal impairment.

Current literature supports the safety of group II gadolinium-based contrast agents in patients with chronic renal insufficiency, a common comorbidity in patients with TAA. Although nephrogenic systemic fibrosis remains a concern in clinical practice, few if any nonconfounded cases of nephrogenic systemic fibrosis have been seen with group II agents. Ferumoxytol has emerged as an alternative to gadolinium-based agents given its safety in renal insufficiency and lack of heavy-metal deposition in the body. Ferumoxytol is an ultrasmall superparamagnetic iron oxide particle approved by the Food and Drug Administration for use in patients with chronic kidney disease for the treatment of iron deficiency anemia, which is used off-label as an MRA contrast agent with high relaxivity and long intravascular half-life (14–21 hours).

FINDINGS, PATHOLOGY, AND DIAGNOSTIC CRITERIA
Aneurysm Morphology, Cause, and Extent

Although maximal diameter is the primary metric used to guide patient management, there are other features of aneurysm morphology that give insight into potential aneurysm etiology and are important for surgical planning. The first step in assessing TAA is determination of the dilated segment (ascending or descending). Occasionally both the ascending and descending segments are dilated, although typically dilation is most severe at one segment. Dilation of the aortic arch is usually seen in association with ascending or descending the arch dilation is contiguous with an adjacent ascending or descending, where aortic aneurysm and the degree of arch dilation is lesser than the primary aneurysm. Isolated aortic arch aneurysms are uncommon and are strongly associated with atherosclerosis. Beyond simply describing TAA anatomy, there are clear associations between the location of aneurysm and the cause. Recent research has shown that embryologic origin of aortic smooth muscle cells varies by aortic segment, suggesting that aneurysm morphology may be related heterogeneity in smooth muscle cell distribution, especially in genetic aortopathy.[30]

Another key distinction in aneurysm morphology is whether the aneurysm is fusiform or saccular. Fusiform (spindle-shaped) morphology describes an aneurysm that gradually tapers at each end of the aneurysm to a normal diameter, with the distribution of wall dilation being circumferential. The fusiform morphology is most indicative of a true aneurysm (ie, all three aortic wall layers are intact), and is most commonly seen with degenerative and genetically mediated TAAs. Conversely, saccular aneurysms tend to have more abrupt transition points with the adjacent uninvolved aorta, present as a more discrete and eccentric outpouching of the aortic wall, and often have an area of narrowing at their base (the "neck"), which leads to the body the aneurysm. A saccular aneurysm morphology is most suggestive of aortic pseudoaneurysm (ie, less than three aortic wall layers remain intact), and common etiologies include penetrating atherosclerotic ulcer (PAU), mycotic/infectious, iatrogenic, and post-traumatic.

Key Imaging Findings that Suggest Specific Cause and Risk

Although there is significant overlap in TAA morphology between different subgroups, there are imaging findings that suggest specific etiologies and risks, which are important to consider when planning treatment strategies. Fusiform dilation of the ascending aorta is most commonly associated with degenerative TAA; however, it can also be seen with genetically mediated TAA. When aortic dilation predominantly affects the aortic root, aortic-related connective tissue disorders (CTD), such as Marfan syndrome (mutated fibrillin-1 gene), should be strongly considered. This pattern of aortic root dilation is termed "annuloaortic ectasia" (AAE) (Fig. 5A), and is classically associated with Marfan syndrome and describes proximal aortic dilation that involves the annulus, sinuses, and proximal ascending aorta, resulting in loss of the normal waist-like contour of the STJ. Annular dilation often results in substantial aortic insufficiency and thus surgical repair of AAE must not only repair aortic root dilation but also resize the aortic annulus (ie, annuloplasty) if the native aortic valve is to be preserved. Vascular Ehlers-Danlos syndrome (vEDS) is a specific aortic-related CTD caused by mutations in the COL3A1 gene. vEDS leads to the development of arterial aneurysms at a young age, often resulting in rupture/dissection. Imaging manifestations of vascular EDS are similar to that of Marfan syndrome, and can include TAA (often with AAE) and ectasia and dissection of the principal aortic branches (eg, visceral aneurysms).[31] Loeys-Dietz syndrome (LDS) is an extremely rare CTD that results in aortic abnormalities similar to Marfan syndrome and vEDS, although patients with LDS are generally considered the most severe of the genetically mediated TAAs and complications present at early ages and smaller aortic diameters. Although imaging findings in LDS also include ascending aneurysm (often with AAE) and dissection, a characteristic unique to LDS is severe tortuosity of the vertebral arteries, and the degree of tortuosity has been shown to correlate with increasing severity of disease (Fig. 5B). Given the variable severity of disease in aortic-related CTDs, different maximal aortic diameter thresholds have been used to trigger surgical repair with the most aggressive repair thresholds of 4.0 to 4.5 cm for repair in patients with LDS and threshold in the range of 4.5 to 5.0 for vEDS and Marfan syndrome.[1] Although most CTDs have other nonvascular manifestations (eg, musculoskeletal, craniofacial, cardiac) aortic aneurysm is a leading cause of morbidity and mortality in these populations, specifically because of the substantially higher rates of aortic dissection compared with the general population.[32] Although not classically considered a CTD, patients with bicuspid aortic valve develop TAA and dissection at a significantly higher rate than the general population and experience accelerated degeneration of their aortic wall integrity, a phenomenon termed bicuspid valve aortopathy. Patterns of ascending TAA in BAV are variable, but most commonly there is pronounced dilation of greater curvature (the

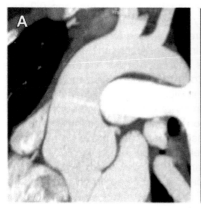 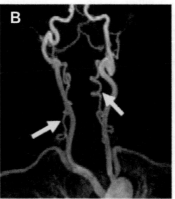 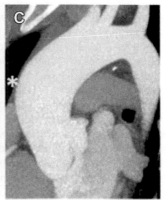

Fig. 5. (*A*) Coronal reformat demonstrating the typical shape of annuloaortic ectasia in a patient with Marfan syndrome. (*B*) Severe tortuosity of the vertebral arteries (*arrows*) as seen in Loeys-Dietz syndrome. (*C*) Bicuspid aortic valve associated ascending TAA with maximal dilation at the midascending level along the greater curvature (*asterisk*).

convexity) of the ascending aorta (**Fig. 5**C). A smaller proportion of bicuspid valve aortopathy patients demonstrate a root-dilation phenotype and have clinical characteristics more similar to classic aortic-related CTDs.[33]

Inflammatory disease of the thoracic aorta can result in aortitis and secondary TAA. Classic imaging findings of aortitis include thickening of the aortic wall (often best seen by MR imaging) with periadventitial enhancement and edema, often resulting in stranding of the periaortic fat on imaging.[34] The wall thickening of aortitis is typically circumferential, which can help differentiate from aortic wall thickening related to atherosclerosis, which is largely eccentric. Extensive intimal calcification can be seen in chronic ("burned out") aortitis, and also tends to be more diffuse and circumferential than typically seen with atherosclerosis. Fluorodeoxyglucose (FDG) PET/CT is useful for confirming aortitis in depicting the full extent of involvement, with areas of active disease typically demonstrating avid FDG uptake (atherosclerotic disease typically shows low-level or no FDG uptake). The two most common forms of noninfectious aortitis include Takayasu arteritis and giant cell arteritis, which can usually be easily differentiated by patient age and clinical presentation; Takayasu is seen in young (<40) women and giant cell arteritis is seen in older patients (>50) and is associated with polymyalgia rheumatica and temporal arteritis. Both Takayasu and giant cell arteritis can result in TAA, but a unique feature of Takayasu is the propensity for the aortic wall inflammation that in the chronic phase results in medial fibrosis and progressive stenosis, most commonly affecting the proximal aortic arch vessels, although involvement of the entire thoracoabdominal aorta and its principal branches is seen. Infectious causes of aortitis are rare in the developed world and are usually seen either in the setting of endocarditis/bacteremia resulting in development of an infectious nidus within the aortic wall (typically at an area of atherosclerotic plaque), or in the postoperative/iatrogenic setting.

Atherosclerotic plaque results in a spectrum of abnormalities that may result in aortic pseudoaneurysm. The earliest manifestation of inflammatory atherosclerotic plaque is termed ulcerated plaque, where there is erosion of the fibrous cap of the aortic atheroma, but without violation of the internal elastic lamina (IEL; which separates the intima from the media). Once plaque erosion extends through the IEL, the process is pathologically termed a PAU. Although the IEL is not able to be resolved by imaging, it is typically assumed that if there is bulging of the outer aortic wall/adventitia on imaging, that the IEL is disrupted and a PAU is present.

Small PAUs are commonly seen on contrast-enhanced imaging, and although there is a significant lack of data regarding the natural history and associated risks of small PAUs, they are generally thought to have an indolent course and the minority result in complications (<15%) or significant aortic enlargement (~25%).[35] Specific surveillance guidelines for small PAUs are lacking, but typical management involves imaging surveillance with CTA or MRA. When PAUs enlarge to the point of extending significantly (>2 cm) beyond the aortic wall and assume a more saccular morphology, they are often termed pseudoaneurysms, and have a much more aggressive disease course characterized by rapid growth and development of complications (eg, rupture). Aortic pseudoaneurysm are typically managed surgically, most commonly using endovascular techniques in the descending thoracoabdominal aorta.

Imaging Features and Findings that Imply Risk

A comprehensive imaging assessment of TAA requires accurate description of secondary findings that imply elevated risk of complications, because such features could significantly change the patient's course of treatment. Although not an imaging feature, pain is a key symptom in aortic disease, and patients presenting with chest pain thought to be related to TAA, PAU, or other aortic abnormality are generally treated with surgical repair regardless of aortic diameter or other imaging features. Other important high-risk imaging features include:

1. Interval growth is an important feature of TAA imaging assessment that needs to be accurately assessed and described when multiple imaging studies are available. TAA growth rates are highly variable, ranging between 0.2 and 4.2 mm/y.[36] Growth rates of greater than 5 mm/y are considered an indication for surgical repair in current American Heart Association guidelines,[5] although in practice a 10 mm/y rate is more commonly used given the substantial variability in diameter measurements. Accurate measurement of TAA growth requires careful attention on the part of the radiologist to ensure that measurements are made in a similar fashion between multiple studies, ideally using multiplanar reformats.

2. IMH is a cause of acute aortic syndrome and is characterized by a hematoma that forms within the medial layer of the aortic wall. IMH is considered a dissection variant, is classified similarly, and typically requires urgent surgical repair.

3. Aneurysm rupture or leak is most commonly seen in descending thoracoabdominal aneurysms and is uncommon in ascending TAA without associated type A dissection. CT findings of rupture/leak include: aortic fat stranding, high-density periaortic fluid collection, pleural/pericardial effusion (often hemorrhagic), and rarely aortic contrast extravasation.

WHAT THE REFERRING PHYSICIAN NEEDS TO KNOW

TAA is a surgical disease as there are yet to be any proven medical therapies to slow disease progression or prevent aortic complications. Thus, imaging evaluations need to aid in the determination of surgical candidacy and inform repair strategy if surgical indications are present. The imaging report in TAA should include the following important features:

1. Maximal diameter is the primary metric used to determine TAA management. It is of utmost importance that imagers accurately measure and report maximal aortic diameter in all patients with TAA, and diameter measurements should be performed using double-oblique reformats rather than on axial images to improve measurement accuracy and minimize measurement variability. When multiple imaging studies are available, it is important for imagers to assess and report TAA stability, ideally performing measurements of maximal diameter with the same measurement technique over multiple prior studies if available.
2. Extent of the aortic disease has important implications for surgical management. Specifically, in ascending TAA description of whether aortic dilation involves the root and/or arch has important implications for surgeons given that the repair of these segments requires additional expertise and advanced surgical techniques, more challenging surgical techniques, and implies additional surgical risk. In descending TAA, it is helpful to report the proximity of the dilated descending thoracic aorta to the left subclavian artery, because this determines the availability of a proximal landing zone for endovascular repair, and the distal extent of the aneurysm, because involvement of the abdominal aorta and visceral branches implies additional technical demands and risks.
3. Imaging assessment of the aortic valve is useful in informing patient management because concomitant aortic valve disease is not uncommon with TAA. Specifically, it should be noted if there is a significant degree of aortic valve

leaflet calcification (raising the possibility of aortic stenosis). Also if image quality permits assessment of aortic valve morphology, it is important to note evidence of bicuspid aortic valve. Bicuspid aortic valve is often better characterized by CT than echocardiography, and is associated with higher risk of progressive TAA growth and dissection.
4. A qualitative assessment of atherosclerotic severity, nature (calcified vs noncalcified), and distribution are useful for guiding aggressiveness of medical therapy and can inform the risk of atheroembolic stroke during surgical repair.
5. The presence of secondary findings that imply heightened risk (eg, PAU, IMH, rapid growth) should be explicitly conveyed in the impression section of the report.

SUMMARY

High-quality aortic imaging plays a central role in the management of patients with TAA. CTA and MRA are the most commonly used techniques for TAA diagnosis and imaging surveillance, with each having unique strengths and limitations that should be weighed when deciding patient-specific applications. Although there are a wide range of potential etiologies for TAA (genetic, degenerative, and inflammatory), most of these diseases are managed based on measurement of maximal aortic diameter. To ensure optimal patient care, imagers must be familiar with potential sources of artifact and measurement error, and dedicate effort to ensure high-quality and reproducible aortic measurements are generated. A complete imaging report should not only describe aortic dimensions, but also provide a complete description of the extent of the disease, detail morphologic features that suggest a specific TAA etiology, and emphasize secondary imaging features that imply additional risk.

DISCLOSURE

The authors have no relevant disclosures.

REFERENCES

1. Brownstein AJ, Ziganshin BA, Kuivaniemi H, et al. Genes associated with thoracic aortic aneurysm and dissection: an update and clinical implications. Aorta (Stamford) 2017;5(1):11–20.
2. McClure RS, Brogly SB, Lajkosz K, et al. Epidemiology and management of thoracic aortic dissections and thoracic aortic aneurysms in Ontario, Canada: a population-based study. J Thorac Cardiovasc Surg 2018;155(6):2254–64.e4.

3. Mori M, Bin Mahmood SU, Yousef S, et al. Prevalence of incidentally identified thoracic aortic dilations: insights for screening criteria. Can J Cardiol 2019;35(7):892–8.

4. Elefteriades JA, Farkas EA. Thoracic aortic aneurysm clinically pertinent controversies and uncertainties. J Am Coll Cardiol 2010;55(9):841–57.

5. Hiratzka LF, Bakris GL, Beckman JA, et al. 2010 ACCF/AHA/AATS/ACR/ASA/SCA/SCAI/SIR/STS/SVM guidelines for the diagnosis and management of patients with Thoracic Aortic Disease: a report of the American College of Cardiology Foundation/American Heart Association Task Force on Practice Guidelines, American Association for Thoracic Surgery, American College of Radiology, American Stroke Association, Society of Cardiovascular Anesthesiologists, Society for Cardiovascular Angiography and Interventions, Society of Interventional Radiology, Society of Thoracic Surgeons, and Society for Vascular Medicine. Circulation 2010;121(13):e266–369.

6. Erbel R, Aboyans V, Boileau C, et al. 2014 ESC guidelines on the diagnosis and treatment of aortic diseases: document covering acute and chronic aortic diseases of the thoracic and abdominal aorta of the adult. The Task Force for the Diagnosis and Treatment of Aortic Diseases of the European Society of Cardiology (ESC). Eur Heart J 2014;35(41): 2873–926.

7. Agarwal PP, Chughtai A, Matzinger FR, et al. Multidetector CT of thoracic aortic aneurysms. Radiographics 2009;29(2):537–52.

8. Hager A, Kaemmerer H, Rapp-Bernhardt U, et al. Diameters of the thoracic aorta throughout life as measured with helical computed tomography. J Thorac Cardiovasc Surg 2002;123(6):1060–6.

9. Davis AE, Lewandowski AJ, Holloway CJ, et al. Observational study of regional aortic size referenced to body size: production of a cardiovascular magnetic resonance nomogram. J Cardiovasc Magn Reson 2014;16(1):9.

10. Freeman LA, Young PM, Foley TA, et al. CT and MRI assessment of the aortic root and ascending aorta. AJR Am J Roentgenol 2013;200(6):W581–92.

11. McComb BL, Munden RF, Duan F, et al. Normative reference values of thoracic aortic diameter in American College of Radiology Imaging Network (ACRIN 6654) arm of National Lung Screening Trial. Clin Imaging 2016;40(5):936–43.

12. American College of Radiology. ACR Appropriateness Criteria. Available at: https://acsearch.acr.org/list. Accessed February 1, 2020.

13. Asch FM, Yuriditsky E, Prakash SK, et al. The need for standardized methods for measuring the aorta: multimodality core lab experience from the GenTAC registry. JACC Cardiovasc Imaging 2016;9(3):219–26.

14. Bireley WR 2nd, Diniz LO, Groves EM, et al. Orthogonal measurement of thoracic aorta luminal diameter using ECG-gated high-resolution contrast-enhanced MR angiography. J Magn Reson Imaging 2007;26(6):1480–5.

15. Diaz-Pelaez E, Barreiro-Perez M, Martin-Garcia A, et al. Measuring the aorta in the era of multimodality imaging: still to be agreed. J Thorac Dis 2017; 9(Suppl 6):S445–7.

16. Roos JE, Willmann JK, Weishaupt D, et al. Thoracic aorta: motion artifact reduction with retrospective and prospective electrocardiography-assisted multidetector row CT. Radiology 2002;222(1):271–7.

17. de Heer LM, Budde RP, Mali WP, et al. Aortic root dimension changes during systole and diastole: evaluation with ECG-gated multidetector row computed tomography. Int J Cardiovasc Imaging 2011;27(8):1195–204.

18. Mao SS, Ahmadi N, Shah B, et al. Normal thoracic aorta diameter on cardiac computed tomography in healthy asymptomatic adults: impact of age and gender. Acad Radiol 2008;15(7):827–34.

19. Murphy DT, Blanke P, Alaamri S, et al. Dynamism of the aortic annulus: effect of diastolic versus systolic CT annular measurements on device selection in transcatheter aortic valve replacement (TAVR). J Cardiovasc Comput Tomogr 2016; 10(1):37–43.

20. Tam MD, Laycock SD, Brown JR, et al. 3D printing of an aortic aneurysm to facilitate decision making and device selection for endovascular aneurysm repair in complex neck anatomy. J Endovasc Ther 2013; 20(6):863–7.

21. Yoshioka K, Tanaka R. MRI and MRA of aortic disease. Ann Vasc Dis 2010;3(3):196–201.

22. Bashir MR, Bhatti L, Marin D, et al. Emerging applications for ferumoxytol as a contrast agent in MRI. J Magn Reson Imaging 2015;41(4):884–98.

23. Tandon A, James L, Henningsson M, et al. A clinical combined gadobutrol bolus and slow infusion protocol enabling angiography, inversion recovery whole heart, and late gadolinium enhancement imaging in a single study. J Cardiovasc Magn Reson 2016; 18(1):66.

24. François CJ, Tuite D, Deshpande V, et al. Unenhanced MR angiography of the thoracic aorta: initial clinical evaluation. Am J Roentgenology 2008; 190(4):902–6.

25. Gopal A, Grayburn PA, Mack M, et al. Noncontrast 3D CMR imaging for aortic valve annulus sizing in TAVR. JACC Cardiovasc Imaging 2015;8(3):375–8.

26. Ho D, Squelch A, Sun Z. Modelling of aortic aneurysm and aortic dissection through 3D printing. J Med Radiat Sci 2017;64(1):10–7.

27. Zoli S, Trabattoni P, Dainese L, et al. Cumulative radiation exposure during thoracic endovascular aneurysm repair and subsequent follow-up. Eur J Cardiothorac Surg 2012;42(2):254–9 [discussion: 259–60].

28. Flors L, Leiva-Salinas C, Norton PT, et al. Endoleak detection after endovascular repair of thoracic aortic aneurysm using dual-source dual-energy CT: suitable scanning protocols and potential radiation dose reduction. AJR Am J Roentgenol 2013; 200(2):451–60.

29. ACR manual on contrast media. Available at: https://www.acr.org/Clinical-Resources/Contrast-Manual. Accessed February 6, 2020.

30. Sawada H, Chen JZ, Wright BC, et al. Heterogeneity of aortic smooth muscle cells: a determinant for regional characteristics of thoracic aortic aneurysms? J Transl Int Med 2018;6(3):93–6.

31. Zilocchi M, Macedo TA, Oderich GS, et al. Vascular Ehlers-Danlos syndrome: imaging findings. AJR Am J Roentgenol 2007;189(3):712–9.

32. Weinsaft JW, Devereux RB, Preiss LR, et al. Aortic dissection in patients with genetically mediated aneurysms: incidence and predictors in the GenTAC registry. J Am Coll Cardiol 2016;67(23):2744–54.

33. Norton E, Yang B. Managing thoracic aortic aneurysm in patients with bicuspid aortic valve based on aortic root-involvement. Front Physiol 2017;8:397.

34. Restrepo CS, Ocazionez D, Suri R, et al. Aortitis: imaging spectrum of the infectious and inflammatory conditions of the aorta. Radiographics 2011;31(2):435–51.

35. Nathan DP, Boonn W, Lai E, et al. Presentation, complications, and natural history of penetrating atherosclerotic ulcer disease. J Vasc Surg 2012;55(1):10–5.

36. Oladokun D, Patterson BO, Sobocinski J, et al. Systematic review of the growth rates and influencing factors in thoracic aortic aneurysms. Eur J Vasc Endovasc Surg 2016;51(5):674–81.

Preoperative Planning for Structural Heart Disease

Michael R. Harowicz, MD[a], Amar Shah, MD, MPA[b], Stefan L. Zimmerman, MD[c],*

KEYWORDS

- TAVR • LAA occlusion • TMVR • Structural heart disease

KEY POINTS

- Pre-procedural computed tomography (CT) for structural heart disease is crucial to provide the interventionalist with information for vascular access approach, device selection, device sizing, and risk stratification.
- Proper orientation to the plane of the aortic annulus during systole on pre–transcatheter aortic valve replacement cardiac CT is important for accurate annular measurements for device sizing.
- Evaluation of left atrial appendage morphology, depth, and presence of thrombus are critical before intervention to assess feasibility of appendage occlusion and device sizing.
- Transcatheter mitral valve replacement device development is an area of ongoing investigation with preoperative assessment of the mitral annulus with cardiac CT playing an imperative role.

BACKGROUND

Aortic stenosis (AS) is a common disease with prevalence increasing with age, and affecting 4% of the population older than 85.[1] Although the disease has a spectrum of severity, untreated symptomatic severe AS carries a markedly high mortality. Historically, a major problem for a large subset of these patients was that treatment with open surgical valve replacement was contraindicated or risky because of multiple comorbidities.[2] The development of transcatheter aortic valve replacement (TAVR) has given patients who would otherwise be exposed to high-risk surgery or limited to medical management a safe alternative for intervention. Recent trials have also expanded TAVR utilization to patients who are of intermediate and low risk for open surgery. These studies demonstrate that TAVR procedures perform equally well as surgery in these populations. Preoperative imaging with computed tomography (CT) has been a crucial step in the development and optimization of TAVR outcomes and is a requirement for presurgical planning for TAVR approach and device sizing.

Devices

There are 2 families of devices with Food and Drug Administration (FDA) approval for use in TAVR: the Edwards Sapien valve (Edwards Lifesciences, Irvine, CA) and the Medtronic CoreValve (Medtronic, Minneapolis, MN). Both devices have undergone several device updates since initial introduction. The major innovations include a reduction in the diameter of the delivery sheath and introducing skirts to reduce paravalvular leak (PVL). The additional major device characteristics,

[a] Russell H. Morgan Department of Radiology and Radiological Science, Johns Hopkins University School of Medicine, Johns Hopkins Hospital, 601 North Caroline Street, Room 4223, Baltimore, MD 21287, USA; [b] Department of Radiology, Donald and Barbara Zucker School of Medicine at Hofstra/Northwell, 300 Community Drive, Manhasset, NY 11030, USA; [c] Russell H. Morgan Department of Radiology and Radiological Science, Johns Hopkins University School of Medicine, Johns Hopkins Hospital, 600 North Wolfe Street, Halsted B180, Baltimore, MD 21287, USA
* Corresponding author.
E-mail address: stefan.zimmerman@jhmi.edu

Radiol Clin N Am 58 (2020) 733–751
https://doi.org/10.1016/j.rcl.2020.02.005

Table 1
Transcatheter aortic valve replacement device characteristics

	Sapien Valve	CoreValve
Sizing method	Area	Perimeter
Expansion technique	Balloon-expandable	Self-expandable
Material	Bovine pericardial tissue	Porcine pericardial tissue
Components	Polyethylene terephthalate skirt at the base of Sapien III, which decreases PVL	Covered segment with flared end
Sizes, mm	20, 23, 26, 29	23, 26, 29, 31
Valve location	Annular	Supra-annular
Trial showing efficacy/noninferiority to SAVR	PARTNER A, B, II, III[3–7]	CoreValve Extreme Risk and High Risk trials; SURTAVI,[8–10] CoreValve Low Risk trial[11]
Primary method of delivery	Transfemoral access	Transfemoral access

Abbreviations: PARTNER, the placement of aortic transcatheter valves; PVL, paravalvular leak; SAVR, surgical aortic valve replacement; SURTAVI, surgical replacement and transcatheter aortic valve implantation.

however, have remained unchanged and are presented in **Table 1**. Examples of these TAVR devices are shown in **Fig. 1**.

IMAGING
Modalities

CT imaging provides a comprehensive assessment pre-TAVR. The first trials evaluating the efficacy of TAVR used echocardiography (echo) for device sizing; however, CT has been shown to have multiple advantages over echo pre-TAVR.[4,5] Several studies have shown that the rate of PVL is lower when CT measurements are used for device sizing as compared with echo.[12–15] This can be explained by the fact that 3-dimensional (3D) volumetric CT datasets allow visualization of the entire aortic annulus, permitting accurate area and perimeter measurements, whereas by 2D-echo, annular size is calculated from a single diameter measurement obtained from the parasternal long axis view, which underestimates true annular size. Underestimation of annular

measurements leads to undersizing and PVL, which has significant implications, because PVL has been shown to increase mortality in TAVR patients.[3]

The other major role of CT for preoperative planning in TAVR is identifying the optimal route for vascular access. Most commonly, the TAVR device is introduced using a delivery sheath via the femoral arteries. Marked atherosclerotic disease, small vessel size, and/or vessel tortuosity may interfere with the ability of the interventionalist to access the femoral vessels or increase the risk of vascular complications, such as vessel rupture or dissection. CT angiography is used to image the entirety of the aorta, the proximal great vessels, and the ilio-femoral vasculature, allowing the interventionalist to plan for the safest approach. Vessel diameters of 6 mm or greater are typically sufficient for the newest generation devices. In addition to vessel size, calcification and tortuosity are assessed. Severe tortuosity, particularly if the tortuous vessel is stiff due to calcification, could make it very difficult to deliver the device sheath.

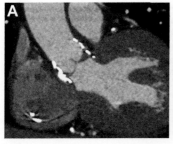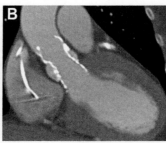

Fig. 1. (*A*) Sapien valve. Examples of TAVR. Edwards Sapien valve with incidental valve leaflet thrombus. (*B*) CoreValve. Examples of TAVR. Medtronic CoreValve.

If the characteristics of the femoral arteries do not allow viable vascular access, then a direct surgical cut-down to the iliac arteries or subclavian access are the preferred secondary options. In patients with severe vascular disease of both the iliacs and subclavians, direct access into the ascending aorta and transapical access through the apex of the left ventricle have been used.

In some patients with anaphylaxis to iodinated contrast or severe renal dysfunction, CT angiography may not be an option. In these cases, noncontrast MR imaging of the heart, with cine image of the left ventricular outflow tract (LVOT) and aortic valve as well as noncontrast 3D MR angiography of the thoracic aorta can be performed. Evaluation of the abdominal and pelvic vasculature could be performed with noncontrast MR angiography or could be performed with noncontrast CT of the abdomen and pelvis to evaluate external vessel diameters.[16]

Computed Tomography Parameters

Recommended parameters and protocol information for pre-TAVR CT are included in **Table 2**. CT should be performed on a multidetector, wide-area, high-pitch scanner, commonly a 256-slice or 320-slice scanner. CT protocol should include an electrocardiography (ECG) gated cardiac CT followed by a nongated CT angiography chest, abdomen, pelvis with iliofemoral runoff. Thin-slice reconstructions allow for high-resolution images when orienting to the annulus. The limiting factor is access, as not all institutions have this type of scanner of available and instead use a 64-slice scanner. An alternative protocol using a 64-slice scanner is presented in **Table 3**. All imaging should be done supine.

Contrast

Iodinated contrast is needed for thorough assessment of the heart and vascular anatomy. Contrast should be injected through a wide-bore intravenous catheter, typically in the antecubital fossa, at a rapid rate of injection of 5 to 7 mL/s, followed by a 40-mL saline flush delivered at the same rate. The saline flush is important, as it helps clear contrast in the ipsilateral subclavian vein, which otherwise may produce streak artifact limiting evaluation of the ipsilateral subclavian artery. Contrast dose, region of interest (ROI) location, and ROI trigger thresholds are presented in **Tables 2** and **3**. Contrast dose can be reduced depending on glomerular filtration rate.

Electrocardiogram Gating

ECG gating is a vital part of the CT because it helps obtain the best-quality images possible of the heart and aortic root. Retrospective gating acquires images throughout multiple cardiac cycles and is generally recommended when available. Although retrospective gating results in increased radiation exposure as opposed to prospective (step and shoot) gating, it has the advantage of allowing for ECG editing in patients with unexpected arrhythmias, often salvaging an otherwise limited examination. For some scanners that do not permit use of retrospective gating, prospective gating with a wide imaging window can be used. Use of dose modulation helps to limit radiation exposure, only using full radiation dose for acquisition of images during the portion of the cardiac cycle that is of interest. For pre-TAVR CT, this is typically 30% to 80% of the R-R interval; however, can be narrowed to 20% to 40% of the R-R interval at institutions where only systolic-phase images are acquired. Imaging of the systolic-phase pre-TAVR is crucial, as this is when the aortic root is maximally distended and is the phase for which annular measurements should be obtained.[17–19] Annular measurements in a phase other than maximal distention risks device undersizing. In some institutions, annular measurements

Table 2
CT protocol for 256-slice or 320-slice scanner

Study	ECG Gating	Contrast Dose	ROI Location	ROI Trigger Threshold	FOV	Tube Potential	Recons
Cardiac CT	Retrospective or prospective	80–120 mL	Mid ascending aorta	250 HU	Heart	100–120 kV	Volumetric 0.5–0.75 mm
CTA CAP runoff	Nongated, immediately following cardiac CT	No additional contrast	None	None	Open	100–120 kV	Volumetric 0.5–1.0 mm

Abbreviations: CAP, chest, abdomen, pelvis; CT, computed tomography; CTA, CT angiography; ECG, electrocardiography; FOV, field of view; HU, Hounsfield units; recons, reconstructions; ROI, region of interest.

Table 3
CT protocol for 64-slice scanner

Study	ECG Gating	Contrast Dose	ROI Location	ROI Trigger Threshold	FOV	Tube Potential	Recons
Cardiac CT	Retrospective or prospective	1st injection of 80 mL	Mid ascending aorta	90–125 HU	Heart	100–120 kV	Iterative 0.5–0.75 mm
CTA CAP runoff	Nongated	2nd injection of 50 mL	Descending aorta	90–125 HU	Open	100–120 kV	Iterative 0.5–1 mm

Abbreviations: CAP, chest, abdomen, pelvis; CT, computed tomography; CTA, CT angiography; ECG, electrocardiography; FOV, field of view; HU, Hounsfield units; recons, reconstructions; ROI, region of interest.

are obtained in the systolic phase selected by the scanner as the most motion free ("best systolic") and the measurements of the sinuses and coronary heights are obtained in the most motion-free diastolic phase. Other institutions use systolic and diastolic measurements at a set phase of the cardiac cycle (commonly 20% and 70%) for measurements. Annular measurements must be obtained in systole; however, there is no guideline recommendation for measurements of the sinuses of Valsalva and coronary heights, which is up to local institutional preference.[20]

Troubleshooting with Computed Tomography

There are several conditions that can limit CT quality, which limits assessment pre-TAVR, particularly for device sizing. Examples of these issues with proposed solutions are presented in **Table 4**.

Pre–transcatheter Aortic Valve Replacement Assessment

The following measurements/characteristics are standardly reported on pre-TAVR CT:

- Aortic valve morphology (tricuspid vs bicuspid)

- Maximum and minimum aortic annulus diameter
- Annulus mean diameter
- Annulus perimeter and area
- Ascending aorta diameter 40 mm above the annulus
- Sinus of Valsalva diameters and heights
- Sinotubular junction diameter
- Ostial heights of the main coronary arteries
- Ideal fluoroscopic angle (C-arm angulation)
- Iliofemoral artery minimum luminal diameter
- Presence and severity of annular calcification

Aortic Annulus

Although all of the measurements listed in the preceding section play an important role in TAVR, aortic annular measurements are the most critical, as these will influence device sizing. To achieve the proper annulus orientation, a double-oblique method is used to demonstrate the plane of the most basal attachment points of the 3 aortic cusps, known as the basal ring, which is the correct plane for annular measurements.[22] An example of orienting to the aortic annulus is shown in **Fig. 2**, with annular measurements in **Fig. 3**.

Table 4
Factors limiting CT

Scenario	CT Limitation	Proposed Solution
Cardiac arrhythmias	Image misregistration	ECG editing, prospective systolic gating[21]
Suboptimal contrast bolus (due to contrast extravasation, IV size, and/or poor patient hemodynamics)	Poor contrast opacification or mistimed examination	Use of large-bore IV, reduce ROI trigger threshold, divide examination into 2 parts, low kVp imaging
Poor patient breath-holding ability	Motion artifact	Reduce coverage of cardiac CT to focus on aortic valve, reducing scan length

Abbreviations: CT, computed tomography; ECG, electrocardiography; IV, intravenous catheter; ROI, region of interest.

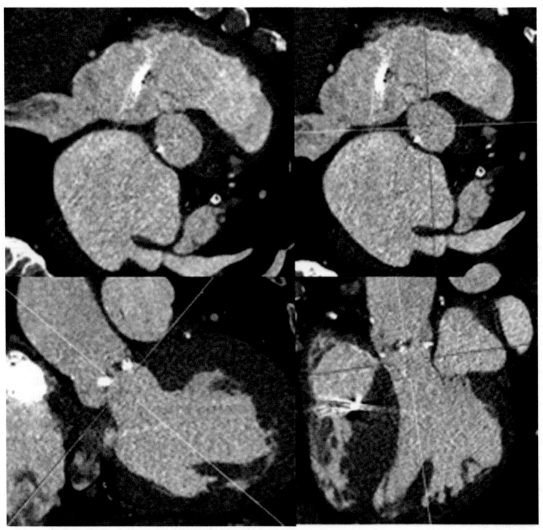

Fig. 2. Aortic annulus orientation. Multiplanar reconstruction showing orientation to the aortic annulus. Crosshairs should be placed in the annulus (*top left*) with adjustments made in the axial (*top right*), coronal (*bottom left*), and sagittal (*bottom right*) planes.

Annular measurements can be done manually, semiautomatically, or with automated software from one of multiple vendors. Specifically, perimeter and area can be measured using freehand contour, polygon tools, attenuation-based contour detection, and cubic spline interpolation; however, it is important to note that methods producing straight or jagged lines risk inaccurate measurements, as the annulus is smooth and ovoid. Smoothing tools should be applied in these situations to improve precision. Use of contouring tools is important, and manual caliper measurements should not be used for overall annular measurements.[20] Contouring in the presence of annular calcifications can be challenging for accurate sizing. At our institution, the contour is drawn bisecting the calcium.

The aortic annulus is a dynamic structure, with maximum dimensions during systole.[17–19] The annular measurements must be performed during systole to minimize the risk of device undersizing. Both area and perimeter are reported, as the Sapien valve uses area for device sizing, whereas CoreValve sizing is based on perimeter.

Aortic Valve Morphology

The role of TAVR in patients with a bicuspid aortic valve has been an area of controversy. Patients with bicuspid valves were initially excluded from early major device trials, and most data on the role of TAVR in patients with bicuspid valves stems from nonrandomized registry data. Although some studies have shown similar outcomes between

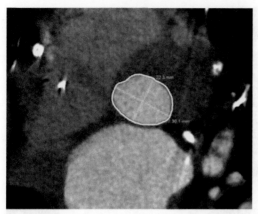

Fig. 3. Aortic annulus measurements. Short axis view of the aortic annulus with maximum and minimum diameters shown with blue lines. Yellow line outlines the annular perimeter.

patients with tricuspid and bicuspid aortic valves, others have shown higher rates of PVL and lower rates of device success in patients with a bicuspid aortic valve.[23–25] Evaluating bicuspid aortic valves before the TAVR procedure can be difficult. Annular measurements can be more challenging, particularly in patients with a valve morphology containing 2 hinge points on the annulus. Care must be taken to perform annular measurements at the base of the valve leaflet insertions. More information on characterization of bicuspid valve morphology based on the number/presence of commissures and raphes can be found in Jilaihawi and colleagues.[24]

Coronary Ostia Heights

The Sapien valve has covered metal struts seated at the level of the aortic annulus. The coronary ostia height measurement (shown in Fig. 4) is important because of the potential risk of these struts obstructing the coronary artery, following placement leading to reduced myocardial perfusion. Coronary occlusion, although rare, can occur in fewer than 1% of TAVR procedures, and has been more frequently reported with the Edward Sapien device.[26,27] An ostial height less than 12 mm does not necessarily preclude TAVR placement; however, increases the risk of coronary artery obstruction.[28,29] The CoreValve device design is associated with a lower risk of coronary obstruction due to an uncovered portion that sits above the level of the valve allowing for retrograde blood flow around the covered portion and into the coronary ostia.

Sinus of Valsalva

The Sinus of Valsalva (SOV) is the anatomic dilatation of the aortic root superior to the annulus and leaflets. Although size of the SOV varies throughout the cardiac cycle, there is no consensus if SOV measurements should be done during systole or diastole. This structure is also relevant to coronary artery obstruction because during TAVR the diseased leaflets are pushed superiorly and laterally by the transcatheter heart valve (THV) into the SOV. There is potential for ostial obstruction in patients with shallow sinuses, when bulky leaflet calcification is displaced by the device over the ostia. SOV diameters ≥30 mm are desired to minimize risk of coronary artery obstruction.[29] Examples of SOV heights are shown in Fig. 5.

Sinotubular Junction

The sinotubular junction (STJ) is the demarcation between the SOV and the more tubular aortic configuration, with the STJ height defined as the measurement from the annulus to the most inferior point of the STJ. The STJ and annulus are commonly not parallel, which is why the

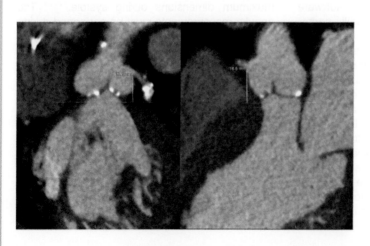

Fig. 4. Coronary ostia heights. Coronary ostia heights for left (*left image*) and right coronary ostia (*right image*) shown with blue lines.

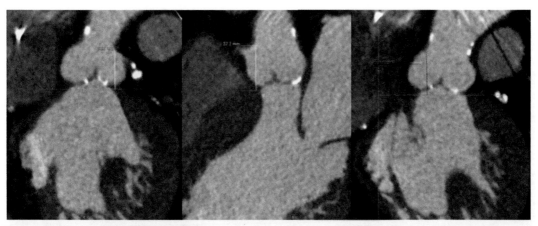

Fig. 5. SOV heights. SOV height for left (*left image*), noncoronary cusp (*middle image*), and right coronary cusps (*right image*).

measurement is specifically to the most inferior aspect of the STJ. The STJ diameter should be measured using a transverse, double-oblique plane aligned with the STJ. This measurement is essential, particularly when a balloon-expandable device is being considered, because if the STJ height is low, an STJ diameter less than device diameter increases the risk for STJ injury.[20]

Calcification

Calcium assessment of the aortic root is relevant because evidence suggests that severe subannular calcification is associated with an increased risk of annular rupture and PVL.[30,31] In addition, calcification of the leaflets and STJ can also affect device deployment. Currently, both qualitative and quantitative methods for assessing degree of annular and subannular calcification are performed. A qualitative calcium assessment scores the calcification ranging from mild-moderate-severe. Quantitative assessment of aortic leaflet calcification can be helpful for evaluation of patients for whom there is equivocal echocardiographic data for AS severity. Agatston scoring of the atrioventricular leaflet can be used to differentiate severe AS from moderate AS in patients with conflicting echo measurements, with supporting evidence from Pawade and colleagues[31] showing that Agatston score is a powerful discriminator of severe AS.

Ideal Fluoroscopic Angle (C-Arm Angulation)

The ideal fluoroscopic angle describes the optimal angle of device deployment when under fluoroscopy and is acquired with software analysis of pre-TAVR CT. Use of this calculation has multiple advantages, as it may reduce fluoroscopic time,

thereby reducing radiation exposure and also reducing contrast load.[32,33] Due to the limited motion of the C-arm, providing alternative angles is recommended when the cranial or caudal angle is >25°. Patient positing of the chest needs to be the same during CT and fluoroscopy for the derived calculation to be applicable, which can make reproducibility challenging.

Device Oversizing

Just as undersizing poses risks to the patient, device oversizing risks annular rupture, which is associated with a high mortality. Risk of annular rupture increases as degree of oversizing increases, but is particularly high when oversizing is greater than 20%.[34] Although some degree of oversizing is desired for the THV, the degree of ideal oversizing is device-specific. Device oversizing is calculated using the following equation: Oversizing [%] = (THV nominal measurement/ annular measurement − 1) × 100. Device oversizing is typically not addressed in the radiographic report but rather a decision that is made by the operator in collaboration with device representatives.

Iliofemoral Artery Minimum Luminal Diameter

Vessel luminal diameter (shown in **Fig. 6**) is key to ensure that vascular access of the iliofemoral vessels with the device delivery sheath is possible. Measurements should be performed in a plane perpendicular to vessel trajectory using curved planar reconstructions from an automated software analysis tool. A qualitative assessment of atherosclerotic calcification also should be done.

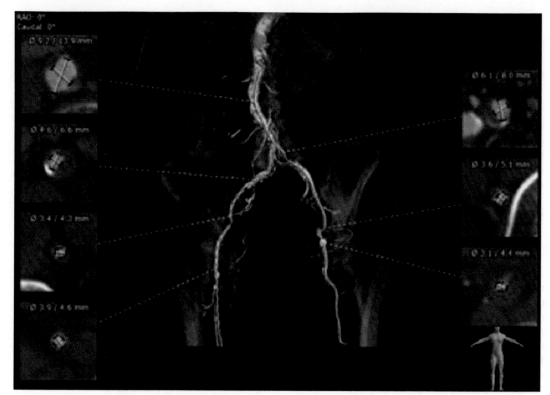

Fig. 6. Iliofemoral vessels. Luminal diameters of the aorta, iliac vessels, and femoral vessels are shown.

Valve-In-Valve

The utilization of bioprosthetic heart valves as an alternative to mechanical heart valves has been increasing since the early 2000s.[35] Bioprosthetic valves degenerate over time, often requiring an additional intervention. The transcatheter valve-in-valve technique was approved for high-risk and extreme-risk patients that are ineligible for surgical aortic valve replacement.[36,37] The prosthetic valve device size is typically reported by the manufacturer using the outer diameter; however, the inner diameter of the surgical ring is the measurement of interest before intervention, as these are the "annular" dimensions that the newly implanted THV will be occupying. Pre-TAVR assessment focuses on identifying the narrowest portion of the prosthetic valve, typically a complete or partial rigid metal ring on which the valve leaflets are suspended. The perimeter and area of this ring are measured and define the size of the THV device that can be placed within the prosthetic valve. This technical procedure comes with significant risk, carrying approximately 3 times the risk of coronary artery obstruction compared with traditional TAVR.[28,38] To help assess the risk for coronary artery obstruction, the virtual THV to coronary ostia measurement was developed, which measures the distance between the expected THV frame to the coronary ostia.[39] This measurement is helpful in patients with a stented surgical valve, with the coronary ostia positioned inferior to the level of the stent posts, as a distance less than 4 mm puts patients at high risk for coronary artery obstruction.[38] Examples of valve-in-valve TAVR and measurements are shown in **Fig. 7**.

LEFT ATRIAL APPENDAGE OCCLUSION
Background

In the United States, the prevalence of stroke is approximately 3% of the adult population, equating to roughly 7 million individuals.[40] One-third of strokes are ischemic, which can be caused by atherosclerosis of the cerebral circulation, occlusion of cerebral small vessels, or cardiac embolism.[41,42] Atrial fibrillation accounts for 15% to 20% of strokes due to thrombus formation, which can embolize and cause ischemic stroke.[43] In patients with nonvalvular atrial fibrillation, 90% of thrombi are formed in the left atrial appendage (LAA).[44] Anticoagulation has been the mainstay for stroke prevention of in these patients; however, the use of anticoagulants comes with a nontrivial risk of bleeding. Multiple studies have shown the

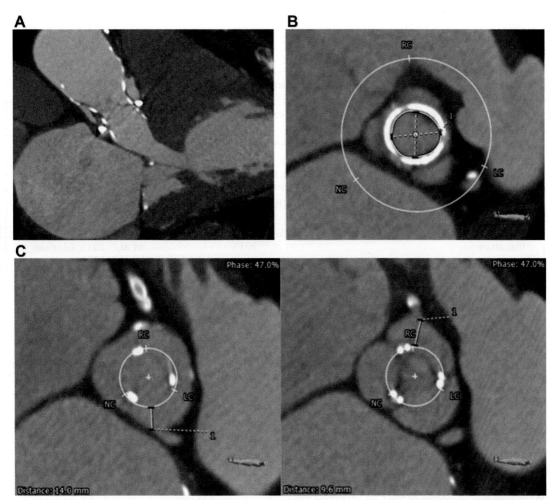

Fig. 7. (A) Valve-in-valve TAVR. Valve-in-valve TAVR. Example of valve-in-valve technique with TAVR within a surgical aortic valve replacement. (B) Inner ring. Inner ring diameters (*dashed lines*) and perimeter (*solid inner white circle*). (C) Virtual THV to coronary ostia. Virtual THV (*inner white circle*) to aortic coronary ostia distance for left coronary ostia (*left image*) and right coronary ostia (*right image*). LC, left coronary cusp; NC, noncoronary cusp; RC, right coronary cusp.

safety and efficacy of LAA occlusion (LAAO) as an alternative treatment and current guidelines recommend use of LAAO in patients with a high bleeding risk and contraindication to anticoagulation.[45–49] Initial studies for sizing for LAAO were done using transesophageal echo; however, CT is being increasingly used for pre-intervention assessment, as studies have shown that CT provides good correlation of sizing with intraprocedural imaging with decreased complications.[50,51]

Devices

There are 3 devices with FDA approval for LAAO, which include the Watchman (Boston Scientific, Marlborough, MA), Amplatzer Cardiac Plug (ACP) (St Jude Medical, St Paul, MN), and Amulet device

(St Jude Medical, St Paul, MN), and the WaveCrest Occluder is currently under clinical investigation. All 3 devices work by plugging the atrial appendage orifice and creating a seal that prevents thrombi from moving out of the LAA. Device characteristics are discussed in **Table 5** with an example of LAA after occlusion in **Fig. 8**.

Imaging

Similar to the CT protocol outlined for TAVR, preoperative CT for LAAO should include a contrast-enhanced, retrospectively ECG-gated cardiac CT, followed by a CT chest, abdomen, pelvis with runoff; 256-slice or 320-slice scanner with wide-area and high-pitch acquisition is preferred. The aforementioned guidelines for use of iodinated

Table 5
LAAO device characteristics

	Watchman	ACP	Amulet
Sizing method	Anatomic orifice	Echocardiographic orifice	Echocardiographic orifice
Expansion technique	Self-expanding	Self-expanding	Self-expanding
Material	Nitinol frame	Nitinol frame	Expanding polytetrofluoroethylene
Components	Fixation barbs and polyester covering	Lobe and disk connected by central waist	Lobe and disk connected by central waist
Sizes (mm)	21, 24, 27, 30, 33	16, 18, 20, 22, 24, 26, 28, 30	16, 18, 20, 22, 25, 28, 31, 34
Relevant literature	PROTECT AF,[52] PREVAIL[47]	Tzikas et al,[53] 2016, Urena et al,[54] 2013	Freixa et al,[55] 2014; Lam et al,[56] 2015; Gloekler et al,[57] 2015, ongoing Amplatzer Amulet LAA Occluder Trial
Primary method of delivery	Trans-septal	Trans-septal	Trans-septal

Abbreviations: ACP, Amplatzer cardiac plug; LAAO, left atrial appendage occlusion device; PREVAIL, prospective randomized evaluation of the Watchman Left Atrial Appendage Closure device in patients with atrial fibrillation versus long-term warfarin therapy; PROTECT AF, percutaneous closure of the left atrial appendage versus warfarin therapy for prevention of stroke in patients with atrial fibrillation.

contrast are also applicable to pre-LAAO CT. ROI should be placed in the left atrium with a trigger threshold of 80 to 130 HU.[58–60] CT is preferred, as echo has been shown to underestimate orifice diameters.[61] CT is also more helpful for assessing the variable morphologies of the LAA, described in detail in the following sections, which can impact suitability for device placement.

Delayed phase imaging

A major difference in pre-LAAO CT as opposed to pre-TAVR is the acquisition of delayed images with a second cardiac CT performed 30 to 180 seconds after the initial scan. The purpose of the delayed phase is to help exclude the presence of cardiac thrombus, which is a contraindication for LAAO. Based on the literature, single-phase cardiac CT has a variable sensitivity, specificity, and positive predictive value for cardiac thrombus; however, has a high negative predictive value of 96% to 100%.[62] The use of dual-phase CT consistently increases sensitivity, specificity, and positive predictive value for thrombus detection, approaching 100% in several studies.[63–65] Mixing artifact and thrombus will both appear as an intracardiac hypodensity on early-phase imaging; however, an intracardiac hypodensity also present on delayed phase is suspicious for thrombus. An example of mixing artifact and thrombus is shown in **Fig. 9**.

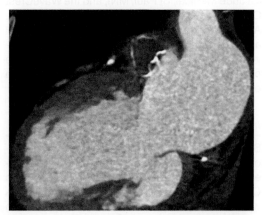

Fig. 8. LAAO device. LAA with occlusion device in position.

Pre-LAAO assessment

The following measurements/characteristics are standardly reported on pre-LAAO CT:

- LAA morphology
- LAA echocardiographic orifice maximum/minimum diameter, perimeter, and depth
- LAA anatomic orifice maximum/minimum diameter, perimeter, and depth

A 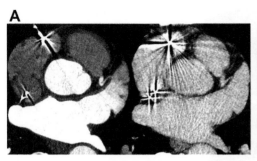 **B**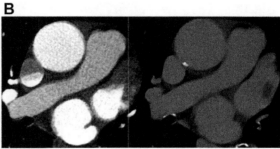

Fig. 9. (*A*) Mixing artifact on delayed phase imaging. Delayed phase imaging of LAA. Arterial phase shows heterogenous densities in the LAA (*left image*), and delayed scan shows no thrombus. (*B*) Thrombus on delayed phase imaging. Arterial phase shows heterogeneous densities in the LAA, and delayed scan shows a persistent hypodensity representing thrombus.

Table 6
LAA morphology

Morphology	Description	Special Considerations
Chicken wing	Multilobed with dominant lobe and sharp bend	"Usable length" determines LAAO feasibility
Windsock	Single dominant lobe without a bend	None
Cactus	Multilobed with dominant central lobe	None
Broccoli/cauliflower	Short, multilobed without dominant lobe	Generally unsuitable for LAAO

Abbreviations: LAA, left atrial appendage; LAAO, transcatheter left atrial appendage occlusion.

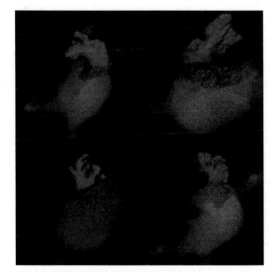

Fig. 10. LAA morphologies. The 4 LAA morphologies are shown with chicken wing (*top left*), windsock (*top right*), cactus (*bottom left*), and broccoli/cauliflower (*bottom right*).

- Proximity to adjacent structures to the LAA orifice (left pulmonary arteries/veins, left circumflex artery, mitral annulus)
- Presence of thrombus

Morphology
The LAA has several different morphologies, which affect feasibility of LAAO, sizing, and risk of thrombus formation. The 4 described morphologies are presented in **Table 6** and **Fig. 10**. Chicken wing morphology is the most common, and broccoli/cauliflower morphology is the least common.[66–68]

The usable length is the depth from the LAA orifice to the sharp bend in the chicken wing–type LAA morphology and is important because the sharp bend limits the depth of the LAA that is accessible for the occlusion device. Usable length that is less than the maximal diameter of the LAA orifice is a contraindication for LAAO.[46]

Left atrial appendage orifice
A double-oblique method using multiplanar reconstruction (shown in **Fig. 11**) is used to orient

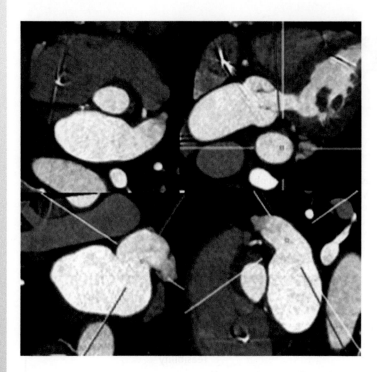

Fig. 11. LAA orifice orientation. Multiplanar reconstruction showing orientation to the LAA orifice. Crosshairs should be placed in the LAA orifice (*top left*) with adjustments made in the axial (*top right*), coronal (*bottom left*), and sagittal (*bottom right*) planes.

to the LAA orifice, which is bound by the left pulmonary veins superiorly and the mitral valve inferiorly. Measurements used for device sizing are device dependent. The Watchman uses the anatomic orifice diameters for sizing, which is defined as the intersection of the smooth walled left atrium and the trabeculated wall of the LAA. An example of anatomic orifice diameters is shown in **Fig. 12**. Depth is measured as the distance from the central point of the orifice to the apex of the main lobe (depending on LAA morphology). Depth should be measured in coronal and sagittal views with the longer of the 2 depths used (**Fig. 13**).[69] The depth needs to be

as deep as the device diameter to be able to accommodate the device.

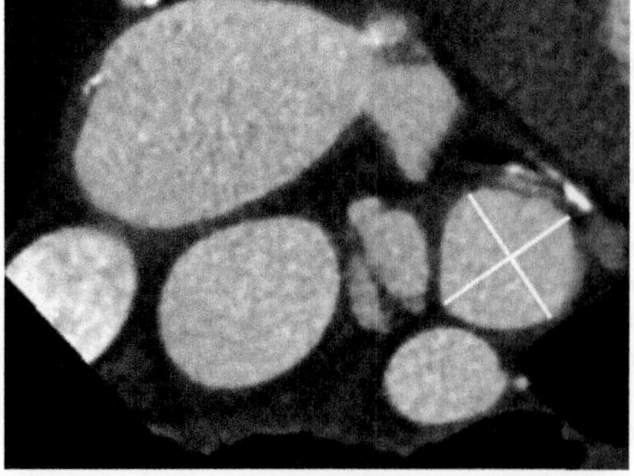

The ACP and Amulet use echocardiographic orifice diameters for sizing, which is the plane between the left circumflex coronary artery, which resides in the atrioventricular groove, and the edge of the pulmonary vein ridge at the superior aspect of the orifice. When using the ACP or Amulet devices, the device landing zone is 10 to 12 mm distal to the orifice.

Because of the variable morphologies of the LAA, it may be challenging to achieve a plane in which both the pulmonary vein ridge and the circumflex artery are both well visualized. Software can be used to assist with orientation and measurement analysis.

Other considerations

Any abnormality of the interatrial septum should be mentioned, as all current devices are delivered trans-septally. Proximity of adjacent structures to the LAA, including the left circumflex artery, pulmonary veins, pulmonary arteries, and mitral annulus, are essential, as device deployment can cause injury to these structures. The left superior pulmonary vein is especially vulnerable to being narrowed or obstructed when the orifice is near the LAA orifice.[69] Close proximity of the pulmonary artery to the LAA orifice risks pulmonary artery rupture causing postoperative hemopericardium.

Fig. 12. LAA orifice diameters. White lines show the maximum and minimum diameters for the LAA anatomic orifice.

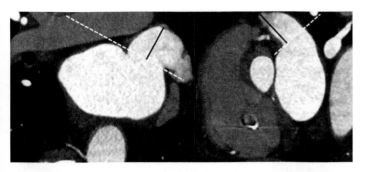

Fig. 13. LAA depth. LAA depth (*black lines*) should be measured in coronal (*left image*) and sagittal (*right image*) from the LAA orifice (*white dotted lines*) as deep as possible. The longer of the 2 depths should be used.

TRANSCATHETER MITRAL VALVE REPLACEMENT
Background

Mitral valve (MV) disease is common, with a prevalence of approximately 10% in patients older than 75 years.[69] MV regurgitation, which is the most common MV disease, affects up to 15% of the population older than 50.[70,71] Prakash and colleagues[72] showed that moderate or severe MV regurgitation was associated with an increase in the risk of death and recurrent hospitalization for heart failure. Similar to TAVR, open MV repair was the standard surgical approach, performed through a sternotomy; however, a significant portion of the patient population with MV disease requiring surgical repair has an unacceptably high surgical risk for open repair. The development of transcatheter MV replacement (TMVR) may provide an alternative treatment option for these patients. TMVR is an area of ongoing research investigation, with several clinical trials under way; as such, there are no set imaging standards and there are no FDA-approved TMVR devices to date.

Imaging

The protocol for pre-TMVR evaluation is very similar to that for pre-TAVR, with a multidetector, wide-area, high-pitch CT scanner being the ideal assessment. Retrospective ECG gating is recommended for cardiac CT for a thorough evaluation of the mitral apparatus throughout the cardiac cycle. As with TAVR, thin-slice reconstructions are critical to obtain accurate annular measurements. Major differences are as follows:

- ROI for trigger threshold should be placed in the left atrium for optimal opacification of the mitral apparatus
- CTA chest, abdomen, and pelvis with runoff of the femoral vessels can be considered, as trans-septal device delivery poses similar vascular access risks as TAVR
- CTA runoff may not be needed when intervention is planned with transapical device delivery

Devices

Although there are numerous devices under current investigation for TMVR, no devices have been approved by the FDA for clinical use at this time. These devices vary widely in the structure, material composition, key measurements for device sizing, available sizes, and delivery approach (trans-septal vs transapical). Details can be obtained by reviewing individual research protocols. An example of a TMVR is shown in **Fig. 14**.

Pre–transcatheter Mitral Valve Replacement Assessment

The following measurements/characteristics are standardly reported on pre-TMVR CT:

- MV annulus perimeter
- MV annulus diameter (middle scallop of anterior leaflet to posterior leaflet)

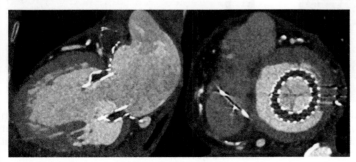

Fig. 14. TMVR. Example of TMVR. Patient also has an LAAO, which is partially seen.

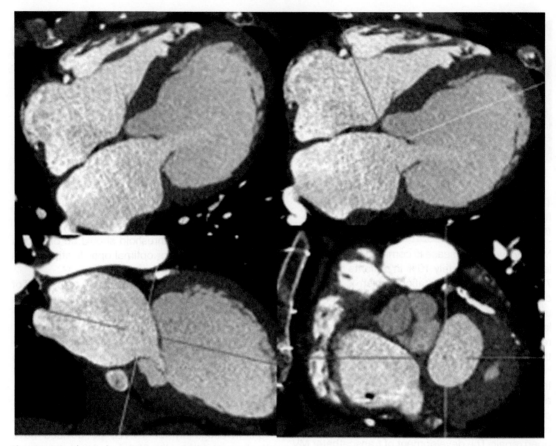

Fig. 15. Mitral annulus orientation. Multiplanar reconstruction showing orientation to the mitral annulus. Crosshairs should be placed in the mitral annulus (*top left*) with adjustments made in the axial (*top right*), coronal (*bottom left*), and sagittal (*bottom right*) planes.

- MV annulus diameter commissure to commissure
- Aorto-mitral angle
- Presence and severity of calcification

- Minimum LVOT area after simulating TMVR device
- Proximity of left coronary artery and coronary sinus to the mitral annulus

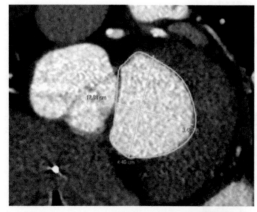

Fig. 16. Mitral annulus measurements. Mitral annulus maximum and minimum diameters shown with blue lines. Outer blue tracing outlines the annular perimeter.

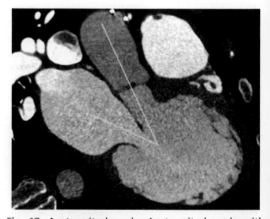

Fig. 17. Aorto-mitral angle. Aorto-mitral angle with one ray placed in the long axis of the aortic root and the other ray placed in the long axis of the mitral annulus trajectory.

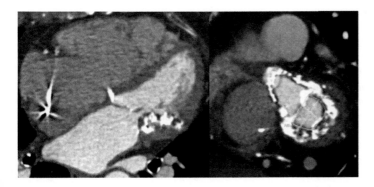

Fig. 18. Heavily calcified mitral annulus. Heavily calcified mitral annulus being evaluated for TMVR. Measurements are shown in right image.

Mitral valve annulus

The inherent structure of the nonplanar, saddle-shaped MV annulus makes accurate orientation and assessment challenging. The posterior aspect of the annulus is clearly defined as the confluence of the left atrium, left ventricle, and posterior MV leaflet insertion. The standard definition of the anterior aspect of the annulus is unclear and an area of dispute.[72] As such, multiple techniques have been described in the literature, with the proposed method by Blanke and colleagues[73–75] to use a D-shaped annulus by excluding the anterior horn of the MV at the level of the fibrous trigones possibly being the most commonly used in practice. An example of orienting to the mitral annulus is shown in **Fig. 15**. Once the view of the annulus is obtained, the perimeter and diameter measurements can be performed (**Fig. 16**). As with TAVR, smoothing software should be applied for accurate measurements.

Aorto-mitral angle

The aorto-mitral angle (shown in **Fig. 17**) is helpful in assessing risk for LVOT obstruction and is measured by placing one ray parallel to the aortic root and the other ray parallel with the mitral valve trajectory. The closer this angle is to 90°, the higher the risk of LVOT obstruction.[76,77]

Calcification

Calcification of the mitral annulus should be qualitatively assessed, as severe annular calcification can be a contraindication to TMVR. Off-label use of TAVR devices in the mitral position for patients with mitral valve disease and either a heavily calcified mitral annulus or a bioprosthetic heart valve in place is an option for patient management. The stiff nature of the annulus when heavily calcified allows for placement of THV. Valve-in-valve technique can be used when there is a bioprosthetic valve in place. When either of these approaches is planned, the inner diameters of either the calcified annulus or the surgical ring, previously

discussed in the valve-in-valve TAVR section, can be used to determine the size of the THV for implantation. The low profile of the Sapien device is advantageous in these scenarios, decreasing the risk of LVOT obstruction. An example of pre-TMVR measurements of a heavily calcified MV is shown in **Fig. 18**.

Other considerations

There are additional factors that contribute to risk of LVOT obstruction including small LV cavity size and hypertrophy of the interventricular septum. Use of software to simulate TMVR device placement and to calculate the minimum LVOT area throughout the cardiac cycle can be useful in determining risk for LVOT obstruction. Although there are no current guidelines, this is an area of ongoing investigation. Close proximity of the annulus to the left circumflex artery and the coronary sinus increases risk for injury to these structures after device deployment.

SUMMARY

Cardiac CT plays a critical role in pre-procedural planning for transcatheter interventions in structural heart disease. Radiologists should be familiar with recommended CT protocols, necessary measurements, and analysis software to provide the interventional team optimal support. Catheter-based cardiac therapies are part of a rapidly growing and evolving field that will likely see further refinements in TAVR and LAAO technique and the introduction of approved TMVR devices in the near future.

DISCLOSURE

The authors have nothing to disclose.

REFERENCES

1. Stewart BF, Siscovick D, Lind BK, et al. Clinical factors associated with calcific aortic valve disease.

Cardiovascular Health Study. J Am Coll Cardiol 1997;29(3):630–4.

2. Nathaniel S, Saligram S, Innasimuthu AL. Aortic stenosis: an update. World J Cardiol 2010;2(6):135–9.

3. Rodes-Cabau J, Pibarot P, Suri RM, et al. Impact of aortic annulus size on valve hemodynamics and clinical outcomes after transcatheter and surgical aortic valve replacement: insights from the PARTNER Trial. Circ Cardiovasc Interv 2014;7(5): 701–11.

4. Leon MB, Smith CR, Mack M, et al. Transcatheter aortic-valve implantation for aortic stenosis in patients who cannot undergo surgery. N Engl J Med 2010;363(17):1597–607.

5. Smith CR, Leon MB, Mack MJ, et al. Transcatheter versus surgical aortic-valve replacement in high-risk patients. N Engl J Med 2011;364(23):2187–98.

6. Leon MB, Smith CR, Mack MJ, et al. Transcatheter or surgical aortic-valve replacement in intermediate-risk patients. N Engl J Med 2016;374(17):1609–20.

7. Mack MJ, Leon MB, Thourani VH, et al. Transcatheter aortic-valve replacement with a balloon-expandable valve in low-risk patients. N Engl J Med 2019;380(18):1695–705.

8. Reardon MJ, Van Mieghem NM, Popma JJ, et al. Surgical or transcatheter aortic-valve replacement in intermediate-risk patients. N Engl J Med 2017; 376(14):1321–31.

9. Popma JJ, Adams DH, Reardon MJ, et al. Transcatheter aortic valve replacement using a self-expanding bioprosthesis in patients with severe aortic stenosis at extreme risk for surgery. J Am Coll Cardiol 2014;63(19):1972–81.

10. Adams DH, Popma JJ, Reardon MJ, et al. Transcatheter aortic-valve replacement with a self-expanding prosthesis. N Engl J Med 2014;370(19): 1790–8.

11. Popma JJ, Deeb GM, Yakubov SJ, et al. Transcatheter aortic-valve replacement with a self-expanding valve in low-risk patients. N Engl J Med 2019; 380(18):1706–15.

12. Jilaihawi H, Kashif M, Fontana G, et al. Cross-sectional computed tomographic assessment improves accuracy of aortic annular sizing for transcatheter aortic valve replacement and reduces the incidence of paravalvular aortic regurgitation. J Am Coll Cardiol 2012;59(14):1275–86.

13. Jabbour A, Ismail TF, Moat N, et al. Multimodality imaging in transcatheter aortic valve implantation and post-procedural aortic regurgitation: comparison among cardiovascular magnetic resonance, cardiac computed tomography, and echocardiography. J Am Coll Cardiol 2011;58(21):2165–73.

14. Mylotte D, Dorfmeister M, Elhmidi Y, et al. Erroneous measurement of the aortic annular diameter using 2-dimensional echocardiography resulting in inappropriate CoreValve size selection: a retrospective comparison with multislice computed tomography. JACC Cardiovasc Interv 2014;7(6): 652–61.

15. Binder RK, Webb JG, Willson AB, et al. The impact of integration of a multidetector computed tomography annulus area sizing algorithm on outcomes of transcatheter aortic valve replacement: a prospective, multicenter, controlled trial. J Am Coll Cardiol 2013;62(5):431–8.

16. Wang J, Jagasia DH, Kondapally YR, et al. Comparison of non-contrast cardiovascular magnetic resonance imaging to computed tomography angiography for aortic annular sizing before transcatheter aortic valve replacement. J Invasive Cardiol 2017;29(7):239–45.

17. Blanke P, Russe M, Leipsic J, et al. Conformational pulsatile changes of the aortic annulus: impact on prosthesis sizing by computed tomography for transcatheter aortic valve replacement. JACC Cardiovasc Interv 2012;5(9):984–94.

18. Hamdan A, Guetta V, Konen E, et al. Deformation dynamics and mechanical properties of the aortic annulus by 4-dimensional computed tomography: insights into the functional anatomy of the aortic valve complex and implications for transcatheter aortic valve therapy. J Am Coll Cardiol 2012;59(2): 119–27.

19. Murphy DT, Blanke P, Alaamri S, et al. Dynamism of the aortic annulus: effect of diastolic versus systolic CT annular measurements on device selection in transcatheter aortic valve replacement (TAVR). J Cardiovasc Comput Tomogr 2016; 10(1):37–43.

20. Blanke P, Weir-McCall JR, Achenbach S, et al. Computed tomography imaging in the context of transcatheter aortic valve implantation (TAVI)/transcatheter aortic valve replacement (TAVR): an expert consensus document of the Society of Cardiovascular Computed Tomography. J Cardiovasc Comput Tomogr 2019;13(1):1–20.

21. Srichai MB, Barreto M, Lim RP, et al. Prospective-triggered sequential dual-source end-systolic coronary CT angiography for patients with atrial fibrillation: a feasibility study. J Cardiovasc Comput Tomogr 2013;7(2):102–9.

22. Piazza N, de Jaegere P, Schultz C, et al. Anatomy of the aortic valvar complex and its implications for transcatheter implantation of the aortic valve. Circ Cardiovasc Interv 2008;1(1):74–81.

23. Yoon S-H, Bleiziffer S, De Backer O, et al. Outcomes in transcatheter aortic valve replacement for bicuspid versus tricuspid aortic valve stenosis. J Am Coll Cardiol 2017;69(21):2579–89.

24. Jilaihawi H, Chen M, Webb J, et al. A bicuspid aortic valve imaging classification for the TAVR era. JACC Cardiovasc Imaging 2016;9(10):1145–58.

25. Yousef A, Simard T, Webb J, et al. Transcatheter aortic valve implantation in patients with bicuspid aortic valve: a patient level multi-center analysis. Int J Cardiol 2015;189:282–8.

26. Arai T, Lefèvre T, Hovasse T, et al. Incidence and predictors of coronary obstruction following transcatheter aortic valve implantation in the real world. Catheter Cardiovasc Interv 2017;90(7):1192–7.

27. Shatila W, Krajcer Z. A cardiologist's nightmare: coronary obstruction during transcatheter aortic valve implantation: how to identify patients at highest risk for this complication. Catheter Cardiovasc Interv 2017;90(7):1198–9.

28. Ribeiro HB, Webb JG, Makkar RR, et al. Predictive factors, management, and clinical outcomes of coronary obstruction following transcatheter aortic valve implantation: insights from a large multicenter registry. J Am Coll Cardiol 2013;62(17):1552–62.

29. Barbanti M. Avoiding coronary occlusion and root rupture in TAVI - the role of pre-procedural imaging and prosthesis selection. Interv Cardiol 2015;10(2):94–7.

30. Hansson NC, Norgaard BL, Barbanti M, et al. The impact of calcium volume and distribution in aortic root injury related to balloon-expandable transcatheter aortic valve replacement. J Cardiovasc Comput Tomogr 2015;9(5):382–92.

31. Pawade T, Clavel M-A, Tribouilloy C, et al. Computed tomography aortic valve calcium scoring in patients with aortic stenosis. Circ Cardiovasc Imaging 2018;11(3):e007146.

32. Binder RK, Leipsic J, Wood D, et al. Prediction of optimal deployment projection for transcatheter aortic valve replacement. Circ Cardiovasc Interv 2012;5(2):247–52.

33. Gurvitch R, Wood DA, Leipsic J, et al. Multislice computed tomography for prediction of optimal angiographic deployment projections during transcatheter aortic valve implantation. JACC Cardiovasc Interv 2010;3(11):1157–65.

34. Barbanti M, Yang TH, Rodes Cabau J, et al. Anatomical and procedural features associated with aortic root rupture during balloon-expandable transcatheter aortic valve replacement. Circulation 2013;128(3):244–53.

35. Isaacs AJ, Shuhaiber J, Salemi A, et al. National trends in utilization and in-hospital outcomes of mechanical versus bioprosthetic aortic valve replacements. J Thorac Cardiovasc Surg 2015;149(5):1262–9.e3.

36. Wenaweser P, Buellesfeld L, Gerckens U, et al. Percutaneous aortic valve replacement for severe aortic regurgitation in degenerated bioprosthesis: the first valve in valve procedure using the corevalve revalving system. Catheter Cardiovasc Interv 2007;70(5):760–4.

37. Webb JG. Transcatheter valve in valve implants for failed prosthetic valves. Catheter Cardiovasc Interv 2007;70(5):765–6.

38. Ribeiro HB, Rodés-Cabau J, Blanke P, et al. Incidence, predictors, and clinical outcomes of coronary obstruction following transcatheter aortic valve replacement for degenerative bioprosthetic surgical valves: insights from the VIVID registry. Eur Heart J 2017;39(8):687–95.

39. Blanke P, Soon J, Dvir D, et al. Computed tomography assessment for transcatheter aortic valve in valve implantation: the Vancouver approach to predict anatomical risk for coronary obstruction and other considerations. J Cardiovasc Comput Tomogr 2016;10(6):491–9.

40. Ovbiagele B, Nguyen-Huynh MN. Stroke epidemiology: advancing our understanding of disease mechanism and therapy. Neurotherapeutics 2011;8(3):319–29.

41. Adams HPJ, Bendixen BH, Kappelle LJ, et al. Classification of subtype of acute ischemic stroke. Definitions for use in a multicenter clinical trial. TOAST. Trial of Org 10172 in acute stroke treatment. Stroke 1993;24(1):35–41.

42. Krishnamurthi RV, Feigin VL, Forouzanfar MH, et al. Global and regional burden of first-ever ischaemic and haemorrhagic stroke during. Lancet Glob Health 2013;1(5):e259–81.

43. Go AS, Hylek EM, Phillips KA, et al. Prevalence of diagnosed atrial fibrillation in AdultsNational implications for rhythm management and stroke prevention: the AnTicoagulation and Risk Factors In Atrial Fibrillation (ATRIA) Study. JAMA 2001;285(18):2370–5.

44. Blackshear JL, Odell JA. Appendage obliteration to reduce stroke in cardiac surgical patients with atrial fibrillation. Ann Thorac Surg 1996;61(2):755–9.

45. Reddy VY, Sievert H, Halperin J, et al. Percutaneous left atrial appendage closure vs warfarin for atrial fibrillation: a randomized clinical Trialleft atrial appendage closure vs warfarin for atrial fibrillation left atrial appendage closure vs warfarin for atrial fibrillation. JAMA 2014;312(19):1988–98.

46. Holmes DR, Reddy VY, Turi ZG, et al. Percutaneous closure of the left atrial appendage versus warfarin therapy for prevention of stroke in patients with atrial fibrillation: a randomised non-inferiority trial. Lancet 2009;374(9689):534–42.

47. Holmes DR, Kar S, Price MJ, et al. Prospective randomized evaluation of the watchman left atrial appendage closure device in patients with atrial fibrillation versus long-term warfarin therapy: the PREVAIL trial. J Am Coll Cardiol 2014;64(1):1–12.

48. Cruz-González I, González-Ferreiro R, Freixa X, et al. Left atrial appendage occlusion for stroke despite oral anticoagulation (resistant stroke). Results from the Amplatzer Cardiac Plug registry. Rev

Esp Cardiol (Engl Ed) 2020. https://doi.org/10.1016/j.rec.2019.02.013.

49. Kirchhof P, Benussi S, Kotecha D, et al. 2016 ESC guidelines for the management of atrial fibrillation developed in collaboration with EACTS. Eur Heart J 2016;37(38):2893–962.

50. Sievert H, Bayard YL. Percutaneous closure of the left atrial appendage: a major step forward editorials published in JACC: cardiovascular interventions reflect the views of the authors and do not necessarily represent the views of JACC: Cardiovascular Interventions or the American College of Cardiology. JACC Cardiovasc Interv 2009;2(7):601–2.

51. Clemente A, Avogliero F, Berti S, et al. Multimodality imaging in preoperative assessment of left atrial appendage transcatheter occlusion with the Amplatzer Cardiac Plug. Eur Heart J Cardiovasc Imaging 2015;16(11):1276–87.

52. Fountain RB, Holmes DR, Chandrasekaran K, et al. The PROTECT AF (WATCHMAN left atrial appendage system for embolic PROTECTion in Patients with Atrial Fibrillation) trial. Am Heart J 2006; 151(5):956–61.

53. Tzikas A, Shakir S, Gafoor S, et al. Left atrial appendage occlusion for stroke prevention in atrial fibrillation: multicentre experience with the AMPLATZER Cardiac Plug. Eurointervention 2016;11(10): 1170–9.

54. Urena M, Rodes-Cabau J, Freixa X, et al. Percutaneous left atrial appendage closure with the AMPLATZER cardiac plug device in patients with nonvalvular atrial fibrillation and contraindications to anticoagulation therapy. J Am Coll Cardiol 2013; 62(2):96–102.

55. Freixa X, Abualsaud A, Chan J, et al. Left atrial appendage occlusion: initial experience with the Amplatzer Amulet. Int J Cardiol 2014;174(3):492–6.

56. Lam SCC, Bertog S, Gafoor S, et al. Left atrial appendage closure using the Amulet device: an initial experience with the second generation amplatzer cardiac plug. Catheter Cardiovasc Interv 2015;85(2):297–303.

57. Gloekler S, Shakir S, Doblies J, et al. Early results of first versus second generation Amplatzer occluders for left atrial appendage closure in patients with atrial fibrillation. Clin Res Cardiol 2015;104(8): 656–65.

58. Rajwani A, Nelson AJ, Shirazi MG, et al. CT sizing for left atrial appendage closure is associated with favourable outcomes for procedural safety. Eur Heart J Cardiovasc Imaging 2017;18(12):1361–8.

59. Kwong Y, Troupis J. Cardiac CT imaging in the context of left atrial appendage occlusion. J Cardiovasc Comput Tomogr 2015;9(1):13–8.

60. Jaguszewski M, Manes C, Puippe G, et al. Cardiac CT and echocardiographic evaluation of peri-device flow after percutaneous left atrial appendage closure using the AMPLATZER cardiac plug device. Catheter Cardiovasc Interv 2015;85(2):306–12.

61. Wang Y, Di Biase L, Horton RP, et al. Left atrial appendage studied by computed tomography to help planning for appendage closure device placement. J Cardiovasc Electrophysiol 2010;21(9): 973–82.

62. Romero J, Cao JJ, Garcia MJ, et al. Cardiac imaging for assessment of left atrial appendage stasis and thrombosis. Nat Rev Cardiol 2014;11:470.

63. Hur J, Kim YJ, Lee H-J, et al. Left atrial appendage thrombi in stroke patients: detection with two-phase cardiac CT angiography versus transesophageal echocardiography. Radiology 2009; 251(3):683–90.

64. Zou H, Zhang Y, Tong J, et al. Multidetector computed tomography for detecting left atrial/left atrial appendage thrombus: a meta-analysis. Intern Med J 2015;45(10):1044–53.

65. Lazoura O, Ismail TF, Pavitt C, et al. A low-dose, dual-phase cardiovascular CT protocol to assess left atrial appendage anatomy and exclude thrombus prior to left atrial intervention. Int J Cardiovasc Imaging 2016;32(2):347–54.

66. Di Biase L, Santangeli P, Anselmino M, et al. Does the left atrial appendage morphology correlate with the risk of stroke in patients with atrial fibrillation? Results from a multicenter study. J Am Coll Cardiol 2012;60(6):531–8.

67. Ismail TF, Panikker S, Markides V, et al. CT imaging for left atrial appendage closure: a review and pictorial essay. J Cardiovasc Comput Tomogr 2015;9(2): 89–102.

68. Korsholm K, Jensen JM, Nielsen-Kudsk JE. Cardiac computed tomography for left atrial appendage occlusion: acquisition, analysis, advantages, and limitations. Interv Cardiol Clin 2018;7(2):229–42.

69. Wang DD, Eng M, Kupsky D, et al. Application of 3-dimensional computed tomographic image guidance to WATCHMAN implantation and impact on early operator learning curve: single-center experience. JACC Cardiovasc Interv 2016;9(22): 2329–40.

70. Nkomo VT, Gardin JM, Skelton TN, et al. Burden of valvular heart diseases: a population-based study. Lancet 2006;368(9540):1005–11.

71. Nishimura RA, Vahanian A, Eleid MF, et al. Mitral valve disease—current management and future challenges. Lancet 2016;387(10025):1324–34.

72. Prakash R, Horsfall M, Markwick A, et al. Prognostic impact of moderate or severe mitral regurgitation (MR) irrespective of concomitant comorbidities: a retrospective matched cohort study. BMJ Open 2014;4(7):e004984.

73. Blanke P, Dvir D, Cheung A, et al. Mitral annular evaluation with CT in the context of transcatheter

mitral valve replacement. JACC Cardiovasc Imaging 2015;8(5):612–5.

74. Blanke P, Dvir D, Cheung A, et al. A simplified D-shaped model of the mitral annulus to facilitate CT-based sizing before transcatheter mitral valve implantation. J Cardiovasc Comput Tomogr 2014; 8(6):459–67.

75. Abdelghani M, Spitzer E, Soliman OII, et al. A simplified and reproducible method to size the mitral annulus: implications for transcatheter mitral valve replacement. Eur Heart J Cardiovasc Imaging 2017;18(6):697–706.

76. Theriault-Lauzier P, Mylotte D, Dorfmeister M, et al. Quantitative multi-slice computed tomography assessment of the mitral valvular complex for transcatheter mitral valve interventions part 1: systematic measurement methodology and inter-observer variability. Eurointervention 2016;12(8): e1011–20.

77. Murphy DJ, Ge Y, Don CW, et al. Use of cardiac computerized tomography to predict neo-left ventricular outflow tract obstruction before transcatheter mitral valve replacement. J Am Heart Assoc 2017; 6(11):e007353.

Four-dimensional-flow Magnetic Resonance Imaging of the Aortic Valve and Thoracic Aorta

Fatemehsadat Jamalidinan, PhD[a,b], Ali Fatehi Hassanabad, MD[b], Christopher J. François, MD[c], Julio Garcia, PhD[a,b,d,e],*

KEYWORDS

- MRI • Flow imaging • 4D-flow MRI • Wall shear stress • Vorticity • Helicity • Viscous energy loss
- Turbulent kinetic energy

KEY POINTS

- Four-dimensional (4D)-flow magnetic resonance imaging (MRI) provides a comprehensive analysis of complex blood flow in the aortic valve and thoracic aorta..
- Recent advances in 4D flow MRI have shortened scanning time, improved pre-processing analysis, and visualization tools, thereby facilitating its clinical feasibility.
- 4D flow MRI facilitates the assessment of aortic and valve diseases using multiplanar visualization, flexible retrospective flow quantification (forward flow, reverse flow, regurgitant fraction, and peak velocity), 3D blood flow velocity visualization and advanced research metrics (flow displacement, wall shear stress, and turbulent kinetic energy).

INTRODUCTION

Knowledge of cardiovascular anatomy and hemodynamic function is vital for detecting, diagnosing, and managing cardiovascular diseases. A comprehensive understanding of these factors is essential for delivery of optimal clinical care. Cardiac magnetic resonance imaging (MRI) is a valuable clinical tool because of its wide field of view, unlimited scanning planes, and excellent tissue contrast. Therefore, it is ideal for the assessment of cardiovascular anatomy and function.[1,2] The growing number of patients with cardiovascular diseases requires a detailed analysis of complex blood flow patterns in the whole heart and great vessels, thus allowing a better understanding of the underlying pathologic mechanisms.

Flow Imaging with Magnetic Resonance Imaging: From Two-dimensional to Four-dimensional

Phase-contrast (PC) MRI can be clinically used to quantify and visualize blood flow. This technique provides an opportunity for calculating a range of unique hemodynamic parameters that help clinicians and researchers improve lesion analysis

[a] Department of Radiology, Cumming School of Medicine, University of Calgary, 1403 - 29 Street Northwest, Calgary, AB T2N 2T9, Canada; [b] Department of Cardiac Sciences, Cumming School of Medicine, University of Calgary, 1403 - 29 Street Northwest, Calgary, AB T2N 2T9, Canada; [c] Department of Radiology, University of Wisconsin, 600 Highland Avenue, Madison, WI 53792, USA; [d] Libin Cardiovascular Institute of Alberta, University of Calgary, Calgary, Alberta, Canada; [e] Alberta Children's Hospital Research Institute, University of Calgary, 1403 - 29 Street Northwest, Calgary, AB T2N 2T9, Canada
* Corresponding author. Foothills Medical Centre - SSB #0700 - 1403 29th Street Northwest, Calgary, AB T2N 2T9, Canada.
E-mail address: julio.garciaflores@ucalgary.ca

Radiol Clin N Am 58 (2020) 753–763
https://doi.org/10.1016/j.rcl.2020.02.008

and diagnosis.[3–8] Conventional two-dimensional (2D) PC-MRI encodes only the time-resolved component of blood velocity that is perpendicular to or within the imaging plane and is a well-established technique to quantify blood flow.[3,9] However, peak blood flow velocity can be underestimated if the acquisition plane is not orthogonal to the vessel of interest or misplaced.[5,10–12] Therefore, minimizing these deleterious effects should improve any underestimation and subsequent interpretation based thereon. One strategy for reducing extrapolation operator inaccuracy is to consider all 3 principal velocity directions (V_x, V_y, V_z) inside the vessel of interest (2D PC-MRI and 3 directions of encoding) and then the magnitude of the total velocity can be calculated by $V = \sqrt{(V_x^2 + V_y^2 + V_z^2)}$.[5,11,12] Alternatively, three-dimensional (3D) spatial encoding allows the acquisition of isotropic high spatial resolution and thus raises the possibility of measuring and visualizing blood flow at any location of 3D volume without restrictions to predefined imaging planes.[4,5,7,13] As such, the number of potential applications of four-dimensional (4D)-flow MRI has increased in recent years.[3,5,14] In the past, the acquisition time of 4D-flow MRI was long, which made it challenging for use in routine clinical settings.[5] However, recent developments in sparse sampling techniques have significantly shortened overall acquisition time to the clinically acceptable scan times (<10 minutes).[3,15,16] The ability to provide comprehensive information on complex blood flow changes in cardiovascular disease

and thus to derive advanced hemodynamic parameters has allowed 4D-flow MRI to be a useful tool in routine clinical practice. A summary of these properties is provided in **Table 1**.

Aortic Four-dimensional Flow

Time-resolved 3-directional 3D velocity (4D-flow) data, acquired using the cardiovascular MRI (CMR) parameters detailed in **Table 2**, provide important information regarding intra-aortic blood flow and aortic valve function. Four-dimensional-flow MRI can be performed using axial, sagittal, or coronal oblique 3D volume. However, for assessment of aortic blood flow, 4D-flow MRI is usually obtained by using respiratory motion compensation and electrocardiogram (ECG) gating with full volumetric coverage of the thoracic aorta (including left ventricular outflow tract, ascending aorta, arch, and descending aorta) in an oblique-sagittal orientation. The generated 4 time-resolved (cine) 3D datasets are composed of magnitude data depicting anatomic structures and 3 time series velocity datasets representing the 3D blood flow velocities (V_x, V_y, V_z). A schematic showing the setup and acquisition of 4D-flow MRI of the aorta is shown in **Fig. 1**.

Four-dimensional-flow Magnetic Resonance Imaging: Three-dimensional Blood Flow Visualization and Quantification

Four-dimensional-flow MRI raw data are often affected by artifacts caused by Maxwell terms,

Table 1
Four-dimensional-flow magnetic resonance imaging

Parameter	4D-Flow MRI
Velocity encoding	Three-directional, full 3D velocity vector field
Respiration control	Navigator gating, bellows, self-gating techniques
Total scan time	5–8 min (dependent on heart rate, efficiency of respiration control, type of acceleration imaging)
Anatomic coverage	3D + time, modify for thoracic aorta and left ventricular outflow tract coverage, whole-heart coverage for congenital disease
Data analysis	Dedicated software packages for 3D flow visualization and quantification of standard MRI flow parameters
Flow visualization	3D (pathlines, streamlines), complex flow 3D patterns viewed dynamically
Basic flow quantification	Retrospective analysis at any location within the acquired volume (peak velocity, net flow, regurgitant fraction)
Advanced hemodynamic quantification	Wall shear stress, flow displacement, 3D pressure difference maps, turbulent kinetic energy, viscous energy loss, vortex/helix flow

Table 2
Technical parameters of four-dimensional-flow measurement

Parameter	Ranges	Comments
ECG gating	Prospective or retrospective	Retrospective preferred: • Avoid sequence interruption • Cover entire RR interval
Respiration control	Navigator gating, bellows	• Mitigate breathing artifact • Increases scan time by 20%–50%
Spatial resolution	2.0–2.5 mm³	• Improving (increasing) spatial resolution increases total scan time • At least 5–6 voxels in vessel of interest are needed for accurate flow quantification
Temporal resolution	35–50 ms	• Improving (decreasing) temporal resolution increases total scan time
V$_{ENC}$	150–400 cm/s	• V$_{ENC}$>expected maximum velocity • Optimal V$_{ENC}$ values can be selected using a V$_{ENC\text{-}SCOUT}$
Flip angle	7°–15°	• Postgadolinium contrast 4D-flow MRI requires higher flip angles
Field of view	192–320 × 176–320 × 16–174 mm³	• It should cover the region of interest
Acceleration factor	Parallel imaging with R = 2–3	• Increased acceleration (higher R) reduces scan time but may also affect velocity and image quality • Advanced parallel imaging techniques may allow acceleration with up to R = 5–8
Acquisition time (standard)	5–10 min	• Total scan times depend on heart rate and respiration control efficiency • Based on standard protocols currently available for main MR systems manufacturers
Acquisition time (advanced)	2–5 min	• Based on new multidimensional imaging acceleration techniques (compressed sensing, k-t undersampling)

Abbreviation: ECG, electrocardiogram, V$_{ENC}$, velocity encoding; V$_{ENC\text{-}SCOUT}$, standard 2D phase-contrast testing to obtain optimal velocity encoding without aliasing.

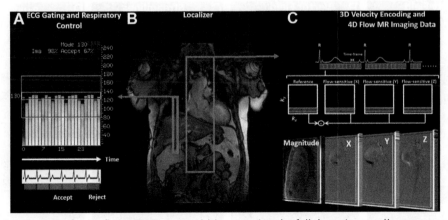

Fig. 1. Data acquisition for 4D-flow MRI. Data acquisition covering the full thoracic aorta (*large orange rectangle* [*B*]) is acquired using ECG gating and respiratory control (*A*) using diaphragm navigator gating (*small orange rectangle* (*B*). 3D velocity encoding (*C*) is used to obtain velocity-sensitive phase images, which are subtracted from reference images to calculate blood flow velocities along all 3 spatial dimensions (X, Y, Z) and averaged magnitude visualizing anatomy over the cardiac cycle.

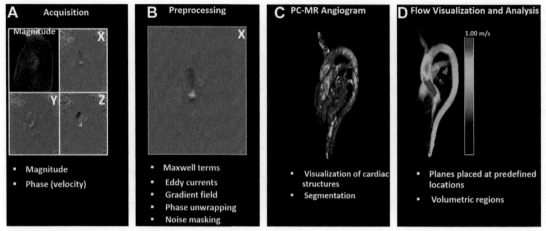

Fig. 2. Preprocessing and visualization. Acquired images with blood flow phase velocities along all 3 spatial dimensions (*X, Y, Z*) and averaged magnitude (*A*) are preprocessed by applying multiple corrections (*B*). A PC angiogram is calculated to visualize the cardiac structures, which can be used for individual segmentation of vessels (*C*). The generated PC-MR angiogram and/or segmentation can be used to mask the velocity field for appropriate visualization and analysis using planes or volumetric regions of interest (*D*). In this example, a 58-year-old healthy volunteer is presented.

eddy currents, and phase wraps caused by velocity aliasing (**Fig. 2**). Therefore, noise-removing techniques should be used as the preprocessing step to improve the accuracy of flow quantification and visualization. After noise removal, the data should be segmented to extract the explicit geometric representation of the underlying object (cardiac or vascular).[12] Then 4D-flow MRI data can be used to quantify potentially useful clinical parameters to evaluate cardiovascular function, including basic parameters such as flow volume, retrograde flow velocity, and peak velocity.[12] Advanced

hemodynamic parameters, such as wall shear stress (WSS),[3] pulse wave velocity (PWV),[17] turbulent kinetic energy (TKE),[18] and 3D pressure difference,[19] can also be quantified.

In 4D-flow CMR data, each voxel includes information about the blood flow vector over the cardiac cycle. Therefore, the resultant 3D blood flow is the vector sum of the blood flow vectors of adjacent voxels, which can be visualized by 3D flow visualization strategies, including particle traces (ie, streamlines and pathlines) (**Fig. 3**). Streamlines are curves tangent to the instantaneous velocity

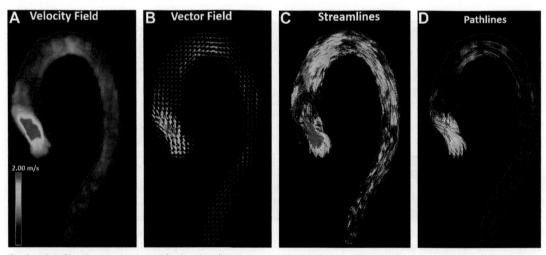

Fig. 3. Visualization strategies. Velocity visualization at peak systole in a 76-year-old patient with mild aortic stenosis. (*A*) the velocity field in the entire thoracic aorta, and (*B*) the corresponding vector field. (*C*) Volumetric streamlines at peak systole and (*D*) pathlines over the cardiac cycle.

vector that can be used to represent the flow field pattern at that given instant within the cardiac cycle (**Fig. 4**). However, pathlines approximate the trajectories that particles follow in a dynamic flow, so they can be used to show the periodic temporal pattern of the blood flow over 1 or multiple cardiac cycles. These visualization methods have been used in several aortic and valvular clinical applications.[3,12,20]

DIAGNOSTIC CRITERIA

Four-dimensional-flow MRI has become an important tool in the clinical evaluation of a wide spectrum of various vascular fields. Blood flow velocity quantification was recently used to evaluate velocity patterns in the cerebral arteries,[21,22] liver and portal vein,[23] renal artery,[24] peripheral arterial disease,[25] pulmonary artery,[26] congenital heart disease,[27–29] intracardiac flow visualization,[30] and aortic diseases.[31–33] This article focuses on the clinical applications of 4D-flow MRI for the hemodynamic assessments of thoracic aorta and aortic valvular diseases.

Acute Thoracic Aortic Syndromes

Acute aortic syndromes are life-threatening aortic diseases and include aortic dissection (AD; **Fig. 5**), intramural hematoma, penetrating aortic ulcer, aortic pseudoaneurysm, aortic aneurysm leak and rupture, and traumatic aortic transection.[34,35] In general, AD begins with an injury to the intimal layer of the aorta, resulting in blood flowing in between intima and media and creating a false lumen (FL). This aberrant blood flow may cause a rupture through the outer layer of aortic wall (adventitia) causing a life-threatening condition or it may flow through other regions via additional tears in the intima.[34] With time, the FL may block and further weaken the aortic wall.[36] Four-dimensional-flow MRI can be used to understand the complex pathologic changes of aortic dissection.[37,38] Although multidetector computed tomography provides excellent anatomic visualization of AD secondary to its high spatial resolution, it fails to provide information pertaining to the hemodynamics present in the FL and true lumen. Four-dimensional-flow MRI can assess flow patterns and evaluate hemodynamic perturbations in AD.[37,38] This assessment includes determining parameters such as helical flow in the FL (which is related to the rate of aortic expansion and rupture) or FL flow rate (or entry tear size), which is an important marker to evaluate risk stratification of patients with AD.[39–41] Moreover, the number, size, and position of the intimal tears as well as FL thrombosis can be determined using 4D-flow MRI.[39,40]

Aortic Aneurysms

After atherosclerosis, aneurysms are the most frequent disease of the aorta.[34] Abdominal aortic aneurysm and thoracic aortic aneurysms are the most common and significant aortic aneurysms.[34] Blood pumping against the weakened area may cause it to bulge outward. The media layer of aorta has elasticity, which prevents blood pressure from rupturing the wall. Atherosclerosis,[42] inflammatory diseases (eg, Behçet disease, giant cell arteritis, and Takayasu arteritis),[43,44] and genetic connective tissue disorders (eg, Marfan syndrome,

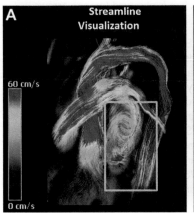
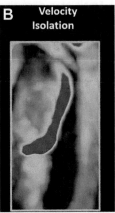
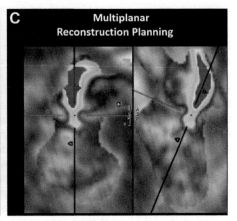

Fig. 4. Mitral insufficiency. Streamline visualization and 3D velocity mapping are used to visualize the location of mitral insufficiency (*A*). (*B*) Velocity isolation of the mitral regurgitant jet. Multiplanar reconstruction of the velocity field can be also used to visualize regurgitant jet (*C*). In this patient (female, 55 years old), the leaflets of the mitral valve are thickened, with evidence of a cleft in the anterior leaflet. There is mild mitral insufficiency with a regurgitation fraction of 15%.

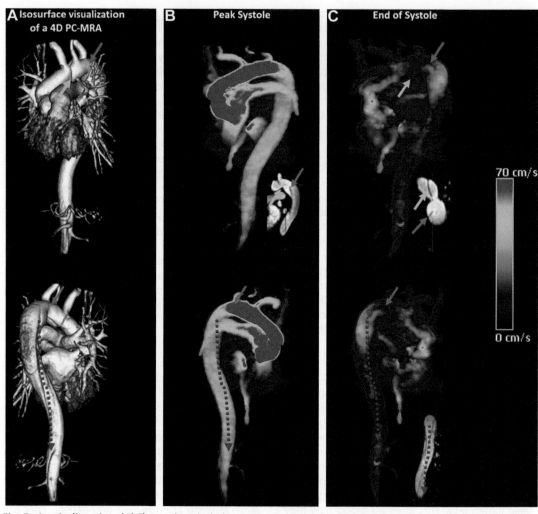

Fig. 5. Aortic dissection. (*A*) Shows the whole-heart PC-MR angiogram (PC-MRA) isosurface visualization of a patient with aortic dissection (male, 43 years old). Flow is visualized at peak systole (*B*) and end systole (*C*). Type III aortic dissection arising at the level of the left subclavian branch (*yellow arrows*) and extending to the length of the descending thoracic aorta (*dotted red arrow*). Small jet in dissection flap is observed (*orange arrows*).

Ehlers-Danlos type IV)[45] can cause the media layer to weaken and result in the breakdown of the aorta. A comprehensive analysis and evaluation of blood flow patterns and WSS based on 4D-flow MRI (Fig. 6) allows improved assessment of factors predisposing to aortic aneurysm rupture.[46] Although 3D WSS mapping allows visualization across multiple subjects, it does not detect abnormal values at the wall. Abnormal values can be addressed using the WSS heatmap concept, which offers the opportunity to quantify the extend regions of altered WSS using a healthy control atlas.[47] WSS heatmaps represent regions of abnormal low or high WSS (ie, outside of 95% confidence interval provided by the control WSS atlas). A recent study showed that regionally abnormal heatmaps in patients with bicuspid aortic valve (BAV) correlated with regional aortic tissue remodeling.[48] BAV showed a reduction WSS during aortic growth, which may indicate a compensatory mechanism to reduce WSS increased forces caused by aortic remodeling.[49] Aortic/valvular interventions induce distinct changes in WSS and the increased number of secondary flow patterns in the ascending aorta.[50,51] Further research is needed to support the value of 4D-flow WSS to predict intervention outcome and inform surgical practice.

Genetic Diseases Affecting the Aorta

Genetic diseases affecting the aorta are mainly divided into 2 categories: syndromic and nonsyndromic. Both are typically autosomal dominant.

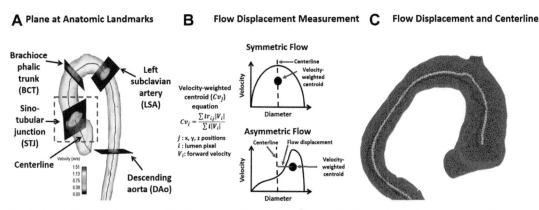

Fig. 6. Aortic flow displacement. (*A*) The automatic creation of analysis planes along the aorta centerline to measure flow displacement (anatomic landmarks can be created for reporting). (*B*) Samples of flow displacement measurements for symmetric and asymmetric flow profiles. (*C*) A patient (male, 65 years old) with severe aortic dilatation (sinus of Valsalva 55 × 53 × 56 mm, sinotubular junction 55 × 58 mm, ascending aorta 46 × 47 mm) and mild aortic stenosis. Volume centerline is shown in blue and flow displacement in red.

One of the most frequent congenital cardiac disorders is BAV, which can be associated with the development of aortic valve dysfunction (aortic valve stenosis and regurgitation) and ascending aorta dilatation.[52–54] Four-dimensional-flow MRI can be used to assess the adverse hemodynamic consequences of BAV, such as altering distribution of aortic blood flow helicity, vorticity, and

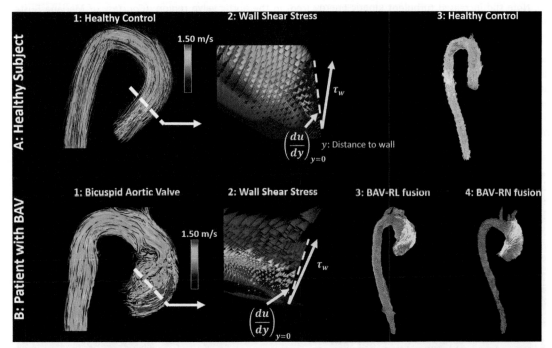

Fig. 7. The white dashed lines represent the location where the sample velocity profile was obtained for a healthy control (*A*) and a patient with BAV (*B*). From these flow profiles, the shear stress rate and blood flow spatial deformation can be estimated. Because no flow occurs through the vessel wall, the speed of the blood flow at the vessel boundary is zero. The near wall region, in yellow, is the boundary layer where WSS forces occur. The WSS expresses the force per unit area exerted in the fluid direction on the local vessel tangent (τ_w). (*A*) The normal blood flow in the proximal ascending aorta of 2 healthy men (ages 37 and 24 years). (*B*) The altered WSS produced by a right-left cusp fusion in a 55-year-old man with a BAV. Column 3 shows right-left (RL) cusp fusions on which flow jet is directed toward the right anterior wall of the ascending aorta producing dilatation of the proximal aorta. Column 4 shows right-noncoronary (RN) cusp fusion on which flow jet is directed toward the posterior wall of the aorta promoting dilatation in the distal aorta within the proximal arch.

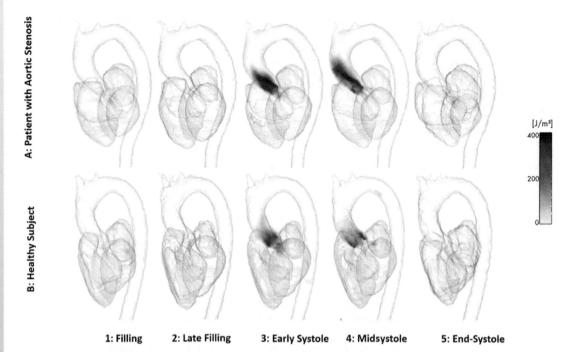

A: Patient with Aortic Stenosis

B: Healthy Subject

[J/m³]
400

200

0

1: Filling   2: Late Filling   3: Early Systole   4: Midsystole   5: End-Systole

Fig. 8. TKE. Temporal evolution of TKE during systole in a patient with aortic stenosis (*A*) and a healthy volunteer (*B*). Note the increased turbulent kinetic energy (*red*) in the aortic valve region. (*Courtesy of* Mariana Busta-mante, Petter Dyverfeldt and Tino Ebbers, Linkoping University, Sweden.)

eccentricity. Some studies compared the blood flow pattern and WSS map in healthy individuals and patients with BAV, and found that the presence of a BAV alters the flow pattern and WSS distribution in the ascending aorta.[55–57] An example of the difference between WSS in a healthy person and that of a patient with BAV is shown in **Fig. 7**. In another study,[58] regional PWV is computed from 4D-flow MRI data to evaluate the ascending aorta stiffness in patients with BAV.[58] Another common form of congenital heart disease is coarctation of the aorta (CoA), which refers to the narrowing of

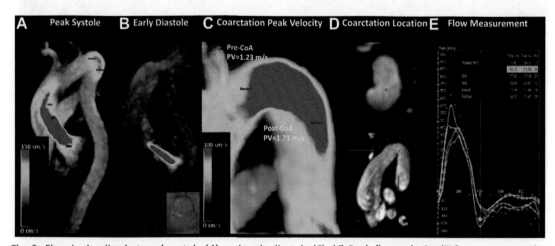

Fig. 9. Flow is visualized at peak systole (*A*) and early diastole (*B*). (*C*) Peak flow velocity (PV) across coarctation (including precoarctation peak velocity and postcoarctation peak velocity). (*D*) The aortic coarctation location. (*E*) Graphs showing flow velocity in the left ventricular outflow tract (LVOT), the aortic sinuses of Valsalva (SOV), mid-ascending aorta (MAA), precoarctation (Pre-CoA) and postcoarctation (Post-CoA). This patient (male, 53 years old) has Sievers type 1/LR BAV with severe aortic insufficiency (regurgitant fraction, 56%), mild stenosis, pseudo-coarctation measuring 21 × 28 mm, and moderate dilatation of the proximal ascending aorta (46 × 46 mm).

the lumen of the thoracic descending aorta.[59,60] The applications of 4D-flow MRI for CoA include quantification of the peak flow velocity, pressure difference of the flow, and TKE in the affected ascending aorta.[61–63] **Fig. 8** shows temporal evolution of TKE within the aortic valve region of a patient with aortic stenosis and a healthy volunteer. This case shows the potential of 4D flow to capture the localized effects of valve lesions (valve type, aortic stenosis, aortic regurgitation) in aortic flow patterns in the entire aorta. Flow disturbances in a patient with BAV with severe aortic insufficiency, mild stenosis, and CoA is shown in **Fig. 9**. Pressure gradients are an important clinical marker for the severity of valve stenosis and aortic coarctation. Although the Bernoulli method is useful for estimating pressure drop, it does not provide the temporal and spatial variations. Alternatively, the 3-directional blood flow velocity field can be used to solve the Navier-Stokes equation (assuming incompressible, laminar newtonian flow). The spatial integration and iterative refinement can be used to obtain a time-resolved 3D pressure difference map.[64,65]

SUMMARY

Advancements made in different imaging modalities have led to tremendous progress in accurately diagnosing various cardiovascular disorders. MRI has played a major role in facilitating precise and customized patient care. Four-dimensional-flow MRI further enhances the diagnostic work-up by providing valuable information with respect to hemodynamic parameters. Its clinical utility has been especially useful in the assessment of flow patterns through the heart and great vessels. Valvular disease leading to aberrant blood flow patterns can be readily and accurately quantified using this method. Previously, long data acquisition time limited the widespread use of MRI in the clinical setting. However, improvements in the technology have greatly reduced collection times. Other obstacles that need further addressing are the cost associated with MRI and accessibility to centers equipped with the appropriate infrastructure.

REFERENCES

1. Patel R, Lim RP, Saric M, et al. Diagnostic performance of cardiac magnetic resonance imaging and echocardiography in evaluation of cardiac and paracardiac masses. Am J Cardiol 2015;117(1): 135–40.
2. Kabir RI, Taru MS, Ullah MA. An Efficient Technique for Detection and Enhancement of Blood Vessels from Cardiac. International Conference on Electrical, Computer and Communication Engineering (ECCE). Bangladesh: Cox'sBazar; 2019. p. 1–6.
3. Garcia J, Barker AJ, Markl M. The role of imaging of flow patterns by 4D flow MRI in aortic stenosis. JACC Cardiovasc Imaging 2019;12(2):252–66.
4. Nayak KS, Nielsen J-F, Bernstein MA, et al. Cardiovascular magnetic resonance phase contrast imaging. J Cardiovasc Magn Reson 2015;17(1):71.
5. Markl M, Schnell S, Wu C, et al. Advanced flow MRI: emerging techniques and applications. Clin Radiol 2016;71(8):779–95.
6. Crandon S, Elbaz MSM, Westenberg JJM, et al. Clinical applications of intra-cardiac four-dimensional flow cardiovascular magnetic resonance: a systematic review. Int J Cardiol 2017;249:486–93.
7. Stankovic Z, Allen BD, Garcia J, et al. 4D flow imaging with MRI. Cardiovasc Diagn Ther 2014;4(2): 173–92.
8. Ota H, Higuchi S, Sun W, et al. Four-dimensional flow magnetic resonance imaging for cardiovascular imaging: from basic concept to clinical application. Cardiovasc Imaging Asia 2018;2(2):85–96.
9. Chelu RG, Wanambiro KW, Hsiao A, et al. Cloud-processed 4D CMR flow imaging for pulmonary flow quantification. Eur J Radiol 2016;85(10): 1849–56.
10. Rose MJ, Jarvis K, Chowdhary V, et al. Efficient method for volumetric assessment of peak blood flow velocity using 4D flow MRI. J Magn Reson Imaging 2016. https://doi.org/10.1002/jmri.25305.
11. Burris NS, Hope MD. 4D flow MRI applications for aortic disease. Magn Reson Imaging Clin 2015; 23(1):15–23.
12. Dyverfeldt P, Bissell M, Barker AJ, et al. 4D flow cardiovascular magnetic resonance consensus statement. J Cardiovasc Magn Reson 2015;17(1):72.
13. Ebbers T. Flow imaging: cardiac applications of 3D cine phase-contrast MRI. Curr Cardiovasc Imaging Rep 2011;4(2):127–33.
14. Vasanawala SS, Hanneman K, Alley MT, et al. Congenital heart disease assessment with 4D flow MRI. J Magn Reson Imaging 2015. https://doi.org/ 10.1002/jmri.24856.
15. Bock J, Töger J, Bidhult S, et al. Validation and reproducibility of cardiovascular 4D-flow MRI from two vendors using 2$\times$ 2 parallel imaging acceleration in pulsatile flow phantom and in vivo with and without respiratory gating. Acta Radiol 2019; 60(3):327–37.
16. Bollache E, Barker AJ, Dolan RS, et al. k-t accelerated aortic 4D flow MRI in under two minutes: Feasibility and impact of resolution, k-space sampling patterns, and respiratory navigator gating on hemodynamic measurements. Magn Reson Med 2018; 79(1):195–207.
17. Wentland AL, Wieben O, François CJ, et al. Aortic pulse wave velocity measurements with

undersampled 4D flow-sensitive MRI: comparison with 2D and algorithm determination. J Magn Reson Imaging 2013;37(4):853–9.

18. Binter C, Knobloch V, Manka R, et al. Bayesian multi-point velocity encoding for concurrent flow and turbulence mapping 2013;1345:1337–45.

19. Bock J, Frydrychowicz A, Lorenz R, et al. In vivo noninvasive 4D pressure difference mapping in the human aorta: Phantom comparison and application in healthy volunteers and patients. Magn Reson Med 2011;1088:1079–88.

20. Fatehi Hassanabad A, Garcia J, Verma S, et al. Utilizing wall shear stress as a clinical biomarker for bicuspid valve-associated aortopathy. Curr Opin Cardiol 2019;34(2):124–31.

21. Sekine T, Takagi R, Amano Y, et al. 4D flow MRI assessment of extracranial-intracranial bypass: qualitative and quantitative evaluation of the hemodynamics. Neuroradiology 2016;58(3):237–44.

22. Wu C, Ansari SA, Honarmand AR, et al. Evaluation of 4D vascular flow and tissue perfusion in cerebral arteriovenous malformations: influence of Spetzler-Martin grade, clinical presentation, and AVM risk factors. Am J Neuroradiol 2015;36(6):1142–9.

23. Stankovic Z. Four-dimensional flow magnetic resonance imaging in cirrhosis. World J Gastroenterol 2016;22(1):89.

24. Wentland AL, Grist TM, Wieben O. Repeatability and internal consistency of abdominal 2D and 4D phase contrast MR flow measurements. Acad Radiol 2013; 20(6):699–704.

25. Frydrychowicz A, Winterer JT, Zaitsev M, et al. Visualization of iliac and proximal femoral artery hemodynamics using time-resolved 3D phase contrast MRI at 3T. J Magn Reson Imaging 2007;25(5): 1085–92.

26. Barker AJ, Roldán-Alzate A, Entezari P, et al. Four-dimensional flow assessment of pulmonary artery flow and wall shear stress in adult pulmonary arterial hypertension: Results from two institutions. Magn Reson Med 2015;73(5):1904–13.

27. Hirtler D, Garcia J, Barker AJ, et al. Assessment of intracardiac flow and vorticity in the right heart of patients after repair of tetralogy of Fallot by flow-sensitive 4D MRI. Eur Radiol 2016. https://doi.org/10.1007/s00330-015-4186-1.

28. Jeong D, Anagnostopoulos PV, Roldan-Alzate A, et al. Ventricular kinetic energy may provide a novel noninvasive way to assess ventricular performance in patients with repaired tetralogy of Fallot. J Thorac Cardiovasc Surg 2015;149(5): 1339–47.

29. Shibata M, Itatani K, Hayashi T, et al. Flow energy loss as a predictive parameter for right ventricular deterioration caused by pulmonary regurgitation after tetralogy of Fallot repair. Pediatr Cardiol 2018; 39(4):731–42.

30. Rodriguez Muñoz D, Markl M, Moya Mur JL, et al. Intracardiac flow visualization: current status and future directions. Eur Heart J Cardiovasc Imaging 2013;1–10. https://doi.org/10.1093/ehjci/jet086.

31. Kari FA, Kocher N, Beyersdorf F, et al. Four-dimensional magnetic resonance imaging-derived ascending aortic flow eccentricity and flow compression are linked to aneurysm morphology. Interact Cardiovasc Thorac Surg 2015;20(5):582–8.

32. Sakata M, Takehara Y, Katahashi K, et al. Hemodynamic analysis of endoleaks after endovascular abdominal aortic aneurysm repair by using 4-dimensional flow-sensitive magnetic resonance imaging. Circ J 2016;80(8):1715–25.

33. Wehrum T, Dragonu I, Strecker C, et al. Aortic atheroma as a source of stroke–assessment of embolization risk using 3D CMR in stroke patients and controls. J Cardiovasc Magn Reson 2017; 19(1):67.

34. Erbel R, Aboyans V, Boileau C, et al. 2014 ESC guidelines on the diagnosis and treatment of aortic diseases: Document covering acute and chronic aortic diseases of the thoracic and abdominal aorta of the adult. The Task Force for the Diagnosis and Treatment of Aortic Diseases of the European Society of Cardiology (ESC). Eur Heart J 2014;35(41):2873–926.

35. Corvera JS. Acute aortic syndrome. Ann Cardiothorac Surg 2016;5(3):188.

36. Trimarchi S, Jonker FHW, van Bogerijen GHW, et al. Predicting aortic enlargement in type B aortic dissection. Ann Cardiothorac Surg 2014;3(3):285.

37. Liu D, Fan Z, Li Y, et al. Quantitative study of abdominal blood flow patterns in patients with aortic dissection by 4-dimensional flow MRI. Sci Rep 2018;8(1):9111.

38. Guo B, Pirola S, Guo D, et al. Hemodynamic evaluation using four-dimensional flow magnetic resonance imaging for a patient with multichanneled aortic dissection. J Vasc Surg Cases Innov Tech 2018;4(1):67–71.

39. Clough RE, Waltham M, Giese D, et al. A new imaging method for assessment of aortic dissection using four-dimensional phase contrast magnetic resonance imaging. J Vasc Surg 2012;55(4): 914–23.

40. de Beaufort HW, Shah DJ, Patel AP, et al. Four-dimensional flow cardiovascular magnetic resonance in aortic dissection: assessment in an ex vivo model and preliminary clinical experience. J Thorac Cardiovasc Surg 2019;157(2):467–76.e1.

41. Cheng Z, Juli C, Wood NB, et al. Predicting flow in aortic dissection: comparison of computational model with PC-MRI velocity measurements. Med Eng Phys 2014;36(9):1176–84.

42. Reed D, Reed C, Stemmermann G, et al. Are aortic aneurysms caused by atherosclerosis? Circulation 1992;85(1):205–11.

43. Erentuğ V, Bozbuğa N, Ömeroğlu SN, et al. Rupture of abdominal aortic aneurysms in Behcet's disease. Ann Vasc Surg 2003;17(6):682–5.

44. Matsumura K, Hirano T, Takeda K, et al. Incidence of aneurysms in Takayasu's arteritis. Angiology 1991; 42(4):308–15.

45. Towbin JA, Casey B, Belmont J. The molecular basis of vascular disorders. Am J Hum Genet 1999;64(3): 678.

46. Ampobasso ROC, Ondemi FRC, Iallon MA V, et al. Evaluation of peak wall stress in an ascending thoracic aortic aneurysm using FSI simulations: effects of aortic stiffness and peripheral resistance 2018;9(4):707–22.

47. van Ooij P, Garcia J, Potters WV, et al. Age-related changes in aortic 3D blood flow velocities and wall shear stress: implications for the identification of altered hemodynamics in patients with aortic valve disease. J Magn Reson Imaging 2015. https://doi.org/10.1002/jmri.25081.

48. Guzzardi DG, Barker AJ, van Ooij P, et al. Valve-related hemodynamics mediate human bicuspid aortopathy. J Am Coll Cardiol 2015;66(8):892–900.

49. Rahman O, Scott M, Bollache E, et al. Interval changes in aortic peak velocity and wall shear stress in patients with bicuspid aortic valve disease. Int J Cardiovasc Imaging 2019. https://doi.org/10.1007/s10554-019-01632-7.

50. Oechtering TH, Sieren MM, Hunold P, et al. Time-resolved 3-dimensional magnetic resonance phase contrast imaging (4D Flow MRI) reveals altered blood flow patterns in the ascending aorta of patients with valve-sparing aortic root replacement. J Thorac Cardiovasc Surg 2019. https://doi.org/10.1016/j.jtcvs.2019.02.127.

51. Bollache E, Fedak PWM, van Ooij P, et al. Perioperative evaluation of regional aortic wall shear stress patterns in patients undergoing aortic valve and/or proximal thoracic aortic replacement. J Thorac Cardiovasc Surg 2018;155(6):2277–86.e2.

52. Capoulade R, Schott JJ, Le Tourneau T. Familial bicuspid aortic valve disease: Should we look more closely at the valve? Heart 2019;105(8):581–6.

53. Farag ES, van Ooij P, Planken RN, et al. Aortic valve stenosis and aortic diameters determine the extent of increased wall shear stress in bicuspid aortic valve disease. J Magn Reson Imaging 2018;48(2): 522–30.

54. Evangelista A, Gallego P, Calvo-Iglesias F, et al. Anatomical and clinical predictors of valve dysfunction and aortic dilation in bicuspid aortic valve disease. Heart 2018;104(7):566–73.

55. Barker AJ, Markl M, Bürk J, et al. Bicuspid aortic valve is associated with altered wall shear stress in the ascending aorta. Circ Cardiovasc Imaging 2012;5(4):457–66.

56. Meierhofer C, Schneider EP, Lyko C, et al. Wall shear stress and flow patterns in the ascending aorta in patients with bicuspid aortic valves differ significantly from tricuspid aortic valves: a prospective study. Eur Heart J Cardiovasc Imaging 2012. https://doi.org/10.1093/ehjci/jes273.

57. Rodríguez-Palomares JF, Dux-Santoy L, Guala A, et al. Aortic flow patterns and wall shear stress maps by 4D-flow cardiovascular magnetic resonance in the assessment of aortic dilatation in bicuspid aortic valve disease. J Cardiovasc Magn Reson 2018;20(1):28.

58. Guala A, Dux-Santoy L, Ruiz-Muñoz A, et al. Is there an instrinsic alteration of aortic mechanical properties in bicuspid aortic valve patients? Regional comparison with tricuspid and marfan patients through 4D flow MRI. J Hypertens 2018;36:e225.

59. Joshi G, Skinner G, Shebani SO. Presentation of coarctation of the aorta in the neonates and the infant with short and long term implications. Paediatr Child Health (Oxford) 2017;27(2):83–9.

60. Nelson JS, Stone ML, Gangemi JJ. Coarctation of the aorta. In: Critical heart disease in infants and children. Elsevier; 2019. p. 551–64.

61. Riesenkampff E, Fernandes JF, Meier S, et al. Pressure fields by flow-sensitive, 4D, velocity-encoded CMR in patients with aortic coarctation. JACC Cardiovasc Imaging 2014;7(9):920–6.

62. Saitta S, Pirola S, Piatti F, et al. Evaluation of 4D flow MRI-based non-invasive pressure assessment in aortic coarctations. J Biomech 2019. https://doi.org/10.1016/j.jbiomech.2019.07.004.

63. Lantz J, Ebbers T, Engvall J, et al. Numerical and experimental assessment of turbulent kinetic energy in an aortic coarctation. J Biomech 2013;46(11): 1851–8.

64. Ebbers T, Wigström L, Bolger A, et al. Estimation of relative cardiovascular pressures using time-resolved three-dimensional phase contrast MRI. Magn Reson Med 2001;45(5):872–9. Available at: http://www.ncbi.nlm.nih.gov/pubmed/11323814.

65. Tyszka JM, Laidlaw DH, Asa JW, et al. Three-dimensional, time-resolved (4D) relative pressure mapping using magnetic resonance imaging. J Magn Reson Imaging 2000;12(2):321–9. Available at: http://www.ncbi.nlm.nih.gov/pubmed/10931596.

Radiologic Imaging in Large and Medium Vessel Vasculitis

Julius Matthias Weinrich, MD[a],*, Alexander Lenz, MD[a],
Gerhard Adam, MD[a], Christopher J. François, MD[b], Peter Bannas, MD[a]

KEYWORDS

- Magnetic resonance imaging • MRA • Vasculitis • PET/CT • Computed tomography
- Giant cell arteritis • Takayasu's arteritis • Large vessel vasculitis

KEY POINTS

- Vasculitides can be classified depending on the size of the predominantly affected vessels.
- Imaging plays a major role in the diagnosis of vasculitis and may help in narrowing down differential diagnoses. Noninvasive imaging has replaced catheter angiography in patients with suspected large- and medium-vessel vasculitis.
- PET and PET/computed tomography enable assessment of disease activity by the increased [18F]-fluorodeoxyglucose uptake of inflamed vessel walls.
- The 2018 European League against Rheumatism recommendations recommend color-coded duplex ultrasound and MR imaging as the first imaging modalities in cranial giant cell arteritis and Takayasu's arteritis.
- The extracranial disease extent of giant cell arteritis and Takayasu's arteritis may be confirmed by PET, computed tomography, MR imaging, or color-coded duplex ultrasound imaging.

INTRODUCTION

Vasculitides are a complex group of diseases sharing the defining feature of inflamed vessel walls. Vasculitides can be categorized based on numerous features such as etiology (infectious vs noninfectious), pathogenesis, clinical manifestations, and genetic predispositions.[1] Consequently, the evaluation of patients with suspected vasculitis can be challenging, because the different forms may result in nonspecific symptoms, which may even overlap with those of other diseases.[2]

A key feature for the classification of vasculitides is based on the size and type of the predominantly affected blood vessels[2] (**Fig. 1**). Radiologic imaging plays a major role in identifying the distribution patterns and extent of the disease.[3] Cross-sectional imaging techniques have gained particular importance in the diagnosis and monitoring of medium- and, especially, large-vessel vasculitides.[4,5] In contrast, cross-sectional imaging techniques are limited by their poor visualization of changes in small vessel vasculitis.[5]

This review discusses the most important imaging modalities and typical findings in large- (**Box 1**) and medium-size vasculitis, implementing current imaging recommendations.

IMAGING MODALITIES
Color-Coded Duplex Ultrasound Examination

Color-coded duplex ultrasound examination allows for assessment of the vessel lumen and wall, including the surrounding perivascular tissues.[4] Compared with other noninvasive imaging modalities, color-coded duplex ultrasound

[a] Department of Diagnostic and Interventional Radiology and Nuclear Medicine, University Medical Center Hamburg-Eppendorf, Martinistraße 52, Hamburg 20251, Germany; [b] Department of Radiology, University of Wisconsin, 600 Highland Avenue, Madison, WI 53792, USA
* Corresponding author.
E-mail address: j.weinrich@uke.de

Radiol Clin N Am 58 (2020) 765–779
https://doi.org/10.1016/j.rcl.2020.02.001

Large vessel vasculitis:
- Takayasu's arteritis
- Giant cell arteritis

Medium vessel vasculitis:
- Kawasaki arteritis
- Polyarteritis nodosa

Small vessel vasculitis:
- *ANCA-associated vasculitis:*
  - Microscopic polyangiitis
  - Granulomatosis with polyangiitis
  - Eosinophilic granulomatosis with polyangiitis
- *Immune complex vasculitis:*
  - Anti–glomerular basement membrane
  - Cryoglobulinemic vasculitis
  - IgA vasculitis
  - Hypocomplementemic urticarial vasculitis

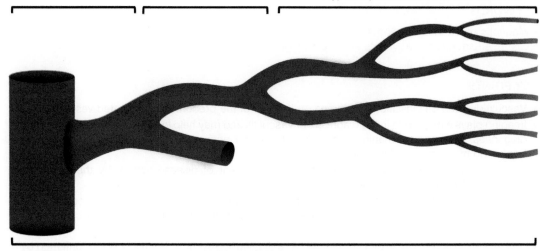

Variable vessel vasculitis:
- Behçet disease
- Cogan's syndrome

Fig. 1. Categories of vasculitides based on vessel size according to the revised Chapel Hill Consensus Conference criteria of 2012.[1] The aorta, large, medium, and small vessels are indicated from left to right. ANCA, antineutrophil cytoplasmic antibody; Ig, immunoglobulin. Note: Single organ vasculitides and vasculitis associated with systemic disease are excluded. (*Adapted from* Jennette JC, Falk RJ, Bacon PA, et al. 2012 Revised International Chapel Hill Consensus Conference Nomenclature of Vasculitides. Arthritis Rheum 2012;65(1):1–11; with permission.)

Box 1
Typical findings in large vessel vasculitis

- Color-coded duplex ultrasound examination: hypoechogenic, noncompressible "halo" sign, stenosis/occlusion/ectasia

- CT, CTA: mural thickening and enhancement, late contrast uptake, stenosis/occlusion/ectasia, surrounding edema/tissue reaction

- MR, MRA: mural thickening and enhancement, late contrast uptake, stenosis/occlusion/ectasia, wall/surrounding edema/tissue reaction

- PET, PET/CT: mural thickening and tracer uptake, stenosis/occlusion/ectasia > surrounding edema/tissue reaction

- CA: stenosis/occlusion/ectasia

---

examination has the highest resolution (0.1 mm), allowing for the detection of inflammatory changes in small arteries.[6]

High-frequency linear transducers with a B-mode frequency of 15 MHz or greater allow for the visualization of small arteries, including the temporal arteries. A B-mode frequency of 7 to 15 MHz should be used for the assessment of extracranial supra-aortic and extremity arteries.[3] A curved array probe with a lower frequency (3.5–5.0 MHz) can be used for assessing large vessels like the aorta and its visceral branches.[4]

Color-coded duplex ultrasound examination does not require ionizing radiation, is widely available, and is less expensive than other cross-sectional imaging modalities. Furthermore, it has been widely used in the assessment of vasculitis, especially of giant cell arteritis (GCA).[6,7] In addition, echocardiography is a favorable screening tool for the detection of coronary artery aneurysms in infants with Kawasaki disease (KD).[8,9] However, ultrasound examinations are operator dependent and of limited value for visualization of the thoracic aorta as well as inflammatory activity in vasculitis.[3]

Computed Tomography Angiography

Computed tomography angiography (CTA) is widely available and allows for accurate depiction of vessel wall changes owing to its excellent spatial resolution and multiplanar reformations.[10] CTA allows visualization of early changes of vasculitis such as arterial wall thickening, contrast enhancement, and the double ring sign on delayed images. The later changes of vasculitis, such as high attenuation or calcification of the arterial wall, are also readily apparent on CTA.[11]

Vasculitic vessel wall changes are usually smoother and more homogeneous than arteriosclerotic lesions and calcifications are less common.[4] In addition, CTA-derived multiplanar reformations enable accurate diameter measurements in case of late complications of vasculitis such as aneurysms or stenoses.[10] CTA is also of high value in the evaluation of other organs when assessing secondary changes caused by vasculitides, such as parenchymal changes, and to rule out alternative diagnoses.

The European League Against Rheumatism (EULAR) task force recommends CTA be performed with multislice scanners and the following parameters: 120 kV tube voltage, tube current time product (mAs) determined by automatic dose modulation, 0.6-mm collimation, and a reconstruction slice thickness between 0.5 and 1.0 mm. The nonionic iodinated contrast agent ($\geq$350 mg/mL) should be body weight adapted (60–120 mL) and injected with a power injector ($\geq$4 mL/s). Imaging should be performed in the arterial phase defined by a bolus-tracking method (threshold of 100 HU) and in the venous phase (50 s after the arterial phase) using electrocardiogram triggering when imaging the thoracic aorta.[3] Newer dual-energy vascular imaging using variable peak kilovoltage can increase vascular attenuation and image quality.[12] In the opinion of the authors, dual-energy CTA should be performed if available. However, there are not enough studies evaluating the impact of dual-energy CTA in patients with vasculitis. In case of suspected involvement of the coronary arteries in medium vessel vasculitis, such as KD, dedicated coronary CTA provides an accurate assessment of the presence of luminal changes of the coronary arteries.[13,14]

Even though most of the arterial vascular system can be evaluated by CTA, its spatial resolution does not allow for the imaging of small vessels (<0.2 mm). Furthermore, CTA uses ionizing radiation and the application of intravenous contrast media is needed.

PET Combined with Computed Tomography or MR Imaging

PET is a functional imaging technique that is, widely used in oncology and has also demonstrated a promising role in the study of vasculitis.[15] Combining PET with CT (PET/CT) or CTA gives additional information on wall thickness and luminal changes. When PET/CT is used for imaging of vasculitis, [^{18}F]-fluorodeoxyglucose (FDG) is intravenously applied.[14] FDG-PET/CT detects glucose uptake from high glycolytic activity of inflammatory cells in inflamed arteries, resulting in a pronounced enhancement of vessel walls (Figs. 2 and 3).[16]

Because patients with vasculitis often present with nonspecific symptoms, use of FDG-PET/CT not only helps to identify a suspected vasculitis, but also other pathologies such as infections or oncologic diseases.[17]

However, FDG-PET/CT is expensive, has a lower availability than other imaging methods, and results in radiation exposure.[10] Because atherosclerosis is also an inflammatory disease, inexperienced readers may misinterpret atherosclerotic lesions as large vessel vasculitis. Of note, the vascular uptake of FDG in vasculitis is typically higher than in atherosclerosis. Even though there are no absolute cut-offs values for distinguishing FDG uptake of vasculitis and atherosclerosis a mild vascular FDG uptake (less than or equal to the FDG uptake of the liver), is not indicative of GCA inflammatory involvement. FDG uptake is commonly estimated by visual qualitative methods, but semiquantitative methods such as the vascular/blood ratio and vascular/liver ratio using standardized uptake values are increasingly being used as well.[15]

Poor spatial resolution, poor distinction of brain activity, and a lack of evidence preclude a recommendation for the use of PET/CT in the assessment of inflammation in cranial arteries.[3]

FDG-PET imaging combined with MR imaging (PET/MR imaging) is a promising new technique that combines the functional information derived from the FDG uptake in PET with the high spatial resolution and soft tissue contrast of MR imaging. However, there is currently only limited information on the clinical impact of PET/MR imaging, and its availability is even lower than that of PET/CT.[18]

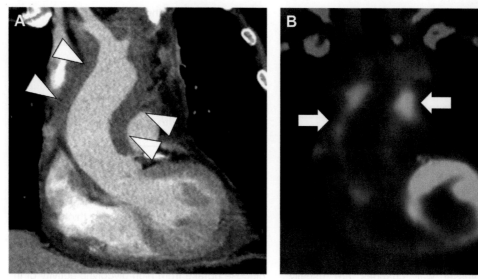

Fig. 2. Giant cell arteritis in a 71-year-old man with involvement of the ascending aorta. (*A*) Coronal contrast-enhanced CT with concentric aortic wall thickening (*arrowheads*). (*B*) Coronal FDG-PET/CT shows corresponding increased FDG-uptake (*arrows*) as an indicator of active disease.

MR Imaging

MR imaging relies on the intrinsic magnetic properties of body tissues and blood in an external magnetic field, enabling imaging without the need of ionizing radiation or nephrotoxic contrast agents.[19] Detailed depiction of the vasculature can be achieved with MR angiography (MRA), which provides excellent image quality with high spatial resolution.[20]

Vasculitis may affect different parts of the vasculature and MRA is an established method for capturing the entire disease extent.[21] MRA is a reliable method for detecting vasculitic changes of large body vessels[21] and superficial cranial arteries.[22] MRA may depict the early inflammatory vasculitic changes with high resolution, including mural thickening and contrast enhancement of the affected vessel (see **Fig. 3**) in addition to luminal stenosis and occlusion.

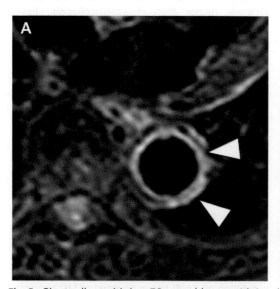

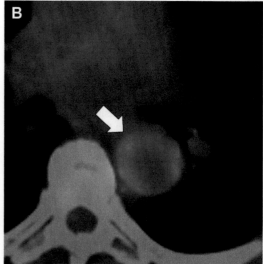

Fig. 3. Giant cell arteritis in a 76-year-old man with involvement of the descending aorta. (*A*) Axial T1-weighted black-blood imaging of contrast-enhanced MR imaging reveals corresponding vessel wall thickening and contrast enhancement (*arrowheads*). (*B*) Axial fused FDG-PET/CT imaging reveals concentric FDG-uptake as an indicator of active disease (*arrow*).

To evaluate as many affected vessels as possible, the scan range should include the aorta and major branches from the carotid bifurcation to the iliac arteries in coronal acquisition, as well as the axillary and brachial arteries.[3,21]

Because MR imaging itself offers technical flexibility, the EULAR task force recommends standardization of MR imaging protocols to produce sensitive, specific and reliable results.[3]

Imaging with 3.0 T scanners rather than 1.5 T scanners is recommended, when available, to obtain the highest resolution, with a minimum 8-channel head and neck coil and 16-channel body coil.[3,19] Settings and technical parameters differ depending on the vasculature to be examined (ie, cranial vessels vs aorta).

Mural inflammation should preferably be assessed using T1-weighted, fat-suppressed, contrast-enhanced sequences and T2-weighted, black blood imaging (eg, navigated 3-dimensional turbo spin echo [TSE], spatial resolution $1.2 \times 1.3 \times 2$ mm^3, repetition time/echo time of 1000/35 ms).[3] In the presence of mural inflammation, T2-weighted TSE sequences can be helpful for edema detection. However, T2-weighted TSE sequences are less sensitive and more prone to artifacts[3,21]

Time-of-flight angiography can be used for assessment of the intracranial arteries.[4,19] Time-resolved contrast-enhanced MRA techniques can be helpful for the evaluation of the large body vessel walls, especially in the case of blood flow alterations owing to stenosis or occlusion.[4] Although time-resolved contrast-enhanced MRA techniques do not allow for the visualization of specific vasculitic changes of the vessel walls, newer sequences like high-resolution T1-weighted 3-dimensional fat-suppressed TSE sequence (volumetric isotropic TSE acquisition) can be combined with contrast-enhanced MRA, which allows simultaneous assessment of lumen and vessel wall.[23] In addition, this 3-dimensional sequence allows for a shorter acquisition time compared with conventional 2-dimensional black blood sequences, as well as multiplanar reconstruction of vessels.

Cardiac MR imaging plays a major role by identifying different patterns of late gadolinium enhancement; it is a common manifestation in several types of vasculitis.[14]

Disadvantages of MRA are the limited availability, long scanning times, dependency on patient's compliance, and relatively high costs.[4]

Catheter Angiography

Catheter angiography (CA) has been the standard in the diagnosis of large vessel vasculitis for several decades.[3] With its high resolution, CA is also still important for the detection of stenoses or microaneurysms in medium-sized vessel vasculitis.[24] In other diseases it has largely been replaced by noninvasive cross-sectional imaging methods. The major limitation of CA is the lack of information regarding the vessel wall and its surrounding tissue. CA is also invasive with a higher procedural risk compared with noninvasive imaging methods. Furthermore, there is limited availability, it is expensive, operator dependent, needs iodinated contrast agents, and comprises exposure to ionizing radiation.[4] Nowadays, the main indication for CA is a part of vascular interventions such as percutaneous transluminal balloon angioplasty or stenting in patients with vascular stenosis.[24]

LARGE VESSEL VASCULITIS

The Revised International Chapel Hill Consensus Conference defines large vessels as the aorta and its major branches, except for the most distal branches.[1] The 2 major vasculitis entities affecting the large vessels are GCA and Takayasu's arteritis (TAK). Even though GCA and TAK have some distinctive imaging features, they are both systemic inflammatory diseases, which might result in variable involvement patterns.[25–29] GCA and TAK also share common histopathologic features, reflecting shared pathways in tissue inflammation.[30]

It has to be noted that an unknown percentage of patients affected by large vessel vasculitis present with atypical involvement of the smaller vessels. This finding is particularly the case in patients with TAK[14,31] where medium-size arteries[1] and coronary arteries might also be involved.

Imaging features of TAK and GCA overlap and are not indicative of 1 disease. Stenosis, occlusion, ectasia, mural and surrounding edema, mural thickening, and contrast enhancement in MR imaging or CT, and FDG uptake in PET/CT can occur in either disease.

The main criteria for diagnosis of either TAK or GCA consist of imaging-based identification of different patterns of vessel involvement, in combination with demographic and clinical information.

Giant Cell Arteritis

GCA is the most common form of systemic vasculitis in patients more than 50 years of age and almost never occurs in younger patients.[32] The incidence is highest in Caucasians with European ancestry and is particularly high in northern European populations.[33] The highest incidence is reported in Denmark with an annual incidence of 76.6 per 100,000, whereas lower incidence rates between 2.2 and 10.0 per 100,000 have been reported in other European countries.[34] The incidence in the United States ranges from 19.8 per 100,000 in a population with a European background[35] to 0.36 per 100,000 in those with African American ancestry.[36]

Even though the etiology of GCA remains inconclusive,[37] recent studies indicate a possible association between GCA and the varicella zoster virus.[38]

Clinical characteristics of GCA are not specific and occur with different frequencies. Headache, scalp tenderness, and jaw claudication are considered as common features (30%–80% of patients) whereas less than 20% of patients present with less common features such as ocular symptoms. Some patients (<5%) may even suffer from infrequent features such as tongue claudication or peripheral neuropathy.[38]

Segmental involvement patterns of the supraaortic vessels, especially of the cranial arteries (superficial temporal and occipital artery) (Fig. 4), are classic features of GCA. Notably, in up to 40% of patients with extracranial GCA there is no involvement of the temporal arteries.[39] Also, GCA tends to have a predilection for the axillary arteries[26] (Fig. 5) and the EULAR task force recommends including these in the color-coded duplex ultrasound examination assessment in patients with suspected predominantly cranial GCA.[3,30]

A dark, hypoechoic circumferential wall thickening called the halo sign is a key lesion defining vasculitis in patients with suspected GCA.[40] Color-coded duplex ultrasound examination has a pooled sensitivity of 77% and a specificity of 96% for diagnosing GCA in the presence of a halo sign in the temporal arteries.[40] Other features assessed by color-coded duplex ultrasound examination are stenoses and occlusions with consecutive alterations of the flow velocity profile.[4]

MR imaging is able to show distinctive changes of cranial arteries such as mural thickening and contrast enhancement, stenosis, occlusion, ectasia, edema, and sequela such as infarction.[4] MR imaging has a similar diagnostic yield as color-coded duplex ultrasound examination, with a sensitivity of 73% and specificity of 82%.[40] The major limitation of both of these imaging modalities is a decreased sensitivity after treatment initiation with glucocorticoids or immunosuppressive medication.[4]

PET/CT scans has a sensitivity of 80% and a specificity of 89% for detection of GCA[41] and a sensitivity of 88% and specificity of 81% in detecting activity associated with large vessel

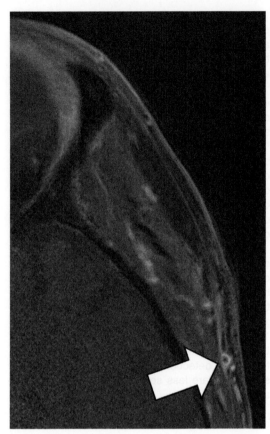

Fig. 4. Giant cell arteritis in a 76-year-old man with involvement of the left superficial temporal artery. Postcontrast fat-suppressed axial T1-weighted MR imaging displays prominent concentric enhancement of the vessel wall of the superficial temporal artery (*arrow*).

vasculitis.[42] However, one of the major limitations in the detection of GCA with PET/CT scan is the decrease of diagnostic accuracy after therapy initiation.[11]

The EULAR task force recommends color-coded duplex ultrasound examination and MR imaging as first-line imaging options in patients with suspected GCA (Table 1).[3] Color-coded duplex ultrasound examination is recommended as the first imaging modality in patients where the suspicion is of predominantly cranial GCA, whereas MR imaging may be used as an alternative if color-coded duplex ultrasound examination is not available or inconclusive. The diagnosis of GCA may be made based on imaging findings alone in patients with high clinical suspicion of the disease. In patients with low clinical probability with no imaging findings, the diagnosis can be considered unlikely.

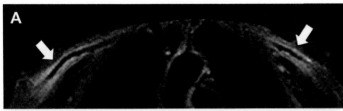
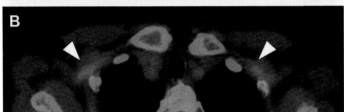

Fig. 5. Giant cell arteritis in a 66-year-old woman with involvement of the axillary arteries. (*A*) Coronal black-blood STIR MR imaging reveals wall thickening of both axillary arteries (*arrows*) with surrounding edema, indicative of active disease. (*B*) Axial FDG-PET/CT imaging reveals high FDG-uptake (*arrowheads*) in the wall of both subclavian arteries, also indicating active disease.

Takayasu's Arteritis

Takayasu's arteritis (TAK) is less common than GCA and affects younger patients (≤40 years) with a female predominance.[14] It was originally diagnosed in Japan and is more common in patients of Asian and African ancestry than European ancestry.[33,43] The reported annual incidences in Western countries range from 0.8 per million in the UK to 2.6 per million in the United States.[44]

The precise etiology of TAK is largely unknown, but inflammatory changes are thought to be caused by an autoimmune disorder.[45]

A broad range in clinical signs and symptoms of at least 1 month's duration are considered characteristic of TAK: limb claudication, pulselessness or pulse differences in limbs, an unobtainable or significant blood pressure difference (>10 mm Hg systolic blood pressure in the limb), fever, neck pain, transient amaurosis, blurred vision, syncope, dyspnea or palpitations.[43]

TAK and GCA overlap in terms of involvement of the aorta and its major branches. TAK may extend from the aortic arch and its major branches from the carotids to the external iliac arteries, including the pulmonary arteries.[37] Also, coronary and pulmonary artery involvement are more frequent in

Table 1
EULAR imaging recommendations[3] in large vessel vasculitis in clinical practice

Vasculitis	Imaging Modality				
	CCDS	CT	PET	MRA	CA
Predominantly cranial GCA	*First-line*	Not recommended for cranial arteries		Alternative if color-coded duplex ultrasound examination is not available or inconclusive	Not recommended
Extracranial GCA	May be used for detection of mural inflammation and/or luminal changes in extracranial arteries				
TAK	Alternative imaging modalities [a]			*First-line*	

Imaging is not routinely recommended for patients in clinical and biochemical remission. MRA, CTA, and ultrasound may be used for long-term monitoring of structural damage, particularly stenosis, occlusion, dilatation, and aneurysm. The frequency of screening as well as the imaging method applied should be decided on an individual basis.
Abbreviations: CCDS, color-coded duplex ultrasound examination; GCA, giant cell arteritis; TAK, Takayasu's arteritis.
[a] Ultrasound examination is of limited value for assessment of the thoracic aorta.
Adapted from Dejaco C, Ramiro S, Duftner C, et al. EULAR recommendations for the use of imaging in large vessel vasculitis in clinical practice. Ann Rheum Dis 2018;77(5):636–43.

TAK than in GCA.[14] The clinical course of TAK typically consists of an inflammatory phase with unspecific systemic symptoms and finally leads to a phase of vascular occlusion with ischemic symptoms such as limb claudication (pulseless disease).[37]

Stenosis secondary to inflammation is a typical feature of TAK, whereas aneurysms occur only in one-third of patients.[43] In addition to the aorta, the subclavian, common carotid, and renal arteries are mainly affected by TAK.[43] Concentric mural thickening of the involved arteries is characteristic and a double ring sign, consisting of an inner low attenuating wall surrounded by an outer high attenuating wall, may be visible in the venous phase (Fig. 6).[10,46]

Late complications result in an occlusive stage with arterial stenosis, occlusion, or aneurysmal dilatation, which may lead to extensive collateral vessels (Fig. 7).[10] Therefore, MRA and CTA should include the aorta and its major branches from the carotid bifurcation to the iliac arteries in coronal acquisition, as well as the axillary and brachial arteries.[3,21]

The choice of imaging in suspected TAK is similar to GCA. However, the temporal arteries are usually spared in patients with TAK, and the role of color-coded duplex ultrasound examination is less important than for patients with suspected GCA.

The EULAR task force recommends MR imaging as the first imaging modality when investigating mural inflammation and luminal vessel changes in patients with suspected TAK. PET/CT scan, CT scan, and ultrasound examination may be used as alternative imaging modalities,[3] although all imaging techniques share similar limitations as in the diagnosis of GCA.[11,17]

MEDIUM VESSEL VASCULITIS

Medium vessel vasculitis predominantly affects the main visceral arteries and their branches.[1,14] In comparison with large vessel vasculitis, inflammation in medium size vessels is more acute and necrotizing, resulting in inflammatory aneurysms and stenosis.[1] Polyarteritis nodosa (PAN) and KD are the 2 main medium vessel vasculitides.

Polyarteritis Nodosa

PAN is a necrotizing arteritis of medium or small arteries, which is typically antineutrophil cytoplasmic antibody negative.[1] PAN is generally found in all age groups, but most commonly in those between 50 and 70 years of age, occurring twice as often in men compared with women.[47] Reported estimates of the annual incidence of PAN in the general population range from 4.6 per million in England to 9.0 per million in the United States.[48]

The etiology of PAN is usually idiopathic, but can be secondary to other causes such as viral infections.[49] A subset of patients suffer from hepatitis B virus-associated PAN.[1,47] However, PAN is becoming a rare disease, which is mainly attributable to the decrease in hepatitis B virus infections,

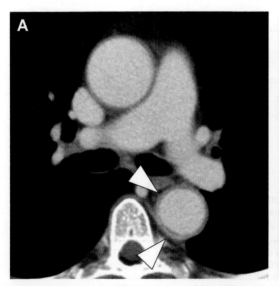
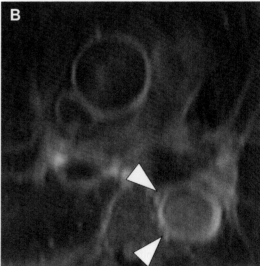

Fig. 6. Takayasu's arteritis in a 63-year-old woman with involvement of the thoracic aorta. (*A*) Axial venous-phase CT shows concentric mural thickening in the ascending and descending aorta with a double ring sign (inner low and outer high enhancement) in the descending aorta (*arrowheads*). (*B*) Axial post-contrast T1-weighted black-blood MR imaging also reveals concentric enhancement of the aortic walls (*B*, *arrowheads*).

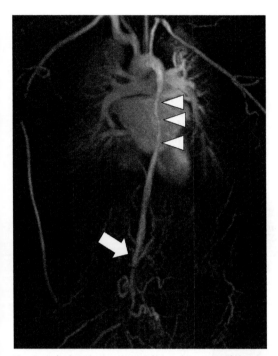

Fig. 7. Takayasu's arteritis with involvement of the descending aorta, left subclavian artery and iliac arteries in a 33-year-old woman. Coronal maximum intensity projection of contrast-enhanced 3D MRA reveals long-distance stenosis of the descending aorta (*arrowheads*) as well as an occlusion of both common iliac arteries which results in extensive collateral vessels (*arrow*).

as well as the increasing recognition and awareness of other systemic necrotizing vasculitides.[49]

The absence of antineutrophil cytoplasmic antibody distinguishes PAN from the small vessel vasculitis microscopic polyangiitis.[10] The main clinical manifestations of PAN include neurologic syndromes (40%–79%), urologic and renal involvement (8%–66%) (**Figs. 8** and **9**), and gastrointestinal tract involvement (14%–44%) (**Fig. 10**).[50]

Characteristic imaging findings of PAN include multiple microaneurysms (1–5 mm) often involving the renal, mesenteric, and hepatic artery branches.[49] Because different stages of the inflammatory process occur simultaneously, vessels with acute necrotizing lesions, alongside fibrotic or healing vessels, might be present.[50] Therefore, microaneurysms often coexist with stenotic lesions.[49]

The presence of microaneurysms can be assessed by CA, CTA, and MRA (see **Figs. 8–10**). The major disadvantage of CA is its invasiveness and inability to depict parenchyma. Although MRA is noninvasive and does not need ionizing

radiation, it is considerably more time consuming, plus additional imaging sequences for evaluation of secondary changes to PAN, such as renal infarctions, require even more time. CTA uses ionizing radiation and iodinated contrast agents. The CTA scan itself is performed quickly and, as well as an arterial phase, a portal venous phase can be acquired to evaluate parenchymal changes. Except for young patients, CTA should be the preferred imaging modality in assessing disease extent in PAN.

A diagnosis of PAN can be established if typical radiographic abnormalities are present.[50] However, image interpretation needs to be conducted by an experienced radiologist to adequately take other structural vasculopathies into consideration, which may lead to multiple aneurysm formations.[50] Fibromuscular dysplasia has to be ruled out as a differential diagnosis, especially in young to middle-aged patients, with a female predominance.[10] Other mimics such as segmental arterial mediolysis or neurofibromatosis type I are possible, but rarer.

Kawasaki Disease

KD is associated with mucocutaneous lymph node syndrome and predominantly affects medium and small arteries in infants and children less than 5 years of age.[1,10] It is more prevalent in Asian populations and has a male dominance.[51] The highest incidence is reported in Japan with 219 cases per million, whereas it ranges between 5 and 15 per million in Europe and 19 per million in the United States.[52] The exact etiology of KD remains unclear; however, it is suggested to be caused by an infectious agent in genetically predisposed children.[8,53]

KD is diagnosed based on clinical criteria—the presence of 5 or more days of fever and at least 4 of the 5 principal clinical features: (1) bilateral bulbar conjunctival injection without exudates, (2) erythema and cracking of lips, strawberry tongue, or erythema of the oral and pharyngeal mucosa, (3) cervical lymphadenopathy (≥1.5 cm in diameter), usually unilateral, (4) rash (maculopapular, diffuse erythroderma or erythema multiforme–like), and (5) erythema and edema of the hands and feet in the acute phase and/or periungual desquamation in the subacute phase.[54]

The coronary arteries are often involved in KD and coronary artery aneurysms develop as a result of coronary vasculitis in about 15% to 25% of untreated patients (**Fig. 11**).[8,55] Coronary artery aneurysms can be classified according to their size (small, <5 mm; medium, 5–8 mm; and large, >8 mm) and shape (saccular or fusiform).[56]

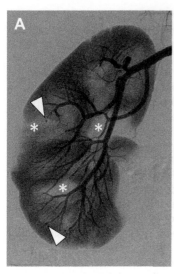
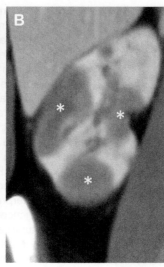

Fig. 8. Polyarteritis nodosa in a 46-year-old woman with involvement of the kidney. (*A*) Digital subtraction angiography of the right kidney shows irregular renal perfusion (*asterisks*) with multiple small microaneurysms in the periphery (*arrowheads*). (*B*) Coronal CT confirms the perfusion defects, corresponding to parenchymal renal infarctions (*asterisks*).

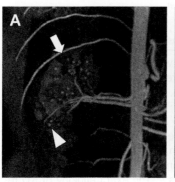
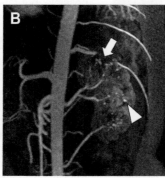

Fig. 9. Polyarteritis nodosa in a 24-year-old man with involvement of the kidney. (*A*, *B*) Magnetic resonance angiography of the kidneys (*A*, *right*; *B*, *left*) shows renal areas of cortical irregularity from multiple infarctions (*A*, *B arrows*) with multiple small microaneurysms in the periphery (*arrowhead*).

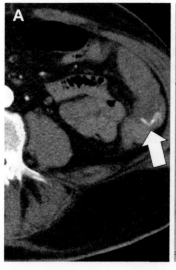
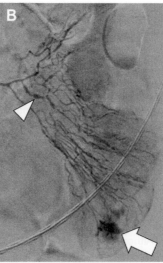

Fig. 10. Polyarteritis nodosa in a 72-year-old man with involvement of the small bowel. (*A*) Axial contrast-enhanced CT arterial-phase imaging shows contrast extravasation corresponding to active intraluminal jejunal bleeding (*arrow*). (*B*) The following therapeutic interventional angiography revealed multiple stenoses and microaneurysms (*arrowhead*) as well as the bleeding (*arrow*).

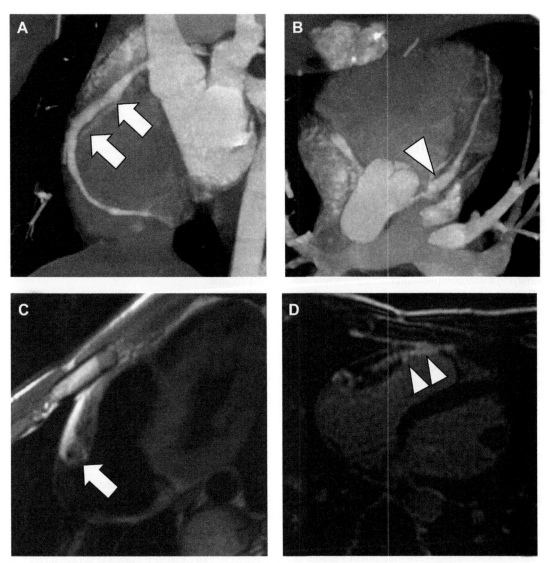

Fig. 11. Kawasaki disease in a 11-year-old boy with involvement of coronary arteries. (*A, B*) Coronary CT angiography with maximum intensity projection of the right coronary artery (*A*) and left anterior descending artery (*B*). Note the aneurysms of the right (*A, arrows*) and left anterior descending artery (*B, arrowhead*). (*C, D*) The patient presented 6 years later with chest pain leading to a cardiac MR image which showed asymmetric wall thickening of the RCA on the double inversion recovery image (*C, arrow*) and abnormal late gadolinium enhancement in the wall of the RCA (*D, arrowheads*).

Large coronary artery aneurysms are associated with a higher risk of complications such as rupture, thrombosis, and stenosis, which possibly lead to myocardial infarction and death.[55,57,58] Coronary artery aneurysms regress in 55% of all patients, although the structural vessel wall changes persist[55,58] and large aneurysms do not regress.[59]

The involvement of other arteries in KD is rare. Aortic root dilation is seen in 8% of patients and associated with greater coronary artery size at diagnosis.[60] Systemic arterial aneurysms occur in approximately 2% of patients with KD, usually those who also have coronary artery aneurysms.[61] Medium-size arteries like the axillary, subclavian, brachial, iliac, and renal arteries are mainly affected. Peripheral aneurysms generally do not require treatment but are associated with the presence of coronary artery aneurysms and indicate more severe vasculitis, which increases the likelihood of cardiac sequelae.[61,62] In rare cases, relevant complications such as peripheral ischemia may occur, although peripheral aneurysms tend to regress.[55,57]

Because coronary artery aneurysms are the most feared complication of KD, imaging of coronary arteries is crucial for the diagnosis and management of patients with KD.[54] Transthoracic echocardiography (TTE) is the primary and most commonly used imaging modality for the detection of aneurysms in KD.[6,54] However, if the initial TTE is performed within the first week of disease onset, it is often normal and does not rule out KD. In addition, TTE has inherent limitations and it becomes progressively more difficult to visualize the distal segments of coronary arteries as a child grows.[54] Even though detection of coronary artery aneurysms and thrombi by TTE has been demonstrated, the sensitivity and specificity for identifying these complications remain unclear.[8,54]

Therefore, multimodality imaging including CTA, MRA/cardiovascular MR imaging, or invasive coronary CA are reasonable choices. The diagnostic approach needs to be customized depending on the clinical setting. In the case of a pulsatile axillary mass, which might indicate a peripheral aneurysm, the whole vasculature needs to be evaluated.[8,54] If visualization by ultrasound examination is not feasible, CTA or MRA/cardiac MR imaging should be performed. Cardiac MR imaging provides information about the coronary anatomy, myocardial ischemia, infarction, inflammation, and function. CTA is an effective alternative and the final choice of modality depends on the availability and expertise of each center.

VARIABLE VESSEL VASCULITIS

Variable vessel vasculitides may affect vessels of any size and types (arteries, veins, and capillaries).[1] Behcet's disease and Cogan's syndrome are the 2 main entities.

Unlike large and medium vessel vasculitides, Behcet's disease is most commonly characterized by thrombotic manifestations, with estimates of prevalence ranging from 10% to 30%, occurring more frequently in male patients.[63] Superficial subcutaneous thrombophlebitis and deep vein thrombosis of the lower limbs are the most common thrombotic events in Behcet's disease; ultrasound examination is the imaging method of choice in these patients. However, the most dangerous complications of vascular Behcet's disease are aneurysms of the pulmonary artery, which can be detected by CTA or MRA.[5,63]

Vasculitis in Cogan's syndrome is only a part of this syndromic disorder, which is primarily characterized by ocular lesions and inner ear diseases. Vasculitic manifestations are highly variable and may include arteritis of any vessel size, aortitis, aortic aneurysms, and aortic and mitral valvulitis.[1]

SMALL VESSEL VASCULITIS

Small vessel vasculitides predominantly affect small intraparenchymal arteries, arterioles, capillaries and venules.[1] Small vessel vasculitis can be divided into 2 categories based on pathogenesis: antineutrophil cytoplasmic antibody-associated vasculitis and immune complex-associated vasculitis.[64]

Antineutrophil cytoplasmic antibody-associated vasculitis can affect both medium and small vessels and includes granulomatosis with polyangiitis, Churg-Strauss syndrome, and microscopic polyangiitis.[1]

Immune complex vasculitides comprise IgA vasculitis, cryoglobulinemic vasculitis, hypocomplementemic urticarial vasculitis (anti-C1q vasculitis), and anti–glomerular basement membrane disease.[1]

Radiologic imaging techniques are particularly useful to diagnose and monitor large and medium vasculitis, but are unable to adequately visualize small vessels.[5] However, imaging findings help to determine disease extent and severity by depicting parenchymal changes such as pulmonary involvement in granulomatosis with polyangiitis (Fig. 12).[2]

Because this review is focused on the role of imaging in large and medium vessels, we do not discuss small vessel vasculitis in detail.

VASCULITIS ASSOCIATED WITH SYSTEMIC DISEASE AND SINGLE ORGAN VASCULITIS

Vasculitis can be associated with or caused by a systemic disease. Common examples of such vasculitides are rheumatoid vasculitis, sarcoidosis vasculitis, or lupus vasculitis.[1] Single organ vasculitis may affect vessels of any size and is by definition restricted to a single organ.[1] Classification can change in patients who demonstrate involvement of other organs during the course of their disease. The involved organ and vessel type are usually included in the name. A distinctive single organ vasculitis of the central nervous system (CNS) is primary CNS vasculitis, which is an idiopathic disorder restricted to the CNS.[65] CNS vasculitis may be secondary to systemic diseases or infections. A diagnosis of primary CNS vasculitis requires a determination that it is not a component of another disease.[1] Recommendations on such focused imaging are beyond the scope of this review.

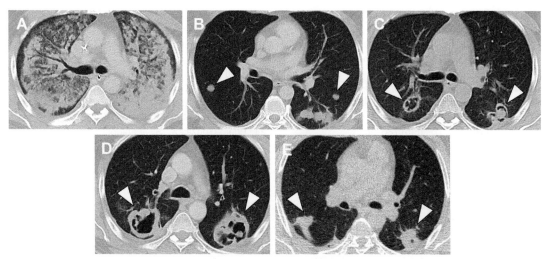

Fig. 12. A 50-year-old woman with granulomatosis with polyangiitis. (A–E). Serial axial CT scans showing serial fluctuations of granulomatosis with polyangiitis nodules. (A) Initial axial CT image shows diffuse bilateral ground-glass and consolidative opacities, compatible with diffuse alveolar hemorrhage. (B) Follow-up CT 3 months later shows formation of bilateral pulmonary nodules (arrowheads). (C, D) Further follow-up CT scans (9 and 12 months) show central cavities as well as an increase in size and wall thickness of the nodules (arrowheads). (E) Finally, size of the pulmonary nodules decreases leaving a scar after treatment (arrowheads).

SUMMARY

Owing to increasing availability and ongoing technological progress, radiologic imaging has gained great importance in the evaluation of vasculitis, particularly in patients with large vessel vasculitis.[4,6] However, establishing a final diagnosis in patients with vasculitis is challenging owing to the inherent complexity of different subtypes of the disease. Inflammation of the vessel wall is a common feature, but different types of vasculitis overlap with other types of vasculitis and other diseases.

Until now, the frequency and choice of imaging modalities for disease monitoring has remained an individual decision.[3] Recently published joint recommendations[3,17] seek to establish standards in imaging of large vessel vasculitis. However, the mentioned recommendations clearly state open issues for future research. In addition, the American College of Rheumatology is currently developing a new evidence-based clinical practice guideline for large and medium vessel vasculitis.[66] The American College of Rheumatology has already pointed out that only a few prospectively validated diagnostic criteria exist and classification criteria should be endorsed instead.[67] Radiologists interpreting imaging studies of patients with suspected vasculitis should be aware of the broad imaging spectrum of different vasculitides and the decrease of sensitivity after treatment initiation.

DISCLOSURE

The authors have nothing to disclose.

REFERENCES

1. Jennette JC, Falk RJ, Bacon PA, et al. 2012 revised international chapel hill consensus conference nomenclature of vasculitides. Arthritis Rheum 2012; 65(1):1–11.
2. Mahmoud S, Ghosh S, Farver C, et al. Pulmonary vasculitis: spectrum of imaging appearances. Radiol Clin North Am 2016;54(6):1097–118.
3. Dejaco C, Ramiro S, Duftner C, et al. EULAR recommendations for the use of imaging in large vessel vasculitis in clinical practice. Ann Rheum Dis 2018; 77(5):636–43.
4. Guggenberger K, Bley T. Imaging in large vessel vasculitides. Rofo 2019;191:1083–90.
5. Pipitone N, Versari A, Hunder GG, et al. Role of imaging in the diagnosis of large and medium-sized vessel vasculitis. Rheum Dis Clin North Am 2013; 39(3):593–608.
6. Muratore F, Pipitone N, Salvarani C, et al. Imaging of vasculitis: state of the art. Best Pract Res Clin Rheumatol 2016;30(4):688–706.
7. Karassa FB, Matsagas MI, Schmidt WA, et al. Meta-analysis: test performance of ultrasonography for giant-cell arteritis. Ann Intern Med 2005;142(5): 359–69.
8. Dietz SM, Tacke CE, Kuipers IM, et al. Cardiovascular imaging in children and adults following

Kawasaki disease. Insights Imaging 2015;6(6): 697–705.

9. Prieto-González S, Arguis P, Cid MC. Imaging in systemic vasculitis. Curr Opin Rheumatol 2015;27(1): 53–62.

10. Hur JH, Chun EJ, Kwag HJ, et al. CT features of vasculitides based on the 2012 International Chapel Hill consensus conference revised classification. Korean J Radiol 2017;18(5):786–98.

11. Versari A, Pipitone N, Casali M, et al. Use of imaging techniques in large vessel vasculitis and related conditions. Q J Nucl Med Mol Imaging 2018;62(1): 34–9.

12. Vlahos I, Chung R, Nair A, et al. Dual-energy CT: vascular applications. AJR Am J Roentgenol 2012; 199(5 Suppl):S87–97.

13. Abbara S, Blanke P, Maroules CD, et al. SCCT guidelines for the performance and acquisition of coronary computed tomographic angiography: a report of the society of Cardiovascular Computed Tomography Guidelines Committee: endorsed by the North American Society for Cardiovascular Imaging (NASCI). J Cardiovasc Comput Tomogr 2016;10(6):435–49.

14. Broncano J, Vargas D, Bhalla S, et al. CT and MR imaging of cardiothoracic vasculitis. Radiographics 2018;38(4):997–1021.

15. Puppo C, Massollo M, Paparo F, et al. Giant cell arteritis: a systematic review of the qualitative and semiquantitative methods to assess vasculitis with 18F-fluorodeoxyglucose positron emission tomography. Biomed Res Int 2014;2014(3):574248.

16. Pipitone NAM, Versari A. Salvarani C Usefulness of PET in recognizing and managing vasculitides. Curr Opin Rheumatol 2018;30(1):24–9.

17. Slart RHJA, Writing group, Reviewer group, et al. FDG-PET/CT(A) imaging in large vessel vasculitis and polymyalgia rheumatica: joint procedural recommendation of the EANM, SNMMI, and the PET Interest Group (PIG), and endorsed by the ASNC. Eur J Nucl Med Mol Imaging 2018;45(7): 1250–69.

18. Einspieler I, Thürmel K, Pyka T, et al. Imaging large vessel vasculitis with fully integrated PET/MRI: a pilot study. Eur J Nucl Med Mol Imaging 2015;42(7): 1012–24.

19. Hartung MP, Grist TM. François CJ Magnetic resonance angiography: current status and future directions. J Cardiovasc Magn Reson 2011;13(1):19.

20. Bannas P, François CJ, Reeder SB. Magnetic resonance angiography of the upper extremity. Magn Reson Imaging Clin N Am 2015;23(3):479–93.

21. Guggenberger KV, Bley TA. Magnetic resonance imaging and magnetic resonance angiography in large-vessel vasculitides. Clin Exp Rheumatol 2018;36:103–7. Suppl 114(5).

22. Bley TA, Wieben O, Uhl M, et al. High-resolution MRI in giant cell arteritis: imaging of the wall of the superficial temporal artery. AJR Am J Roentgenol 2005; 184(1):283–7.

23. Treitl KM, Maurus S, Sommer NN, et al. 3D-black-blood 3T-MRI for the diagnosis of thoracic large vessel vasculitis: a feasibility study. Eur Radiol 2016;27(5):2119–28.

24. Prieto-González S, Espígol-Frigolé G, García-Martínez A, et al. The expanding role of imaging in systemic vasculitis. Rheum Dis Clin North Am 2016;42(4):733–51.

25. Kermani TA, Crowson CS, Muratore F, et al. Extracranial giant cell arteritis and Takayasu arteritis: how similar are they? Semin Arthritis Rheum 2015; 44(6):724–8.

26. Grayson PC, Maksimowicz-McKinnon K, Clark TM, et al. Distribution of arterial lesions in Takayasu's arteritis and giant cell arteritis. Ann Rheum Dis 2012;71(8):1329–34.

27. Maksimowicz-McKinnon K, Clark TM, Hoffman GS. Takayasu arteritis and giant cell arteritis. Medicine 2009;88(4):221–6.

28. Yoshida M, Watanabe R, Ishii T, et al. Retrospective analysis of 95 patients with large vessel vasculitis: a single center experience. Int J Rheum Dis 2016; 19(1):87–94.

29. Furuta S, Cousins C, Chaudhry A, et al. Clinical features and radiological findings in large vessel vasculitis: are Takayasu arteritis and giant cell arteritis 2 different diseases or a single entity? J Rheumatol 2015;42(2):300–8.

30. Koster MJ, Warrington KJ. Classification of large vessel vasculitis: can we separate giant cell arteritis from Takayasu arteritis? Presse Med 2017;46(7–8 Pt 2):e205–13.

31. Kang E-J, Kim SM, Choe YH, et al. Takayasu arteritis: assessment of coronary arterial abnormalities with 128-section dual-source CT angiography of the coronary arteries and aorta. Radiology 2014; 270(1):74–81.

32. Smetana GW, Shmerling RH. Does this patient have temporal arteritis? JAMA 2002;287(1):92–101.

33. Watts RA, Robson J. Introduction, epidemiology and classification of vasculitis. Best Pract Res Clin Gastroenterol 2018;32(1):3–20.

34. Koster MJ, Warrington KJ, Kermani TA. Update on the epidemiology and treatment of giant cell arteritis. Curr Treatm Opt Rheumatol 2016;2(2):138–52.

35. Chandran AK, Udayakumar PD, Crowson CS, et al. The incidence of giant cell arteritis in Olmsted County, Minnesota, over a 60-year period 1950-2009. Scand J Rheumatol 2015;44(3):215–8.

36. Smith CA, Fidler WJ, Pinals RS. The epidemiology of giant cell arteritis. Report of a Ten-Year Study in Shelby County, Tennessee. Arthritis Rheum 1983; 26(10):1214–9.

37. Tracy A, Cardy CM, Carruthers D. Large vessel vasculitides. Medicine 2018;46(2):112–7.

38. Hoffman GS. Giant cell arteritis. Ann Intern Med 2016;165(9):ITC65–80.

39. Brack A, Taboada VM, Stanson A, et al. Disease pattern in cranial and large-vessel giant cell arteritis. Arthritis Rheum 1999;42(2):311–7.

40. Duftner C, Dejaco C, Sepriano A, et al. Imaging in diagnosis, outcome prediction and monitoring of large vessel vasculitis: a systematic literature review and meta-analysis informing the EULAR recommendations. RMD Open 2018;4(1):e000612.

41. Besson FL, Parienti J-J, Bienvenu B, et al. Diagnostic performance of ¹⁸F-fluorodeoxyglucose positron emission tomography in giant cell arteritis: a systematic review and meta-analysis. Eur J Nucl Med Mol Imaging 2011;38:1764–72.

42. Lee S-W, Kim S-J, Seo Y, et al. F-18 FDG PET for assessment of disease activity of large vessel vasculitis: a systematic review and meta-analysis. J Nucl Cardiol 2019;26(1):59–67.

43. de Souza AWS, de Carvalho JF. Diagnostic and classification criteria of Takayasu arteritis. J Autoimmun 2014;48-49:79–83.

44. Richards BL, March L, Gabriel SE. Epidemiology of large-vessel vasculidities. Best Pract Res Clin Rheumatol 2010;24(6):871–83.

45. Espinoza J, Ai S, Matsumura I. New insights on the pathogenesis of Takayasu arteritis: revisiting the microbial theory. Pathogens 2018;7(3) [pii:E73].

46. Park JH, Chung JW, Im JG, et al. Takayasu arteritis: evaluation of mural changes in the aorta and pulmonary artery with CT angiography. Radiology 1995;196(1):89–93.

47. Stanson AW, Friese JL, Johnson CM, et al. Polyarteritis nodosa: spectrum of angiographic findings. Radiographics 2001;21(1):151–9.

48. Guillevin L. Infections in vasculitis. Best Pract Res Clin Rheumatol 2013;27(1):19–31.

49. Forbess L, Bannykh S. Polyarteritis nodosa. Rheum Dis Clin North Am 2015;41(1):33–46, vii.

50. Hernández-Rodríguez J, Alba MA, Prieto-González S, et al. Diagnosis and classification of polyarteritis nodosa. J Autoimmune 2014;48-49:84–9.

51. Burns JC. The riddle of Kawasaki disease. N Engl J Med 2007;356(7):659–61.

52. Uehara R, Belay ED. Epidemiology of Kawasaki Disease in Asia, Europe, and the United States. J Epidemiol 2012;22(2):79–85.

53. Onouchi Y. Genetics of Kawasaki disease: what we know and don't know. Circ J 2012;76(7):1581–6.

54. McCrindle BW, Rowley AH, Newburger JW, et al. Diagnosis, treatment, and long-term management of Kawasaki disease: a scientific statement for health professionals from the American Heart Association. Circulation 2017;135(17):e927–99.

55. Duarte R, Cisneros S, Fernandez G, et al. Kawasaki disease: a review with emphasis on cardiovascular complications. Insights Imaging 2010;1(4):223–31.

56. Liu Y-C, Lin M-T, Wang J-K, et al. State-of-the-art acute phase management of Kawasaki disease after 2017 scientific statement from the American Heart Association. Pediatr Neonatol 2018;59(6):543–52.

57. Rowley AH, Shulman ST. Kawasaki syndrome. Clin Microbiol Rev 1998;11(3):405–14.

58. Kato H, Sugimura T, Akagi T, et al. Long-term consequences of Kawasaki disease. A 10- to 21-year follow-up study of 594 patients. Circulation 1996;94(6):1379–85.

59. Lin M-T, Sun L-C, Wu E-T, et al. Acute and late coronary outcomes in 1073 patients with Kawasaki disease with and without intravenous γ-immunoglobulin therapy. Arch Dis Child 2015;100(6):542–7.

60. Printz BF, Sleeper LA, Newburger JW, et al. Noncoronary cardiac abnormalities are associated with coronary artery dilation and with laboratory inflammatory markers in acute Kawasaki disease. J Am Coll Cardiol 2011;57(1):86–92.

61. Kato H, Inoue O, Akagi T. Kawasaki disease: cardiac problems and management. Pediatr Rev 1988;9(7):209–17.

62. Hoshino S, Tsuda E, Yamada O. Characteristics and fate of systemic artery aneurysm after Kawasaki disease. J Pediatr 2015;167(1):108–12.e1–2.

63. Tomasson G, Monach PA, Merkel PA. Thromboembolic disease in vasculitis. Curr Opin Rheumatol 2009;21(1):41–6.

64. Singhal M, Gupta P, Sharma A. Imaging in small and medium vessel vasculitis. Int J Rheum Dis 2019;22(1):78–85.

65. Abdel Razek AAK, Alvarez H, Bagg S, et al. Imaging spectrum of CNS vasculitis. Radiographics 2014;34(4):873–94.

66. Vasculitis-Guideline-Project-Plan-Large-Medium-Vessel 2018:1–29. Available at: https://www.rheumatology.org/Portals/0/Files/Vasculitis-Guideline-Project-Plan-Large-Medium-Vessel.pdf. Accessed March 18, 2020.

67. Aggarwal R, Ringold S, Khanna D, et al. Distinctions between diagnostic and classification criteria? Arthritis Care Res 2015;67(7):891–7.

Recent Innovations in Renal Vascular Imaging

Arash Bedayat, MD[a],*, Cameron Hassani, MD[a], Ashley E. Prosper, MD[a], Hamid Chalian, MD[b], Pegah Khoshpouri, MD[b], Stefan G. Ruehm, MD[a]

KEYWORDS

- Computed tomography (CT) • Magnetic resonance imaging (MR imaging) • Angiography
- Renal vascular imaging • Renal artery • Renal vein

KEY POINTS

- Computed tomographic angiography and magnetic resonance angiography are appropriate imaging modalities to investigate renal vascular pathologic conditions.
- Technical advances in computed tomography and magnetic resonance have led to improved image quality for evaluation of suspected renal vascular pathologic conditions.
- Knowledge of imaging appearances of different renal vascular pathologic conditions is critical for accurate diagnosis.

INTRODUCTION

Noninvasive imaging of the vascular renal system is a common request in diagnostic radiology. Typical indications include suspected renovascular hypertension, vasculitis, neoplasm, vascular malformation as well as structural diseases of the kidney. Profound knowledge of the renal anatomy, including vascular supply and variants, is mandatory for radiologists and allows for optimized protocolling and interpretation of imaging studies. Aside from renal ultrasound, computed tomography (CT) and magnetic resonance (MR) imaging are commonly requested cross-sectional studies for renal as well as renal vascular imaging. The aim of this article is to discuss basic renal vascular anatomy, common imaging findings as well as current and potential future imaging protocols for various renovascular pathologic conditions.

RENAL ARTERY ANATOMY AND VARIANTS

Right and left renal arteries typically originate from the aorta at the level of the second lumbar vertebral body (L2). The origin of the right renal artery is typically slightly higher than the origin of the left renal artery. The right renal artery is longer than the left renal artery and courses inferiorly posterior to the inferior vena cava (IVC) and the right renal vein before reaching the right renal hilum. The left renal artery is more horizontally oriented and courses posterior to the left renal vein[1,2] (Fig. 1A). The main renal arteries typically are divided into 5 segmental arteries: apical, superior, middle, inferior, and posterior segmental arteries.[1] The segmental arteries further divide into lobar branches.[3] The junction between the anterior two-thirds and posterior one-third of the kidney, known as the Brödel bloodless line of incision, is a relatively avascular plane separating the posterior arterial segment from the other arterial segments. Awareness of this plane can help avoid bleeding complications in percutaneous nephrostomy.[2,4] Before reaching the renal hilum, the renal arteries give rise to a few additional branches, such as the ureteric artery, the inferior adrenal artery, and the capsular artery. As part of

[a] Department of Radiological Sciences, Thoracic and Diagnostic Cardiovascular Imaging, David Geffen School Medicine, University of California Los Angeles (UCLA), 10945 Le Conte Avenue, Suite 3371, Los Angeles, CA 90095, USA; [b] Department of Radiology, Cardiothoracic Imaging, Duke University Medical Center, 2301 Erwin Road, Durham, NC 27710, USA

* Corresponding author.
E-mail address: abedayat@mednet.ucla.edu

Radiol Clin N Am 58 (2020) 781–796
https://doi.org/10.1016/j.rcl.2020.02.010
0033-8389/20/© 2020 Elsevier Inc. All rights reserved.

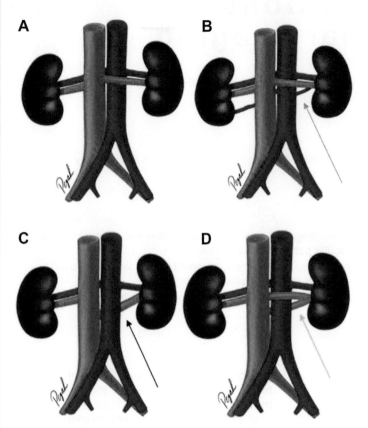

Fig. 1. Normal anatomy and variants of the renal arteries and veins. (*A*) Single bilateral arteries and veins. (*B*) Accessory renal arteries arising from the aorta (*green arrow*). (*C*) Retroaortic left renal vein (*black arrow*). (*D*) Circumaortic left renal vein (*purple arrow*).

the evaluation of pretransplant donor patients, it is important to describe the branching pattern of the first 2 cm of the renal arteries in order to prevent complications related to the vascular anastomosis of the transplant kidney.[2,3]

Accessory renal arteries (**Fig. 1**B) are present in 30% of the individuals and can be found bilaterally in about 10% of the individuals.[1] Accessory renal arteries are much more common in individuals with renal fusion or positional anomalies of the kidneys, including horseshoe kidney or crossed fused renal ectopia.[5,6] Accessory renal arteries usually arise more inferior to the main renal arteries. However, they can arise anywhere between T11 and L4 vertebral bodies. Accessory renal arteries cross anterior to the ureter and can cause obstruction of the ureter.[2]

Aberrant renal arteries (also known as polar renal arteries), in contrast to accessory renal arteries that enter the kidney through the renal hilum, enter the kidney through the renal capsule.[7] Assessment of the exact anatomy of the renal arteries is important before renal donation surgery. The presence of more than 4 renal arteries is considered a relative contraindication for living renal donor surgery.[8]

RENAL VEIN ANATOMY AND VARIATIONS

A single vein typically provides drainage of deoxygenated blood from the kidneys into the IVC bilaterally. However, right and left renal veins are not symmetric, and there are clinically significant variations of the renal vein anatomy.

The right renal vein is typically located anteriorly to the right renal artery at the hilum of the right kidney. It typically courses in an anterior-superior direction toward the lateral aspect of the IVC. Unlike the left renal vein, the right renal vein typically has less anatomic variations and is less likely to have venous tributaries along its course. About 30% of individuals demonstrate more than 1 branch of the right renal vein. In about 6% of individuals, the right adrenal gland vein drains into the right renal vein, which reflects the normal anatomy on the left side. Retroperitoneal veins, such as lumbar veins, drain into the right renal vein in about 3% of individuals.[9,10]

The left renal vein is longer (about 8.5 cm) than the right renal vein (about 2.5 cm) because it passes anterior to the aorta on its transverse course from the left renal hilum to the medial aspect of the IVC. The typical venous tributaries joining the left renal vein before its insertion into the IVC include (1) the left adrenal gland vein, (2) a branch of the inferior phrenic vein that drains into the superior aspect of the left renal vein, (3) the left gonadal vein that drains into the inferior aspect of the left renal vein, and (4) additional tributaries, in about 75% of individuals, to the posterior aspect of the left renal vein from lumbar and hemiazygos veins.[9] A circumaortic left renal vein (Fig. 1C) is the most common anatomic variant of the left renal vein. It is characterized by 2 veins arising from the main left renal vein trunk, with 1 renal vein coursing anterior to the aorta and the other renal vein coursing obliquely inferiorly between the aorta and vertebral bodies; eventually both veins drain into the medial aspect of the IVC. This anomaly can infrequently cause hematuria, proteinuria, or massive bleeding if inadvertently injured during surgery.[11] Another less common renal vein variant is the retroaortic left renal vein (about 3%) (Fig. 1D). Here, the left renal vein courses posterior to the aorta before it drains into the IVC, usually at a lower level than typical for a normal left renal vein insertion. Much less likely, the retroaortic left renal vein drains into the left common iliac vein. The presence of a retroaortic left renal vein has also been associated with proteinuria and hematuria.[12,13]

IMAGING PROTOCOLS
Computed Tomography Imaging

CT is a commonly used imaging modality for the noninvasive assessment of renal vascular anatomy and pathologic condition. The advantages of CT imaging include high-spatial resolution, fast image acquisition, and the availability of volumetric data sets for image processing, such as 3-dimensional maximum intensity projection (3D MIP) as well as multiplanar and curved planar reformations. MIP images are useful for the 3D depiction of small vascular pathologic conditions, such as aneurysms or pseudoaneurysms of the renal arteries and the analysis of the spatial relationship relative to adjacent renal vasculature branches. Curved planar reformations can be beneficial for the assessment of stenotic disease, for example, in tortuous renal arteries. Exposure to ionizing radiation may be a concern in younger patients, who may need to undergo repeated imaging studies. Contrast-associated acute kidney injury following the administration of iodinated contrast agent can occur as a complication particularly in patients with compromised renal function.[14]

A typical imaging protocol for renal vascular imaging using state-of-the-art equipment can be characterized by the following parameters: 120-kVp tube potential (variable depending on patient size with a spectrum ranging from 70 to 150 kV depending on scanner type based on Care kV with a reference setting of 120 kV), CareDose with reference mAs of 200, collimation of 192 × 0.625 mm, pitch of 0.6, and a rotation time of 0.5 second. Field-of-view in z-direction from 2 cm above the level of the kidneys to the level of the aortic bifurcation in the arterial phase and through the entire pelvis including bladder on the venous phase. Patients receive 100 to 150 mL of iodinated contrast material at 4 mL/s injection rate. For arterial phase imaging, bolus tracking with region of interest placed in the aorta approximately 2 cm above the renal arteries with a threshold of 150 HU. Venous phase acquisition with 80-second scanning delay after injection.

The emergence of dual-energy CT technology has provided many opportunities in improving identification and characterization of different pathologic conditions as well as the mitigation of traditional CT imaging artifacts, including beam hardening. Dual-energy technology can provide benefits for renovascular imaging. Using virtual monoenergetic images (at lower peak kilovolt) retrospectively reconstructed from dual-energy datasets, contrast enhancement of the abdominal vasculature can be improved compared with conventional polyenergetic images. Therefore, the use of dual-energy technology offers the potential of contrast dose reduction without compromising image quality, a feature particularly beneficial for patients with poor renal function.[15,16]

Renal Magnetic Resonance Angiography

MR angiography provides a powerful alternative to CT angiography in the evaluation of renal vasculature. Capable of achieving spatial resolution close to that acquired with CT, MR offers the additional benefit of imaging without the use of ionizing radiation.

Both 1.5-T and 3-T systems can be used to achieve high-resolution MR angiograms (MRA). In general, the voxel size should be kept to ≤1 mm³ to optimize spatial resolution.[17] Isotropic voxels are ideal because they enable multiplanar postprocessing and the generation of 3D volumetric renderings.

When adjusting MR acquisition parameters, it is important to be mindful of changes that affect the signal-to-noise ratio (SNR). The acquired voxel size is directly proportional to SNR. As a result, decreasing the voxel size, in isolation, without changing other parameters, will decrease the SNR. Time to acquisition and field strength similarly have proportional effects on the SNR. Because signal is proportional to the square of field strength, whereas noise increases linearly, 3-T MR systems have a theoretic improvement in SNR of up to 2-fold when compared with 1.5-T systems. This gain in SNR at 3-T MR can in turn be used to improve spatial resolution and/or data acquisition speed.[18] Therefore, MR angiography at 3 T is the preferred option for renal vascular imaging, as available.

In addition to the utilization of stronger field strengths, MRA can be improved with the utilization of parallel imaging. Parallel imaging relies on the inherent differences in signal detected by multiple coils, as a result of their position, to obtain spatial information about the object being imaged.[19] The use of spatial information from the coils decreases the number of phase-encoding steps needed, and in turn, decreases the time of image acquisition. Improving acquisition speed decreases the length of breath-holding required and minimizes motion artifact.

An additional consideration in contrast-enhanced renal MRA is the type of contrast used. A benefit in the selection of MR renal angiography as opposed to CT is the ability to avoid iodinated contrast. Many of the patients requiring renal angiography have impaired renal function. Described by the American College of Radiology as a "real, albeit rare, entity," contrast-induced nephropathy (CIN) is the sudden deterioration in renal function that is caused by the intravascular administration of iodinated contrast medium. CIN is a causative diagnosis and a subgroup of post-contrast acute kidney injury.[20] The preponderance of evidence in numerous studies has shown gadolinium contrast agents not to be a cause of CIN when administered at recommended standard doses.[21] Although the potential avoidance of CIN makes contrast-enhanced MR angiography with gadolinium-based contrast agents (GBCA) an attractive diagnostic option, caution must be used in patients with severe, end-stage disease (chronic kidney disease [CKD] 5, growth factor receptor [GFR] <15 mL/min/1.73 m^2) and severe CKD (CKD 4, GFR 15–29 mL/min/1.73 m^2) in whom there is a 1% to 7% risk of developing nephrogenic systemic fibrosis (NSF) after exposure to a class 1 GBCA.[22] If deemed necessary, use of gadolinium-based contrast in patients with impaired renal function should be isolated to group II agents for which the risk of NSF is low or nonexistent.[22]

After the recognition of the small, albeit real risk of NSF with use of GBCA in patients with advanced CKD, interest has developed in the utilization of noncontrast MR angiographic techniques, such as electrocardiogram-gated Fourier fast spin echo and balanced steady-state free precession imaging. Studies have shown that these noncontrast techniques can be a useful first step in evaluating the renal vasculature, serving as a means of triaging patients to a contrast-enhanced examination, as needed.[23,24]

Similar to contrast-enhanced computed tomography angiograms (CTA), when using GBCA contrast-enhanced MRA, the contrast injection should be optimized for the renal arteries. One method of ensuring proper timing is to use a small volume of contrast, for example, 1 mL, as a test bolus, to time the arrival of contrast at the level of the renal arteries. The calculation of time to arrival and execution of optimal imaging timing on a subsequent full-dose contrast administration can be complicated by variations in breath-holding and is prone to human error. For these reasons, the use of time-resolved imaging is commonly used as an alternative with imaging initiated at the same time as the contrast administration. In addition to ensuring optimal bolus timing, time-resolved imaging can be performed, which provides the added benefit of real-time visualization of blood flow, and can prove useful in the detection of arterial stenoses, arteriovenous fistulas, or malformations. The use of a non-CBCA, such as ferumoxytol, may serve as an attractive alternative in patients with severe and end-stage renal disease. Ferumoxytol is based on ultrasmall paramagnetic iron oxide particles. The compound was initially investigated as an MR contrast agent, but ultimately was approved by the Food and Drug Administration (FDA) for the intravenous treatment of anemia in patients with end-stage renal disease.[25,26] Ferumoxytol benefits from both excellent T1-shortening properties and a long intravascular half-life of 14 to 21 hours, allowing for high-resolution steady-state angiography at doses as low as 1 mg/kg up to a total of 510 mg.[27]

Although time-resolved imaging with ferumoxytol is technically feasible, a rapid bolus injection is not advised per FDA recommendations as outlined in the package insert of the compound. The long half-life and resultant steady-state contrast in the blood pool obviates bolus timing in most cases. As with CT angiography, analysis of MR angiographic images is best performed using a 3D postprocessing suite with multiplanar and curved planar reformatting capabilities. 3D volumetric renderings are a powerful visual tool for demonstrating vascular pathologic condition, particularly for the nonradiologist. When high-resolution, isotropic images are acquired, renal MRA can also be 3D printed for surgical planning.

RENAL VASCULAR PATHOLOGIC CONDITION
Renal Artery Stenosis

Renal artery stenosis is the leading cause of secondary hypertension. It is found in 1% to 5% of all patients who suffer from hypertension.[28] The most common cause of renal artery stenosis is atherosclerosis, with the highest prevalence in older male patients.[29] Typically, the proximal 2 cm of the renal artery are affected. This results in a decrease in renal perfusion and consequently an increase in systemic blood pressure owing to activation of renin-angiotensin cascade.[2] Bilateral renal artery stenosis is seen in 30% of affected patients. Other less likely causes of renal artery stenosis include fibromuscular dysplasia (FMD), dissection, embolic disease, vasculitis, or external compression, which are discussed separately.[30,31]

Defining a clinically relevant cutoff for the degree of luminal narrowing is controversial. However, a stenosis exceeding 50% of diameter reduction is typically considered significant, although symptoms may not occur until the stenosis exceeds 70%. It is noteworthy that in a metaanalysis of 947 patients from 113 centers with renal artery stenosis owing to atherosclerosis, there was no difference between medical therapy and renal stenting.[31] Therefore, investigating the presence, cause, and degree of stenosis appears particularly relevant in patients with failure of medical management of hypertension, new-onset hypertension, in young patients and patients with progressive renal insufficiency.[2,30,31]

Renal Doppler ultrasound is frequently used as a first-line imaging modality for the evaluation of renal artery stenosis. However, the diagnostic accuracy of renal Doppler ultrasound is limited for several reasons, including the experience of the technologist or radiologist performing the study, patient's body habitus, or presence of overlying bowel gas. Typically, a stenosis is considered significant if the peak systolic velocity (PSV) exceeds 200 cm/s or if the renal artery PSV/aorta PSV ratio exceeds 3.5:1.[28]

CTA is an excellent choice for the evaluation of the anatomy of the renal arteries with the possibility of providing multiplanar reconstructions (Fig. 2). CTA is a rapid noninvasive technique with higher resolution compared with MRA.[32] The sensitivity and specificity of CTA for the diagnosis of renal artery stenosis exceeding 50% have been reported to be in the range of 88% and 96% and 77% and 98%, respectively.[33,34] Because of its high negative predictive value, a CTA interpreted as normal essentially excludes significant stenotic disease of the renal arteries. A decrease in cortical enhancement, poststenotic dilation, and kidney atrophy are considered secondary findings indicative of significant renal artery stenosis.[35]

Gadolinium-enhanced 3D MRA of the renal arteries or steady-state free precession and arterial spin labeling methods are MR imaging techniques available for the evaluation of renal artery stenosis. Sensitivities and specificities for the diagnosis of renal artery stenosis for MRA have been reported to range between 88% and 100% and 71% and 100%, respectively.[36–38] Other methods currently under investigation are blood-oxygen level–dependent MR imaging to study kidney oxygenation.[39] Advanced MRA techniques have been proposed for artifact-free in-stent lumen visualization.[40] Generally, in patients with an endothelial growth factor receptor less than 30, gadolinium should not be administered because of the risk of NSF.[41]

Renal Artery Entrapment

In young patients with hypertension, a potential underlying cause may be the compression of the proximal portion of any of a renal artery by the psoas musculature or a crus of the diaphragm resulting in a narrowing of the affected renal artery.[42] This entity is typically seen in less than 5% of patients with hypertension.[43] This finding is more likely to involve the left renal artery. The modality of choice to evaluate the relevant anatomy, including course, degree, and length of renal artery compression, is CT angiography.[42] The initial treatment of choice is stenting of the affected artery. However, the success of the procedure may be challenged because of stent failure as a consequence of mechanical forces generated by repetitive muscle contractions, and surgical repair may need to be considered.[44,45]

Renal Artery Dissection

Renal artery dissections can occur as isolated or as part of aortic dissections extending into the renal arteries. Associated clinical symptoms may occur in the form of deteriorated renal function and increase in blood pressure or acute onset of flank pain. Isolated cases are mainly complications of endovascular interventions or sequela of blunt abdominal traumas. Rarely, spontaneous dissections that mainly involve the distal portions of the main renal arteries can occur in patients with FMD, history of cocaine abuse, collagen vascular syndromes such as Ehlers-Danlos or Marfan syndrome, or in the context of cystic medial necrosis.[46,47]

Contrast-enhanced CTA is the modality of choice in the evaluation of a suspected dissection (Fig. 3) to demonstrate the presence and

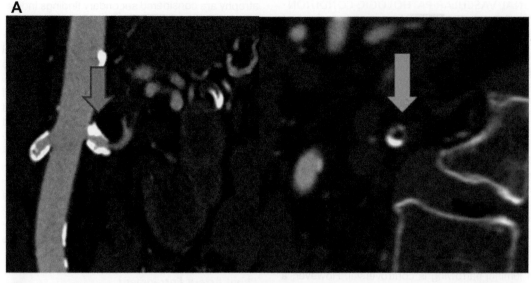

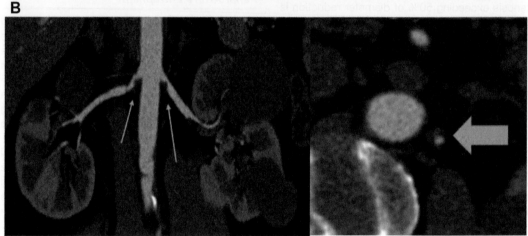

Fig. 2. Renal artery stenosis. (*A*) Coronal reformat demonstrating calcified plaques at the origins of both right and left renal arteries. Reformatted magnified sagittal oblique view demonstrates severe narrowing, which can be exaggerated on CT with blooming artifact. (*B*) Noncalcified plaques at the origins of the renal arteries (*thin arrows*). Circumferential thickening and narrowing of the proximal left renal artery (*thick arrow*).

extension of an intimal flap; however, despite the superior spatial resolution of CTA, small flaps and thrombotic changes of small-caliber vessels may be difficult to visualize.[8] Secondary signs of renal artery dissections include luminal narrowing, abrupt terminating of the vessel, also referred to as vessel cutoff sign, or renal ischemia.[47,48] If the patient is clinically stable, observation and anticoagulation are recommended treatment options. In unstable patients, the treatment of choice is endovascular stent repair.[46,49]

Renal Artery Aneurysm and Pseudoaneurysm

Renal artery aneurysms (RAA) (**Fig. 4**) develop following a weakening of the renal arterial wall

with consequent expansion of the arterial lumen owing to increased intraluminal pressure. RAAs are rare, with an estimated prevalence of 0.1%. They are found mostly in patients with systemic arterial hypertension.[50,51] RAAs tend to be asymptomatic and therefore typically diagnosed incidentally on cross-sectional imaging of the abdomen.[52] When symptomatic, they can be associated with pain, hematuria, and renal infarction. Complications include rupture, thrombosis, and embolism.[53,54] RAAs mostly occur in the main right or left renal artery, most commonly at the site of the renal artery bifurcation.[54] Additional aneurysms originating from visceral arteries can be seen in up to 6.5% of patients with RAAs.[55] On grayscale ultrasound imaging, noncalcified RAAs

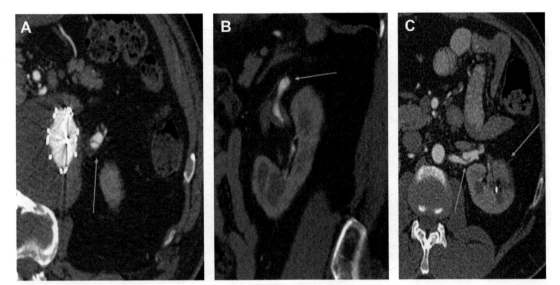

Fig. 3. Axial view of dissected left renal artery in a patient with endovascular repair of abdominal aorta. (*A*) Flap within the left renal artery (*blue arrow*) indicates dissection. (*B*) Sagittal reformat demonstrating same patient. (*C*) Dissection of the left renal artery (*blue arrow*) with hypoenhancement of the upper pole of the left kidney (*green arrow*) indicates ischemia.

appear anechoic, whereas calcified aneurysms may demonstrate increased echogenicity. Doppler sonography can be used to assess the perfusion pattern of RAAs.[48] CT angiography is considered the modality of choice because it allows for the comprehensive assessment of aneurysms in abdomen and pelvis.

Not all patients with RAAs require treatment. The treatment of aneurysms becomes mandatory if there is an increased risk of aneurysmal rupture, often influenced by medical conditions, such as pregnancy, uncontrolled systemic hypertension, or inflammatory diseases like polyarteritis nodosa.[56,57] In otherwise healthy patients, aneurysms larger than 1.5 cm should be treated because the mortality from rupture can amount to 10%. Image-guided endovascular interventions have largely replaced the need for open surgery because they offer lesser invasive treatment with a lower risk of complications.[58] RAAs smaller than 1.5 cm in patients with no risk factors can be monitored by MR angiography or CT angiography in 1 to 2 years with MRA being the more desirable modality because of the lack of ionizing radiation.[57]

Renal artery pseudoaneurysms (**Fig. 5**) typically present as saccular lesions, often arising as a consequence of direct penetrating trauma to the arterial wall and causing contained disruption and extravasation of blood in the adventitia or neighboring tissue.[52,59] On spectral Doppler ultrasound, the characteristic finding is the so-called yin-yang sign, reflecting turbulent flow within the aneurysmal sac as a result of a pressure gradient between artery and pseudoaneurysm. CT angiography is the modality of choice; in patients with impaired renal function, MR angiography without contrast or with a non–gadolinium contrast compound, such as ferumoxytol, may be considered. Pseudoaneurysms larger than 2 cm are considered high risk for rupture and can be treated with transcatheter embolization. Smaller pseudoaneurysms may resolve spontaneously over time.[60] In cases of infectious arteritis, for example, in patients suffering from a renal abscess, pyelonephritis, or septic emboli from a remote infectious site in the body, a subtype of pseudoaneurysm called mycotic aneurysm can develop. This type of pseudoaneurysm is associated with vessel wall thickening and enhancement, often associated with perivascular fluid or fat stranding. Initial treatment strategies typically include intravenous antibiotics; large mycotic aneurysms (>2 cm) or symptomatic cases typically undergo urgent surgical or endovascular repair.[61,62]

Renal Artery Vasculitis

The spectrum of renal artery vasculitis (**Fig. 6**) may range from mild to life-threatening. Vasculitis manifests as an inflammation that typically causes thickening and stenosis of the vessel wall. Renal artery vasculitis is a rare disease that can result in reduced blood flow and ultimately arterial

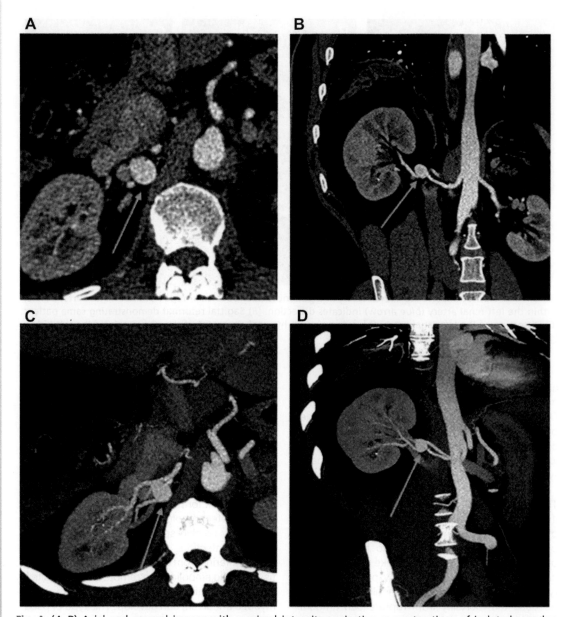

Fig. 4. (*A–D*) Axial and coronal images with maximal intensity projection reconstructions of isolated saccular aneurysm in the midright renal artery from a branching point incidentally noted in a patient.

occlusion and ischemia of the kidney.[63,64] In general, any vessel size or vascular territory in any organ system can be affected. Symptoms may vary depending on the histologic type of inflammation, the organ suffering reduced blood flow, and the extent of involvement.[65]

The originally proposed Chapel Hill classification categorizes the type of vasculitis based on the affected vessel size (small, medium, or large). However, because of substantial overlap and different clinical presentations, more recent classifications focus on both size and disease manifestation.[63,66]

Some forms of vasculitis, such as Kawasaki disease and Henoch-Schonlein purpura (HSP), predominantly occur in children, whereas other forms, such as Takayasu arteritis, a form of large vessel vasculitis, mostly affect adults.[63] Aside from primary forms of vasculitis, there are secondary forms with similar effects on blood vessels and clinical presentation. They can occur as a result of collagen vascular diseases or reflect paraneoplastic complications.[48,67] Renal artery vasculitis may affect the kidney in many ways because of the numerous vessels inside the kidneys as well as the large renal arteries supplying

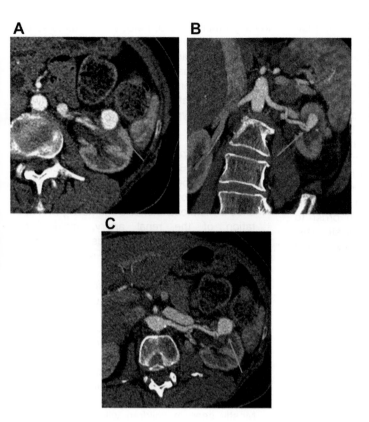

Fig. 5. Pseudoaneurysm following renal biopsy. (*A, C*) Axial CT demonstrates a collection of contrast (*arrow*) in both arterial (*A*) and venous (*C*) phases in the upper pole of the left kidney. (*B*) Coronal CT in same patient demonstrating pseudoaneurysm in the upper pole.

them.[64] The most common types of small vessel vasculitis include microscopic polyarteritis, granulomatosis with polyangiitis, HSP, and cryoglobulinemic vasculitis (associated with hepatitis C).[66] Forms of medium- and large-vessel vasculitis may affect the main renal artery and therefore decrease blood flow to the kidneys.[68] As an example, polyarteritis nodosa, recognized by necrotizing inflammatory lesions and its affinity to involve aorta and its large branches, demonstrates renal artery invasion along with systemic hypertension in 90% of affected patients.[65,69] Other forms of medium- or large-vessel vasculitis involve the renal arteries less frequently, for example, Takayasu arteritis in young adults, giant cell or temporal arteritis in the elderly, and Kawasaki disease in children.[70,71]

Common causes of secondary vasculitis include autoimmune diseases, such as systemic lupus erythematosus (SLE), neurofibromatosis, or amphetamines or cocaine abuse.[67] Renal artery vasculitis may occur in malignancies either as a

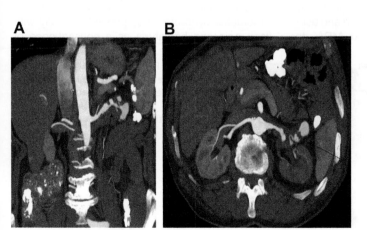

Fig. 6. Renal artery vasculitis. Coronal (*A*) and axial (*B*) images of the left renal artery demonstrates a multilobulated and markedly thick-walled aneurysm with suggestion of flow restriction evidenced by decreased perfusion of the entire left kidney.

paraneoplastic reaction or as a side effect of radiation or chemotherapy.[48]

Whereas Doppler ultrasound can demonstrate decreased flow in renal arteries, PET is capable of directly visualizing inflammatory changes of the vessel wall as a consequence of vasculitis.[67] MR and CT are capable of both directly demonstrating changes of the vessel wall, including increased contrast uptake. MR with the ability of phase contrast angiographic imaging can, in addition, demonstrate altered blood flow in the renal arteries.[72] Infracted renal parenchyma should raise the suspicion of vasculitis, and CT or MR angiography should be considered in order to evaluate vessel wall thickness, edema, stenosis, and renal parenchymal changes. Microaneurysms as a complication of vasculitis may rupture and can form a perinephric hematoma.[73] Both CT and MR angiography can be used to comprehensively evaluate the different aspects of vasculitis, whereas conventional catheter angiography is limited to the display of luminal abnormalities and clot formation in the vessels.[48] Vasculitis is typically treated medically; occasionally, invasive or minimally invasive procedures are necessary to treat complications of vasculitis, such as aneurysms of arterial stenosis, in order to improve end organ function.[74]

Fibromuscular Dysplasia

FMD is an idiopathic, nonatherosclerotic, and noninflammatory disease of the muscular layer of arterial walls, leading to segmental stenosis of small- and medium-sized arteries.[75] FMD (**Fig. 7**) is more common in young women with hypertension, by far, the most frequent presenting symptom. In the ARCADIA (Assessment of Renal and Cervical Artery Dysplasia) study, 77.4% of 469 patients with FMD were hypertensive.[76] The 2014 European FMD Consensus recommended that "patients with FMD should undergo imaging of all vessels from brain to pelvis, at least once and usually with CTA or contrast-enhanced MRA, to identify other areas of FMD, as well as to screen for occult aneurysms and dissections."[77]

The revised classification of FMD based on renal artery lesions was described by Stanley[78] in 1996. This classification is based on the most affected layer of the renal arteries. It is worth mentioning that different types can coexist in the same patient.[79]

1. *The medial type:* This is the most common type and includes 60% to 70% of the FMD cases. In the medial type, the smooth media muscle cells are replaced by fibrous tissue. Imaging appearance is multifocal stenosis alternating with dilatation of the renal artery, making the characteristic string-of-beads appearance. This type is most commonly seen in women aged 30 to 50 years.
2. *The perimedial or subadventitial type*: In this second most common type (10%–20%), the external layer of the media is involved. In this type, the stenoses are more tubular, and interval segments are not exceeding the diameter of the normal renal artery.
3. *The intimal type*: Intimal fibrosis and subendothelial connective tissue proliferation are the underlying pathophysiology in the intimal type. Mostly seen in children with male predominance, the radiologic manifestation of this type of FMD is focal stenosis.[79,80]

Nutcracker Syndrome

The nutcracker syndrome (**Fig. 8**) occurs when there is a compression of the left renal vein between the aorta and superior mesenteric artery, mostly seen in thin and young female patients in their third or fourth decade of life with a history of weight loss. Nutcracker syndrome results in left renal vein hypertension.[81] Nutcracker syndrome can also be associated with a retroaortic left renal vein, causing compression of this vein between the aorta and the adjacent vertebral body.[82,83] Nutcracker syndrome may present clinically with flank pain and hematuria as a consequence of

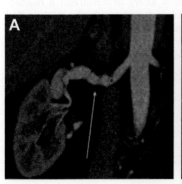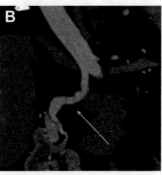

Fig. 7. FMD. Coronal (*A*) and sagittal oblique (*B*) views of the right renal artery demonstrated beaded appearance of the middle portion compatible with FMD (*arrows*).

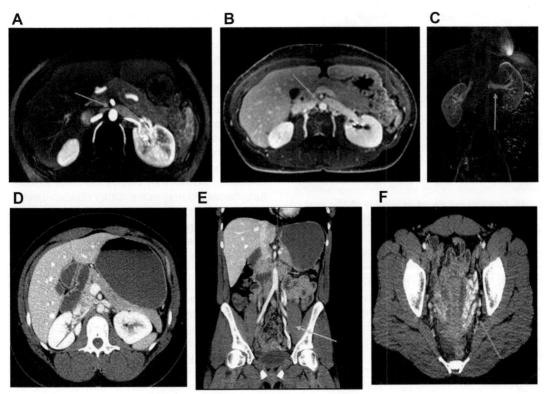

Fig. 8. Nutcracker syndrome. (*A–C*) Axial volumetric interpolated brain examination (VIBE) in arterial (*A*) and venous (*B*) phases and time-resolved MRA (*C*) demonstrate compression of the left renal vein between the aorta and superior mesenteric artery. (*D–F*) Axial (*D*) image of the contrast-enhanced CT of abdomen and pelvis demonstrates compression of the left renal artery between the aorta and superior mesenteric artery. Coronal view (*E*) of the same patient demonstrates a very prominent left gonadal vein. Axial view at the level of pelvis (*F*) demonstrates very prominent pelvic veins in same patient with nutcracker syndrome.

the rupture of thin-walled veins into the collecting system.[84] In addition, pelvic congestion syndrome in women, and varicoceles and variceal veins in the lower extremities have been associated with nutcracker syndrome.[82] Nutcracker syndrome

has also been reported to be associated with superior mesenteric artery syndrome (SMA syndrome). The reduced angle of 35° or less in nutcracker syndrome between the superior mesenteric artery and aorta (normal angle

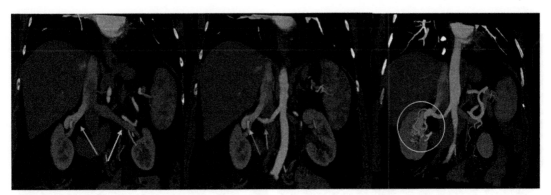

Fig. 9. AVM. Three coronal images demonstrating early filling of the right renal vein on arterial phase (*blue arrow*), nonopacification of the left renal vein on arterial phase (*purple arrow*), similar enhancement of the right renal artery (*red arrow*) and AVM/connection (*orange arrow*), and network of abnormal arteriovenous connections (*white circle*).

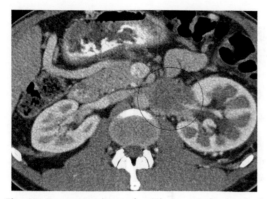

Fig. 10. Contrast-enhanced axial view at the level of kidneys demonstrates occlusion of the left renal vein by a pancreatic mass.

is >45°), which results in a compression of the left renal vein, has been described as the beak sign on CT or MR.[82,85] Aside from the acute angle of less than 35° between the SMA and aorta, often an abrupt narrowing of the left renal vein with proximal dilation is visualized (sensitivity of 91.7% and specificity of 88.9%).[84] As a result of the renal vein narrowing, draining collateral veins may be present mainly in the form of distended paralumbar, gonadal, and hemiazygos veins, which may indicate impaired venous drainage. A ratio of aortomesenteric to hilar diameter of left renal vein of 4.9 or more has been reported to have a sensitivity of 66.7% and specificity of 100% for nutcracker syndrome, respectively. On conventional angiography, a pressure gradient greater than 3 mm Hg between IVC and renal vein has been described in nutcracker syndrome.[83]

The treatment of choice in symptomatic patients is surgical or less-invasive endovascular repair.[82] The spectrum of open surgical interventions consists of renal vein transposition, superior mesenteric artery transposition, renal autotransplantation,

and gonadocaval bypass. Endovascular stent deployment in the renal vein has been proposed; however, complications, such as stent migration, stent occlusion, or fracture, have been reported.[86]

Renal Vascular Malformations

Arteriovenous malformations (AVMs) are abnormal connections between vein and artery that can manifest as fistula (single artery to a dilated vein) or a complex nidus with tortuous channels between single or several arteries and veins called cirsoid.[87,88] When they involve the renal vasculature, hematuria may occur. Other clinical manifestations include high blood pressure, high-output heart failure, and flank pain. Of cases, 75% are acquired mostly as a consequence of renal biopsies, as a consequence of trauma, or as a result of neoplasms. AVMs are more commonly seen in women than in men (3:1), with the right kidney more commonly affected.

CT angiography (**Fig. 9**) is a great tool to identify the feeding artery, nidus, and draining vein, as well as for the detection of complications, including perinephric and subcapsular hematomas. MR angiography can demonstrate the pathologic condition as a flow-void on T2-weighted sequence. Noncontrast MRA can be used in patients with renal failure. The treatment of choice is percutaneous embolization. In complex cases, partial or total nephrectomy can be considered.[89,90]

Renal Vein Thrombosis

Thrombosis of the renal vein (**Figs. 10–12**) is a result of bland versus tumor thrombus. Renal vein thrombosis may manifest as luminal narrowing or total occlusion. Renal vein thrombosis is more common on the left side because of its longer course and drainage of the gonadal vein

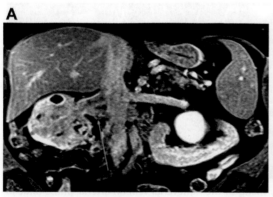
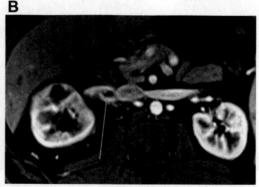

Fig. 11. Coronal T1 3D VIBE postcontrast (*A*) and T1 VIBE axial arterial phase (*B*) views of the right renal vein demonstrating low intensity within the right renal vein compatible with tumor thrombus in a patient with known renal cell carcinoma.

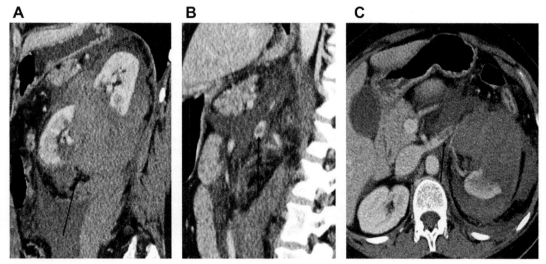

Fig. 12. Renal transection (*A*) in a patient after a motor vehicle accident with renal artery avulsion (*B*) and renal vein thrombus (*C*).

into the left renal vein. Clinical symptoms include gross hematuria, flank pain, and renal failure. Risk factors of bland renal vein thrombosis include glomerulonephritis, collagen vascular disease (SLE), amyloidosis, diabetes, thrombophlebitis, and trauma. Associated complications include renal atrophy, pulmonary embolism, and renal papillary necrosis.

On CT or MR venography, acute renal vein thrombosis presents as a filling defect within a distended renal vein.[2] Other imaging findings include delayed renal cortical enhancement with lack of parenchymal enhancement, enlarged ipsilateral kidney, edema in the renal sinus and perinephric space, and development of collateral veins. The sensitivity and specificity of contrast-enhanced MR venography for the diagnosis of renal vein thrombosis have been shown to be similar to those of CT.[91] Trauma-induced renal vein thrombosis almost invariably manifests with additional renal artery or parenchymal injury.[92,93]

The treatment of choice depends on the underlying cause. In cases of bland thrombus, anticoagulation is the treatment of choice. In cases of glomerulonephritis, nephrotic syndrome, or collagen vascular diseases, steroid and immunosuppression therapy are primary considerations. IVC filter placement may be necessary in cases of advanced tumor thrombus.[94,95]

SUMMARY

Because of dramatic technical improvements in hardware, software, and image analysis algorithms, CT and MR imaging have evolved as the primary imaging modalities for the evaluation of renal artery disease. State-of-the-art MR scanner hardware allows for the acquisition of 3D contrast-enhanced data sets with submillimeter isotropic resolution within a single breath-hold. Short acquisition times enable multisequence imaging protocols for combined morphologic and functional renal imaging, for example, phase-contrast MRA for the determination of abnormal blood flow in renal arteries or veins, time-resolved MR angiographic imaging for the visualization of complex vascular abnormalities, or dynamic renal parenchymal imaging for the detection and characterization of renal mass lesions/abnormalities. Advantages of CT imaging with multidetector technology include the imaging of an extended volume of human anatomy with isotropic spatial resolution of approximately 0.5 mm within only a few seconds. Therefore, CT imaging plays a crucial role in the emergency evaluation of patients with suspected renal vascular injury and allows for comprehensive imaging of additional vascular territories, such as the thoracoabdominal aorta or pulmonary vasculature.

Radiologists play an essential role in guiding physicians to accurately diagnose and treat various clinical entities affecting both kidneys and renal vasculature. A basic understanding of renal vascular anatomy, pathologic condition, and treatment options is important and helps in choosing both adequate imaging modality and protocols for effective diagnostic and therapeutic patient management.

DISCLOSURE

The authors have nothing to disclose.

REFERENCES

1. Standring S, Gray H. Gray's anatomy: the anatomical basis of clinical practice. 40th edition. Edinburgh (Scotland): Churchill Livingstone; 2008.

2. Al-Katib S, Shetty M, Jafri SMA, et al. Radiologic assessment of native renal vasculature: a multimodality review. Radiographics 2017;37(1):136–56.

3. Leslie S, Sajjad H. Anatomy, abdomen and pelvis, renal artery. 2019. Available at: https://www.ncbi.nlm.nih.gov/books/NBK459158/. Accessed March 22, 2020.

4. Dyer RB, Regan JD, Kavanagh PV, et al. Percutaneous nephrostomy with extensions of the technique: step by step. Radiographics 2002;22(3):503–25.

5. Natsis K, Piagkou M, Skotsimara A, et al. Horseshoe kidney: a review of anatomy and pathology. Surg Radiol Anat 2014;36(6):517–26.

6. Glodny B, Petersen J, Hofmann KJ, et al. Kidney fusion anomalies revisited: clinical and radiological analysis of 209 cases of crossed fused ectopia and horseshoe kidney. BJU Int 2009;103(2):224–35.

7. Flors L, Leiva-Salinas C, Ahmad EA, et al. MD CT angiography and MR angiography of nonatherosclerotic renal artery disease. Cardiovasc Intervent Radiol 2011;34(6):1151–64.

8. Falesch LA, Foley WD. Computed tomograpy angiography of the renal circulation. Radiol Clin North Am 2016;54(1):71–86.

9. Bowdino CS, Shaw PM. Anatomy, abdomen and pelvis, renal veins [Internet]. StatPearls. 2019. Available at: http://www.ncbi.nlm.nih.gov/pubmed/30855882. Accessed March 22, 2020.

10. Pozniak MA, Balison DJ, Lee FT, et al. CT angiography of potential renal transplant donors. Radiographics 1998;18(3):565–87.

11. Matsunaga M, Ushijima T, Fukahori M, et al. A circumaortic left renal vein. BMJ Case Rep 2015; 2015:1–2.

12. Karaman B, Koplay M, Öÿzturk E, et al. Retroaortic left renal vein: multidetector computed tomography angiography findings and its clinical importance. Acta Radiol 2007;48(3):355–60.

13. Chuang VP, Mena CE, Hoskins PA. Congenital anomalies of the inferior vena cava. Review of embryogenesis and presentation of a simplified classification. Br J Radiol 1974;47(556):206–13.

14. Davenport MS, Perazella MA, Yee J, et al. Use of intravenous iodinated contrast media in patients with kidney disease: consensus statements from the American College of Radiology and the National Kidney Foundation. Radiology 2020;294(3):660–8.

15. Chalian H, Kalisz K, Rassouli N, et al. Utility of virtual monoenergetic images derived from a dual-layer detector-based spectral CT in the assessment of aortic anatomy and pathology: a retrospective case control study. Clin Imaging 2018;52:292–301.

16. Rassouli N, Chalian H, Rajiah P, et al. Assessment of 70-keV virtual monoenergetic spectral images in abdominal CT imaging: a comparison study to conventional polychromatic 120-kVp images. Abdom Radiol (N Y) 2017;42(10):2579–86.

17. Attenberger UI, Morelli JN, Schoenberg SO, et al. Assessment of the kidneys: magnetic resonance angiography, perfusion and diffusion. J Cardiovasc Magn Reson 2011;13(1):70.

18. Soher BJ, Dale BM, Merkle EM. A review of MR physics: 3T versus 1.5T. Magn Reson Imaging Clin N Am 2007;15(3):277–90.

19. Glockner JF, Hu HH, Stanley DW, et al. Parallel MR imaging: a user's guide. Radiographics 2005;25(5):1279–97.

20. ACR manual on contrast media. Available at: https://www.acr.org/-/media/ACR/Files/Clinical-Resources/Contrast_Media.pdf. Accessed March 22, 2020.

21. Ledneva E, Karie S, Launay-Vacher V, et al. Renal safety of gadolinium-based contrast media in patients with chronic renal insufficiency. Radiology 2009;250(3):618–28.

22. Contrast manual|American College of Radiology. Available at: https://www.acr.org/Clinical-Resources/Contrast-Manual. Accessed March 22, 2020.

23. Braidy C, Daou I, Diop AD, et al. Unenhanced MR angiography of renal arteries: 51 patients. Am J Roentgenol 2012;199(5):W629–37.

24. Yamuna J, Chandrasekharan A, Rangasami R, et al. Unenhanced renal magnetic resonance angiography in patients with chronic kidney disease & suspected renovascular hypertension: can it affect patient management? Indian J Med Res 2017; 146(November):22–9.

25. Spinowitz BS, Kausz AT, Baptista J, et al. Ferumoxytol for treating iron deficiency anemia in CKD. J Am Soc Nephrol 2008;19(8):1599–605.

26. Lu M, Cohen MH, Rieves D, et al. FDA report: ferumoxytol for intravenous iron therapy in adult patients with chronic kidney disease. Am J Hematol 2010; 85(5):315–9.

27. Toth GB, Varallyay CG, Horvath A, et al. Current and potential imaging applications of ferumoxytol for magnetic resonance imaging. Kidney Int 2017; 92(1):47–66.

28. Granata A, Fiorini F, Andrulli S, et al. Doppler ultrasound and renal artery stenosis: an overview. J Ultrasound 2009;12(4):133–43.

29. Creager M, Loscalzo J, Dzau V. Vascular medicine: a companion to Braunwald's heart disease. Philadelphia: Elsevier Saunders; 2006.

30. Textor SC, Lerman L. Renovascular hypertension and ischemic nephropathy. Am J Hypertens 2010; 23(11):1159–69.

31. Cooper CJ, Murphy TP, Cutlip DE, et al. Stenting and medical therapy for atherosclerotic renal-artery stenosis. N Engl J Med 2014;370(1):13–22.

32. Willmann JK, Wildermuth S, Pfammatter T, et al. Aortoiliac and renal arteries: prospective intraindividual comparison of contrast-enhanced three-dimensional MR angiography and multi-detector row CT angiography. Radiology 2003;226(3):798–811.

33. Beregi JP, Elkohen M, Deklunder G, et al. Helical CT angiography compared with arteriography in the detection of renal artery stenosis. Am J Roentgenol 1996;167(2):495–501.

34. Farrés MT, Lammer J, Schima W, et al. Spiral computed tomographic angiography of the renal arteries: a prospective comparison with intravenous and intraarterial digital subtraction angiography. Cardiovasc Intervent Radiol 1996;19(2):101–6.

35. Mounier-Vehier C, Lions C, Devos P, et al. Cortical thickness: an early morphological marker of atherosclerotic renal disease. Kidney Int 2002;61(2):591–8.

36. Kramer U, Wiskirchen J, Fenchel MC, et al. Isotropic high-spatial-resolution contrast-enhanced 3.0-T MR angiography in patients suspected of having renal artery stenosis. Radiology 2008;247(1):228–40.

37. McGregor R, Vymazal J, Martinez-Lopez M, et al. A multi-center, comparative, phase 3 study to determine the efficacy of gadofosveset-enhanced magnetic resonance angiography for evaluation of renal artery disease. Eur J Radiol 2008;65(2):316–25.

38. Soulez G, Pasowicz M, Benea G, et al. Renal artery stenosis evaluation: diagnostic performance of gadobenate dimeglumine-enhanced MR angiography–comparison with DSA. Radiology 2008;247(1):273–85.

39. Niendorf T, Pohlmann A, Arakelyan K, et al. How bold is blood oxygenation level-dependent (BOLD) magnetic resonance imaging of the kidney? Opportunities, challenges and future directions. Acta Physiol (Oxf) 2015;213(1):19–38.

40. Spuentrup E, Ruebben A, Stuber M, et al. Metallic renal artery MR imaging stent: artifact-free lumen visualization with projection and standard renal MR angiography. Radiology 2003;227(3):897–902.

41. Utsunomiya D, Miyazaki M, Nomitsu Y, et al. Clinical role of non-contrast magnetic resonance angiography for evaluation of renal artery stenosis. Circ J 2008;72(10):1627–30.

42. Thony F, Baguet JP, Rodiere M, et al. Renal artery entrapment by the diaphragmatic crus. Eur Radiol 2005;15(9):1841–9.

43. Paven G, Waugh R, Nicholson J, et al. Screening tests for renal artery stenosis: a case-series from an Australian tertiary referral centre. Nephrology 2006;11(1):68–72.

44. Baguet JP, Thony F, Sessa C, et al. Stenting of a renal artery compressed by the diaphragm. J Hum Hypertens 2003;17(3):213–4.

45. Chua SK, Hung HF. Renal artery stent fracture with refractory hypertension: a case report and review of the literature. Catheter Cardiovasc Interv 2009;74(1):37–42.

46. Kanofsky JA, Lepor H. Spontaneous renal artery dissection. Rev Urol 2007;9(3):156–60.

47. Lacombe M. Isolated spontaneous dissection of the renal artery. J Vasc Surg 2001;33(2):385–91.

48. Liu PS, Platt JF. CT angiography of the renal circulation. Radiol Clin North Am 2010;48(2):347–65.

49. Pellerin O, Garçon P, Beyssen B, et al. Spontaneous renal artery dissection: long-term outcomes after endovascular stent placement. J Vasc Interv Radiol 2009;20(8):1024–30.

50. Orion KC, Abularrage CJ. Renal artery aneurysms: movement toward endovascular repair. Semin Vasc Surg 2013;26(4):226–32.

51. González J, Esteban M, Andrés G, et al. Renal artery aneurysms. Curr Urol Rep 2014;15(1):376.

52. Cura M, Elmerhi F, Bugnogne A, et al. Renal aneurysms and pseudoaneurysms. Clin Imaging 2011;35(1):29–41.

53. Down LA, Papavassiliou DV, O'Rear EA. Arterial deformation with renal artery aneurysm as a basis for secondary hypertension. Biorheology 2013;50(1–2):17–31.

54. Henke PK, Cardneau JD, Welling TH, et al. Renal artery aneurysms: a 35-year clinical experience with 252 aneurysms in 168 patients. Ann Surg 2001;234(4):454–63.

55. Rafailidis V, Gavriilidou A, Liouliakis C, et al. Imaging of a renal artery aneurysm detected incidentally on ultrasonography. Case Rep Radiol 2014;2014:1–4.

56. Rundback JH, Rizvi A, Rozenblit GN, et al. Percutaneous stent-graft management of renal artery aneurysms. J Vasc Interv Radiol 2000;11(9):1189–93.

57. Moore W. Vascular and endovascular surgery: a comprehensive review. Philadelphia: Elsevier Saunders; 2006.

58. Nosher JL, Chung J, Brevetti LS, et al. Visceral and renal artery aneurysms: a pictorial essay on endovascular therapy. Radiographics 2006;26(6):1687–704.

59. Jesinger RA, Thoreson AA, Lamba R. Abdominal and pelvic aneurysms and pseudoaneurysms: imaging review with clinical, radiologic, and treatment correlation. Radiographics 2013;33(3):E71–96.

60. Ginat DT, Saad WEA, Turba UC. Transcatheter renal artery embolization: clinical applications and techniques. Tech Vasc Interv Radiol 2009;12(4):224–39.

61. Raman SP, Fishman EK. Mycotic aneurysms: a critical diagnosis in the emergency setting. Emerg Radiol 2014;21(2):191–6.

62. Lee WK, Mossop PJ, Little AF, et al. Infected (mycotic) aneurysms: spectrum of imaging appearances and management. Radiographics 2008;28(7):1853–68.

63. Jennette JC, Falk RJ, Andrassy K, et al. Nomenclature of systemic vasculitides: proposal of an international consensus conference. Radiology 1994; 194(3):187–92.

64. Charles Jennette JC, Falk RJ. The pathology of vasculitis involving the kidney. Am J Kidney Dis 1994;24(1):130–41.

65. Kumar V, Abbas AK, Fausto N, et al. Robbins and Cotran pathologic basis of disease, professional edition: expert consult-online. Robbins and Cotran pathologic basis of disease. Philadelphia: Elsevier Saunders; 2009. p. 487–528.

66. Jennette JC, Falk RJ. Small-vessel vasculitis. N Engl J Med 1997;337(21):1512–23.

67. Sidhu R, Lockhart ME. Imaging of renovascular disease. Semin Ultrasound CT MR 2009;30(4):271–88.

68. Scarpioni R, Poisetti PG, Cristinelli L, et al. Isolated renal giant cell arteritis, not so rare a cause of renal failure? Am J Kidney Dis 2003;41(3):720.

69. Kawashima A, Sandler CM, Ernst RD, et al. CT evaluation of renovascular disease. Radiographics 2000;20(5):1321–40.

70. Takayasu's arteritis : Johns Hopkins Vasculitis Center. Available at: https://www.hopkinsvasculitis.org/types-vasculitis/takayasus-arteritis/. Accessed March 22, 2020.

71. Maritati F, Iannuzzella F, Pavia MP, et al. Kidney involvement in medium- and large-vessel vasculitis. J Nephrol 2016;29(4):495–505.

72. Ozaki K, Miyayama S, Ushiogi Y, et al. Renal involvement of polyarteritis nodosa: CT and MR findings. Abdom Imaging 2009;34(2):265–70.

73. Kissin EY, Merkel PA. Diagnostic imaging in Takayasu arteritis. Curr Opin Rheumatol 2004;16(1):31–7.

74. Weaver FA, Kumar SR, Yellin AE, et al. Renal revascularization in Takayasu arteritis-induced renal artery stenosis. J Vasc Surg 2004;39(4):749–57.

75. Di Monaco S, Lengelé J-P, Heenaye S, et al. Prevalence and characteristics of renal artery fibromuscular dysplasia in hypertensive women below 50 years old. Eur J Clin Invest 2019;49(10):e13166.

76. Plouin PF, Baguet JP, Thony F, et al. High prevalence of multiple arterial bed lesions in patients with fibromuscular dysplasia: the ARCADIA registry (Assessment of Renal and Cervical Artery Dysplasia). Hypertension 2017;70(3):652–8.

77. Gornik HL, Persu A, Adlam D, et al. First international consensus on the diagnosis and management of fibromuscular dysplasia. J Hypertens 2019;37(2):229–52.

78. Stanley J. Renal vascular disease. In: Novik A, Scoble J, Hamilton G, editors. Renal vascular disease. 2nd edition. London: W.B. Saunders; 1996. p. 21–3.

79. Varennes L, Tahon F, Kastler A, et al. Fibromuscular dysplasia: what the radiologist should know: a pictorial review. Insights Imaging 2015;6(3): 295–307.

80. Plouin P, Perdu J, La Batide-Alanore A, et al. Fibromuscular dysplasia. Orphanet J Rare Dis 2007;2(1).

81. Kurklinsky AK, Rooke TW. Nutcracker phenomenon and nutcracker syndrome. Mayo Clin Proc 2010; 85(6):552–9.

82. Ahmed K, Sampath R, Khan MS. Current trends in the diagnosis and management of renal nutcracker syndrome: a review. Eur J Vasc Endovasc Surg 2006;31(4):410–6.

83. Kaufman J, Lee M. Vascular and interventional radiology: the requisites. 2nd edition. Philadelphia: Elsevier Saunders; 2004.

84. Sablón González N, Villalba NL, Parodis López Y, et al. Nutcracker syndrome. Medicina (B Aires) 2019;79(2):150–3.

85. Zhang H, Li M, Jin W, et al. The left renal entrapment syndrome: diagnosis and treatment. Ann Vasc Surg 2007;21(2):198–203.

86. Chen S, Zhang H, Shi H, et al. Endovascular stenting for treatment of nutcracker syndrome: report of 61 cases with long-term followup. J Urol 2011;186(2):570–5.

87. Chimpiri AR, Natarajan B. Renal vascular lesions: diagnosis and endovascular management. Semin Intervent Radiol 2009;26(3):253–61.

88. Tarkington MA, Matsumoto AH, Dejter SW, et al. Spectrum of renal vascular malformation. Urology 1991;38(4):297–300.

89. Cura M, Elmerhi F, Suri R, et al. Vascular malformations and arteriovenous fistulas of the kidney. Acta Radiol 2010;51(2):144–9.

90. Maruno M, Kiyosue H, Tanoue S, et al. Renal arteriovenous shunts: clinical features, imaging appearance, and transcatheter embolization based on angioarchitecture. Radiographics 2016;36(2):580–95.

91. Zhang LJ, Wu X, Yang GF, et al. Three-dimensional contrast-enhanced magnetic resonance venography for detection of renal vein thrombosis: comparison with multidetector CT venography. Acta Radiol 2013;54(10):1125–31.

92. Kau E, Patel R, Shah O. Isolated renal vein thrombosis after blunt trauma. Urology 2004;64(4):807–8.

93. Shariat SF, Roehrborn CG, Karakiewicz PI, et al. Evidence-based validation of the predictive value of the American Association for the Surgery of Trauma kidney injury scale. J Trauma Inj Infect Crit Care 2007;62(4):933–9.

94. Glassock RJ. Prophylactic anticoagulation in nephrotic syndrome: a clinical conundrum. J Am Soc Nephrol 2007;18(8):2221–5.

95. Wu CH, Ko SF, Lee CH, et al. Successful outpatient treatment of renal vein thrombosis by low-molecular weight heparins in 3 patients with nephrotic syndrome. Clin Nephrol 2006;65(6):433–40.

MR Imaging of the Mesenteric Vasculature

Jeremy D. Collins, MD, FSIR

KEYWORDS

- Mesenteric ischemia • MR angiography • MR venography • 4D flow MR imaging • Vasculitis
- Atherosclerosis • Fibromuscular dysplasia • Venous thrombosis

KEY POINTS

- MR angiography is a flexible technique enabling assessment of the arterial and venous vasculature of the abdomen in a single examination.
- MR angiography of the abdomen can be performed using gadolinium-based contrast media or ferumoxytol as a blood pool contrast agent.
- Noncontrast MR angiographic techniques are mature, available across vendor platforms, and enable depiction of the mesenteric arterial vasculature.
- 4D flow MR imaging can be performed simultaneously with MR angiography, adding functional evaluation to the anatomic visualization.
- Common and rare causes of mesenteric ischemia, including atherosclerosis, noninflammatory vasculopathies, vasculitis, dissection, arterial embolization, and mesenteric venous thrombosis are well depicted at MR angiography.

INTRODUCTION

Vascular MR techniques are well suited to evaluate for suspected mesenteric ischemia or to further characterize severity of aortic or mesenteric venous disease leading to mesenteric ischemia. MR techniques useful for this evaluation include contrast-enhanced MR angiography (MRA), phase-contrast imaging, including four-dimensional (4D) flow MR imaging, pseudo–steady-state imaging, noncontrast MR angiographic techniques, and vessel well imaging. MR has advantages over computed tomographic (CT) methods due to the insensitivity of the method for artifacts related to vascular calcifications, the intravascular T1 shortening achievable with lower amounts of administered contrast, flexibility to image the blood vessels in multiple phases of respiration, the ability to simultaneously evaluate the abdominal venous vasculature, and the lack of ionizing radiation. Disadvantages compared with CT include a longer examination time and artifact from ferromagnetic devices in the field of view, including stainless steel endografts and stents, surgical clips, and embolization coils. This review article describes MR techniques of relevance and discusses their role in the assessment of the mesenteric vasculature in patients with suspected mesenteric ischemia.

MR ANGIOGRAPHIC TECHNIQUES
First-Pass MR Angiography

First-pass MRA is a conventional angiographic technique enabling multiphase imaging of the abdominal arterial and venous vasculature.[1] Contrast is administered intravenously followed by a saline flush and the first imaging acquisition is initiated to align acquisition of the central lines of k-space with peak contrast arrival in the abdominal aorta and abdominal aortic branches (**Fig. 1**). This first phase is typically performed with k-space sampling methods that focus on filling the central lines of k-space first, followed by the peripheral lines after peak arterial enhancement in the

Department of Radiology, Mayo Clinic, 200 First Street Southwest, Rochester, MN 55901, USA
E-mail address: collins.jeremy@mayo.edu

Radiol Clin N Am 58 (2020) 797–813
https://doi.org/10.1016/j.rcl.2020.03.001

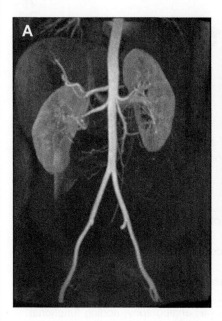
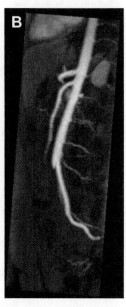

Fig. 1. First-pass MR angiogram. (*A*) Coronal and (*B*) sagittal maximum-intensity projections from a first-pass MR angiogram demonstrating excellent signal-to-noise and wide patency of the mesenteric branches.

vascular territory of interest.[2] MR angiographic techniques rely on the paramagnetic effect of gadolinium with T1 shortening.[3] Using a spoiled gradient recalled echo imaging technique with a short repetition time (TR) increases the conspicuity of the vascular territory of interest. Mask subtraction additionally suppresses unenhanced background tissue improving the signal-to-noise ratio of the vasculature over perivascular fat.[4]

First-pass MR angiographic techniques can be extended to multiple acquisitions, with continued use of the mask subtraction technique for visualization of the late arterial, early venous, and late venous phases of enhancement. These subsequent acquisitions are obtained using a sequential k-space ordering schema as the imaging is obtained after the pass of the peak arterial bolus or during the bolus tail.[5]

First-pass MRA can be obtained with or without electrocardiographic (ECG) gating. ECG gating is necessary to freeze pulsatile motion in the mid-ascending aorta and aortic root, but is not necessary for assessing the arch, descending thoracic aorta, or abdominal aorta. ECG gating for abdominal aortic applications is helpful when imaging structures that change in configuration over the cardiac cycle, such as dissection flaps, pseudoaneurysms, luminal thrombus, or complex atheromas.

Time-Resolved MR Angiography

TR-MRA is an extension of the first-pass MR angiographic technique to enable highly accelerated imaging.[6,7] Although vendors have used different solutions to achieve TR-MRA imaging, the underlying principles are the same. Following complete sampling of the initial imaging volume or mask, the central lines of k-space are updated more frequently than the peripheral lines. All of the sampled k-space data are combined to enable a more frequent update of the entire k-space dataset than would be possible with accelerated methods and complete sampling of k-space alone. The addition of mask subtraction enables efficient review of these TR-MRA angiographic data (Fig. 2). TR-MRA is helpful in identifying the contrast kinetics associated with atherosclerosis and dissection. In addition, the method is simple to perform and does not require careful timing of the onset of the acquisition with contrast arrival in the vascular territory of interest. TR-MRA is often used in conjunction with first-pass MR angiographic techniques as a method to calculate the transit time of contrast from a peripheral vein to the arterial territory of interest while obtaining useful information about vascular pathology.

Pseudo–Steady-State Imaging

The gadolinium-based contrast media available on the market today are classified as extracellular, non-blood pool agents.[8] Other than liver function agents, the gadolinium contrast media equilibrate into the interstitium and are excreted primarily via renal filtration with variable amounts of hepatic and enteric excretion. Despite formulation that does not optimize dwell time of gadolinium contrast media in the arterial and venous

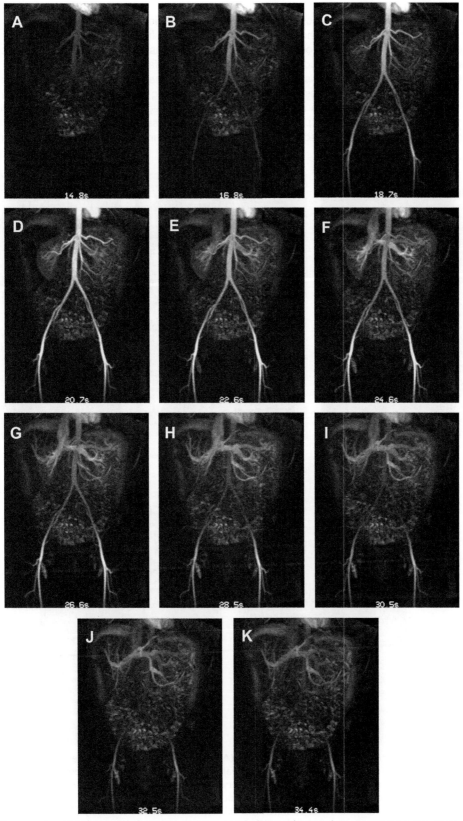

Fig. 2. Time-resolved MR angiogram. Sequential temporal-phase subtracted maximum-intensity projection images (A–K) from a time-resolved MR angiogram demonstrating typical dynamic image quality achievable. This patient demonstrates reflux into the proximal left ovarian vein.

vasculature, vascular contrast concentration enabling effective imaging of the T1 shortening effect extends well beyond the second or third pass of gadolinium. So-called pseudo–steady-state imaging methods take advantage of this prolonged vascular dwell time as the contrast is being excreted, enabling imaging with both arterial and venous territories opacified (**Fig. 3**).[9] Pseudo–steady-state imaging can be performed with either spoiled gradient recalled echo imaging methods, T1-weighted imaging techniques using fat saturation to increase the conspicuity of the vasculature adjacent to fat, or other methods with inversion recovery-based fat suppression. Pseudo–steady-state imaging enables extension of a nonangiographic imaging examination to include a late-phase assessment of the arterial and venous vasculature in an anatomic region of interest.

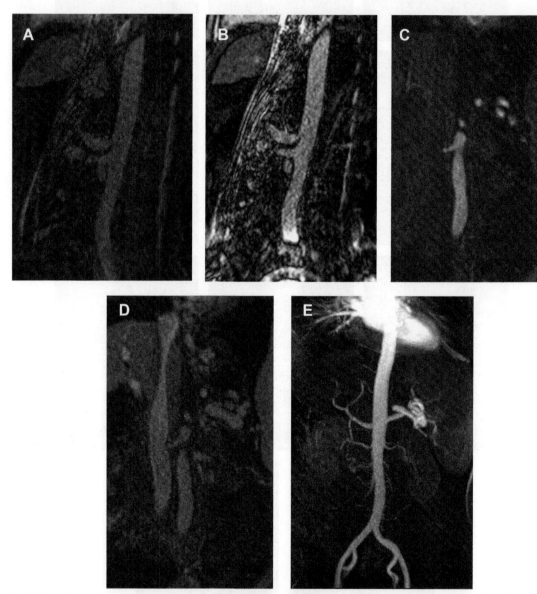

Fig. 3. Pseudo–steady-state MRA. Partition images from (*A*) 3D inversion recovery prepared spoiled gradient recalled echo and (*B*) 3D inversion recovery prepared balanced steady-state free precession MR angiograms through the celiac axis and superior mesenteric artery origins demonstrate celiac axis stenosis on end-expiratory-phase triggered imaging. (*C*) Coronal partition images from first-pass MRA and (*D*) venous-phase first-pass MRA demonstrates mild celiac axis stenosis. (*E*) Coronal maximum-intensity projection image from the first-pass MR angiogram demonstrates the difference in conspicuity of the arterial vasculature compared with pseudo–steady-state imaging.

This approach works well with medium and larger vessels, where clear separation of the artery and accompanying vein(s) is possible. However, this approach is limited where smaller arterial branches are positioned adjacent to variably present paired veins, such as the distal branches of the mesenteric vasculature, along the portal triads, and at the visceral hila. Pseudo–steady-state imaging also precludes any assessment of contrast kinetics as the contrast media is completely dispersed throughout the arterial and venous vasculature. Imaging during the pseudo-steady state is useful to improve the conspicuity of the vasculature for 4D flow MR imaging, further increasing the contrast to noise ratio from perivascular fat and other tissue with short T1 values.[10]

3D ECG-gated techniques with respiratory compensation methods have been developed and championed for pseudo–steady-state imaging.[9] Respiratory compensation methods include respiratory bellows, respiratory navigators, and k-space reordering, with the central lines obtained at end-expiration and peripheral lines obtained at other less consistent portions of the cardiac cycle. Contrast medium in the pseudo-steady state is helpful with these methods as the intravascular T1 shortening effect can be used to take advantage of inversion recovery-based techniques to improve the conspicuity of the vasculature relative to perivascular fat. These techniques use spoiled gradient recalled echo or balanced steady-state free precession methods.[9] Spoiled gradient recalled echo imaging has inherently less signal but is more resistant to off-resonance effects and susceptibility artifacts, useful for applications in the abdomen with air-filled bowel loops.

Steady-State Imaging with Ferumoxytol

Ferumoxytol (Feraheme, AG Pharmaceuticals) is an iron supplement Food and Drug Administration (FDA) approved for iron deficiency anemia.[11–13] Ferumoxytol is an ultrasmall paramagnetic iron oxide with a dextran-derivative coating enveloping the Fe particle core resulting in a particle diameter of approximately 30 nm.[12] The agent is slowly removed from the blood stream by the reticuloendothelial system with a half-life of approximately 14 hours. The long persistence in the blood stream necessitates coordination of other MR imaging tests with ferumoxytol administration[14]; nonangiographic MR imaging should be delayed for 3 days after administration. In addition, ferumoxytol has an FDA black box warning noting the risk of anaphylactoid-type reactions in susceptible patients in whom the agent is administered undiluted at the rate initially recommended by the manufacturer. It is now well recognized that administration of undiluted ferumoxytol unnecessarily increases the risk of treatment-resistant hypotension. Slower administration of dilute ferumoxytol coupled with screening for a history of medication-associated hypotension, resting systolic blood pressure less than 100 mm Hg, and past intolerance of Fe-related medications, while providing both intravenous and oral hydration, has been proven to be safe in clinical practice. The FeraSafe MRI Multi-Center Registry, developed and maintained by investigators from the University of California, Los Angeles, has documented the safe administration of ferumoxytol to more than 500 patients.[15]

Ferumoxytol is administered intravenously and has been shown to act as an effective blood pool contrast agent at 1.5 and 3 T (**Fig. 4**).[16,17]

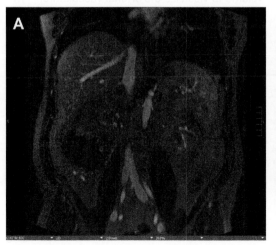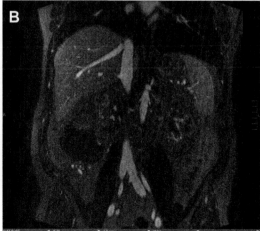

Fig. 4. Feraheme MRA. (*A*) Early steady-state and (*B*) late steady-state MRA with Feraheme. Note the similar appearance of the arterial and venous vasculature. Image (*B*) was obtained 5 minutes after image (*A*).

Ferumoxytol has distinct benefits for MR angiographic and venographic imaging in patients with suspected mesenteric ischemia. Ferumoxytol is typically administered as a slow bolus outside of the magnet with in-room nurse monitoring and subsequent imaging in the steady state. This enables simultaneous high-resolution imaging of the arterial and venous vasculature. Spatial resolution achievable with ferumoxytol is not limited by the short dwell time of high contrast concentration in the arterial vasculature; rather the image quality is primarily limited by the patient's breath-holding ability or respiratory navigator technique used.[18] Ferumoxytol greatly facilitates 4D flow MR imaging by improving the image quality of the accompanying phase-contrast MR angiogram, streamlining data analysis by improving the vascular segmentation step.[19] Simultaneous arterial and venous imaging with adequate spatial resolution to distinguish arteries and veins in close proximity optimizes table time in these patients.[18] Venous and arterial causes of mesenteric ischemia can be assessed simultaneously. What is lost from the dynamic components of the typical MR angiographic study with arterial, late arterial, portal venous, and systemic venous phases can be captured with 4D flow MR imaging. Artifact from bowel motility can be reduced by administering glucagon IV.[20]

In addition, a meal challenge with Ensure can be performed to simulate the physiologic stressors leading to intestinal angina without requiring additional intravenous contrast for imaging after the meal challenge.[21,22] The long half-life of ferumoxytol also enables postinterventional steady-state imaging without administering additional contrast media.

Noncontrast MR Angiographic Techniques

Noncontrast MR angiographic techniques have been developed for peripheral MRA, and modifications of these methods applied to the mesenteric vasculature. The primary impetus for development was concerns around nephrogenic systemic fibrosis and subsequently the low but unknown risk of gadolinium chelate accumulation in patients irrespective of renal insufficiency. With the availability of macrocyclic gadolinium-based contrast and Fe-based contrast media the clinical need for noncontrast MR angiographic techniques is less apparent. Although a comprehensive review of noncontrast MR angiographic methods is beyond the scope of this review, methods useful in the mesenteric arterial system include both bright blood relatively flow-insensitive and bright blood flow-sensitive imaging techniques.[23]

Bright blood flow-insensitive methods

3D balanced steady-state free precession (bSSFP) described above as an imaging strategy for pseudo–steady-state imaging can also be used as a noncontrast MR angiographic technique (Fig. 5). This technique is more commonly used in the chest for noncontrast coronary and thoracic aortic MRA. The relatively bright fat surrounding the vasculature compared with postcontrast techniques and susceptibility artifact from adjacent air-filled bowel loops can limit the overall image quality.

Quiescent interval single shot (QISS) is a robust technique with well-recognized accuracy in the evaluation of abdominal aortic, iliac, and lower extremity peripheral arterial disease.[24] This approach suppresses signal from adjacent veins by using a tracking saturation pulse positioned toward the feet, an inversion pulse for static tissue, and a dedicated fat-suppression pulse.[25] The resultant 2D axial images highlight the arterial signal. The principle limitation of this technique is the slice orientation and requirement for the blood vessel of interest to be orientated nearly orthogonal to the slice. Consequently, the superior mesenteric and inferior mesenteric arteries are well seen but the celiac axis is poorly assessed.[26] When applied in the abdomen, concatenated breath-holds are used to cover the abdominal aorta and mesenteric branches (Fig. 6).

Bright blood flow-sensitive methods

bSSFP inflow enhanced imaging overcomes the limitation of plane positioning described above with QISS.[23] Implemented as a respiratory navigated 3D technique, the pulse sequence relies on saturating static tissue and venous inflow while highlighting fresh signal from arterial inflow into the volume to visualize the arterial vasculature.[27] This approach is well suited to image the mesenteric arteries as well as the celiac axis and its branches (Fig. 7). The inflow time can be lengthened in the presence of disease with reduced distal arterial flow. This method is, therefore, both anatomic and functional, similar to contrast-enhanced methods.

Ancillary techniques

Ancillary imaging techniques include 2D phase-contrast (PC) imaging, 4D flow MR imaging, and vessel wall imaging.

Two-dimensional phase-contrast MR imaging 2D PC imaging has been a useful adjunct for determining the hemodynamic severity of vascular stenosis and flow directionality. 2D PC imaging enables determining peak velocity for estimating pressure gradients, and flow quantification.[28] The

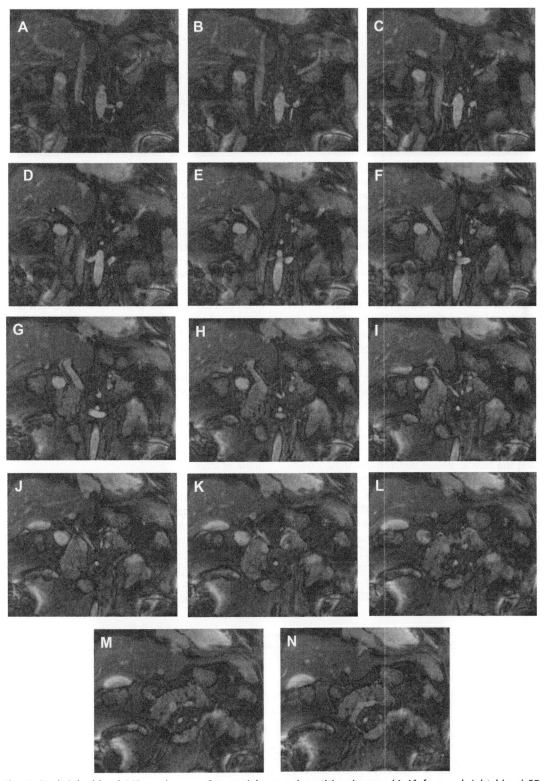

Fig. 5. 3D bright blood MR angiogram. Sequential coronal partition images (*A–N*) from a bright blood 3D balanced steady-state free procession MR angiogram demonstrating the image quality achievable with this technique. The origins of the celiac axis, superior mesenteric artery, and inferior mesenteric artery are well seen, as is the branching of the celiac axis. More distal branches of the superior mesenteric artery are not as well seen. Note the well visualized IVC, portal vein, and superior mesenteric vein branches.

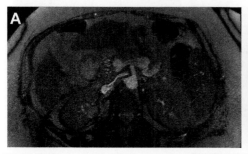
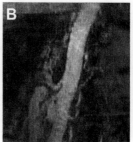
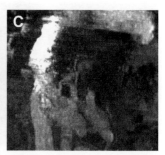

Fig. 6. Quiescent interval single-shot MRA. (*A*) Axial maximum-intensity projection at the superior mesenteric artery origin and (*B*) oblique sagittal maximum-intensity projection showing the proximal celiac axis and superior mesenteric artery origins. (*C*) Oblique coronal maximum-intensity projection image showing the left gastric origin from the celiac axis. Images were obtained with concatenated breath-holds at end-expiration.

2D approach has several notable limitations, including a rectangular voxel with relatively poor through-plane resolution, peak velocity dependence on plane positioning orthogonal to the direction of flow, and appropriate choice of the velocity encoding (VENC) gradient for the vascular territory of interest and approximate severity of vascular disease when present. For example, 2D PC imaging can be used to confirm dynamic stenosis associated with median arcuate ligament syndrome (MALS)-related celiac stenosis by imaging patients in deep inspiration and at end-expiration, demonstrating higher velocities at end-expiration. Flow directionality is also able to be assessed with 2D PC imaging; for example, imaging the flow direction within mesenteric collateral arcades can help confirm the severity of proximal stenoses. 2D PC encodes velocity either in-plane or orthogonal to a plane of interest; both are dependent on plane orientation for accurate velocity estimation. In vitro work has shown that plane malpositioning greater than 20° to the direction of flow in a vessel results in errors in the peak velocity and net flow of greater than 10%.[29] Although so-called tri-directional 2D approaches

with flow encoding in the x-, y-, and z-axis directions can overcome this limitation, the longer breath-hold and limited coverage poses challenges to clinical use. The choice of VENC is important for accurate peak velocity and flow calculations as the velocity noise scales proportionately to the VENC. Underestimating the peak velocity by more than a factor of 2 results in problematic aliasing and erroneous velocity values. Velocity scout imaging is available from multiple vendors to facilitate appropriate VENC selection; review of prior vascular ultrasound studies may also be helpful to identify the correct VENC. The VENC should be matched to just greater than the highest peak velocity expected in the imaging plane of interest.

Four-dimensional flow MR imaging 4D flow MR imaging extends flow imaging into a 3D volume with flow encoding in the x-, y-, and z-directions (**Fig. 8**).[30] The imaging acquisition is ECG gated with either respiratory k-space reordering and/or respiratory navigator gating. 4D flow MR imaging is well suited to assess flow directionality, hemodynamic significance of a vascular stenosis, or

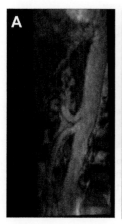
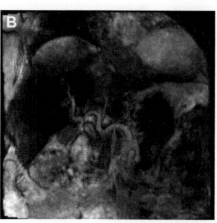

Fig. 7. Balanced steady-state free precession MRA. (*A*) Sagittal maximum-intensity projection at the celiac axis and superior mesenteric artery origins and (*B*) coronal maximum-intensity project image at the common hepatic artery bifurcation. This technique uses a respiratory bellows triggering at end-expiration.

A

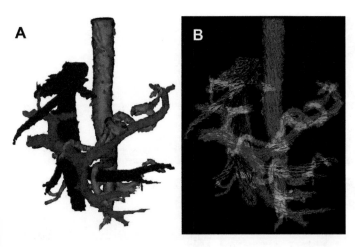

Fig. 8. 4D flow MR imaging. (*A*) Vascular segmentation with the aorta colored red, the mesenteric, splenic, and portal veins colored light purple, and the systemic and hepatic veins blue. (*B*) Pathlines overlaid on the segmented vasculature demonstrates the flow directionality in all of the vasculature.

visualize collateral vascular arcades.[21] 4D flow MR imaging is triggered at end-expiration given the more consistent anatomic positioning at that respiratory phase. At rest, visualizing vascular collaterals is helpful in determining the direction of flow in collateral arcades associated with MALS, although as noted above the demonstration of dynamic changes between inspiration and expiration is helpful. A clinically relevant application of 4D flow MR imaging in patients with suspected mesenteric ischemia includes functional imaging with a meal challenge as described above.[22] Patients are imaged with 4D flow MR imaging at baseline and after 2 cans of Ensure (**Fig. 9**). The resultant changes in mesenteric flow allows determination of clinical severity of celiac axis and mesenteric artery stenoses, thus guiding revascularization. 4D flow MR imaging is also useful in visualizing flow directionality in the mesenteric veins and portal venous system.[21]

Vessel wall imaging Vessel wall imaging is helpful when imaging patients with suspected atherosclerosis, vasculitis, or noninflammatory vasculopathies. These techniques rely on T1-weighted imaging precontrast and postcontrast as well as dark blood-prepared 2D and 3D imaging to isolate vessel wall signal from the adjacent vessel lumen and perivascular tissues (**Fig. 10**). Common pulse sequences include dark blood-prepared T1-weighted and dark blood-prepared T2-weighted fat-saturated imaging.[31] Mural thickness is well assessed with dark blood-prepared T1-weighted imaging; juxta arterial edema is well seen with dark blood-prepared fat-saturated T2-weighted imaging. Mural edema may be appreciated when the wall is adequately thickened to assess mural T2 signal. In addition, 3D T1-weighted imaging techniques are useful when more extended coverage is desired; for example, visualizing all mesenteric branches and the abdominal aorta in

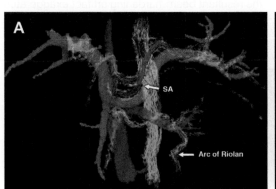

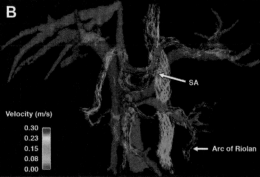

Fig. 9. 4D flow with meal challenge. Images from a 4D flow MR imaging dataset performed before (*A*) and after (*B*) meal challenge demonstrating increased flow through the arc of Riolan (*arrow*). Also, increased flow is noted in the gastroduodenal arcade. (*Reprinted from* Roldan-Alzate A, Francois CJ, Wieben O, et al. Emerging applications of abdominal 4D flow MRI. AJR Am J Roentgenol 2016;207(1):58-66; with permission.)

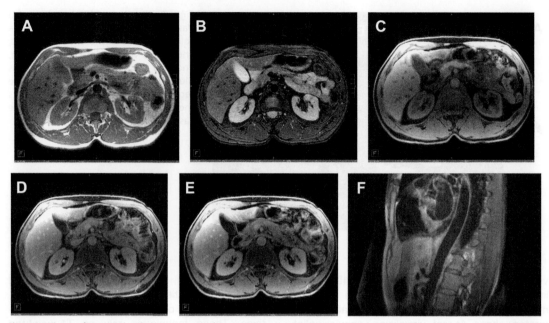

Fig. 10. Tissue characterization sequences for vessel wall imaging. (*A*) Dark blood T1 turbo spin echo, (*B*) dark blood short tau inversion recovery, precontrast (*C*), 1-minute postcontrast (*D*), and 5-minute postcontrast (*E*) 3D T1 fat–water-separated multiecho, and (*F*) 3D respiratory navigator and ECG-gated T1 turbo spin echo imaging demonstrates a normal appearance of the abdominal aortic wall and superior mesenteric artery at the level of the left renal vein.

a single acquisition. 2D or 3D precontrast and post-contrast T1-weighted fat-suppressed techniques are useful in the evaluation of mural inflammation; it is important to standardize the timing of postcontrast acquisitions to adequately capture early and late phases of mural enhancement. Some authors have advocated for delayed enhancement techniques similar to myocardial delayed enhancement methods in the identification of mural fibrosis; however, such approaches are limited in the medium-sized mesenteric vessels.[32]

SPECIFIC CLINICAL ENTITIES
Atherosclerosis

Atherosclerosis of the abdominal aorta and its branches is prevalent with age.[33] When

flow-limiting stenoses involve the origins of all 3 mesenteric branches, the collateral arcades present are no longer able to accommodate the fluctuations in blood flow to the gastrointestinal tract required as part of the normal digestive process. This results in abdominal pain termed "mesenteric angina" that is reproducible and occurs after eating (**Fig. 11**). Although ultrasound, CT angiography and MRA are used in confirming the clinical suspicion of mesenteric arterial stenoses, MRA has several distinct advantages in making this diagnosis. Calcification is a prevalent component of abdominal aortic and branch atherosclerosis; the resultant beam-hardening artifact exaggerates arterial stenoses at CT angiography. Alternative causes for mesenteric ischemia include mesenteric venous thrombosis (see venous thrombosis

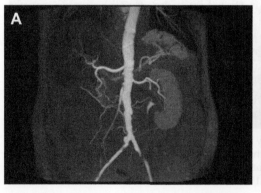

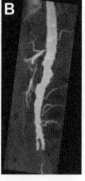

Fig. 11. Chronic mesenteric ischemia. (*A*) Coronal and (*B*) sagittal maximum-intensity projection images of a first-pass MR angiogram demonstrating severe stenosis of the celiac axis and superior mesenteric artery. The inferior mesenteric artery is severely diseased and faintly opacified proximally on the sagittal MR angiogram.

section below), which can be assessed simultaneously at MRA performed with delayed phased imaging. Collateral arterial arcades are well assessed at MRA, an important secondary sign of the severity of arterial stenosis. 4D flow MR imaging can be performed at the same time to confirm the severity of arterial stenosis and demonstrate flow directionality in arterial collaterals.[22]

Abdominal aortic aneurysms often coexist with advanced abdominal aortic atherosclerosis. MRA is well suited to assess the size and extent of abdominal aortic aneurysms, determine the extent of mural thrombus, and evaluate for high-risk features, including peri-aortic inflammation, peri-aortic hematomas, and aneurysms involving other territories, including the internal iliac arteries.[34] Penetrating ulcers also coexist with advanced atherosclerosis; MR is well suited to assess the chronicity of such vascular pathology by assessing the integrity of the adventitia and identifying edema in the surrounding fat.

A limitation of MRA is imaging patients after stainless steel stent placement, after surgery with placement of metallic clips, or after embolization with stainless steel coils. Balloon expandable stents are commonly used in the treatment of mesenteric arterial stenoses; such stents cause susceptibility artifact. Although the stents will not move the in MR imaging environment, the susceptibility artifact precludes assessment of in-stent restenosis and limits evaluation of the adjacent vasculature. When such devices are present, other imaging modalities should be considered, with CT angiography the primary choice when anatomic imaging is desired. Susceptibility artifact from surgical clips adjacent to mesenteric branch vessels can cause pseudostenosis or can preclude visualization of arterial segments. The clip composition and proximity to the vessel of interest are important considerations; reviewing nonangiographic CT imaging is helpful in determining the likely impact on MR angiographic image quality. Some embolization coils are extremely dense on CT but have limited susceptibility on MR imaging; hence, a priori knowledge of the coil composition is critical when considering MRA. Stainless steel embolization coils are commonly used for ureteral embolization and can be used in other vascular applications; when present these cause significant susceptibility artifact and limit visualization of arterial structures far from the coil pack. It is important to remember that conventional contrast-enhanced MR angiographic techniques rely on spoiled gradient recalled echo imaging, which is resistant to local field inhomogeneity. Therefore, nonferromagnetic materials (nitinol alloys, titanium-based

devices) are visible in the MR environment but demonstrate only local susceptibility artifact. Self-expanding nitinol stents in the common iliac arteries are large enough to permit visualization inside the stents. Similarly, endografts with nitinol supporting alloys are well characterized at MRA. In medium or smaller vessels, however, even with the small amount of associated artifact, the lumen of the stent is too small to confidently assess for in-stent restenosis; patency can be inferred, however, by visualization of flow distal to the stented segment. Another benefit of MRA is the lack of artifact from liquid embolics and glues. These materials cause significant artifact on CT angiography as well as conventional digital subtraction angiography.

Less significant artifacts from inferior vena cava (IVC) filters penetrating the cava contacting the abdominal aorta can limit evaluation of adjacent aortic wall. The impact is related to the extent of contact of the IVC filter along the IVC wall adjacent to the abdominal aorta, and the location of penetrating struts relative to abdominal aortic branches. Similarly, other implanted nitinol-based devices adjacent to the aorta limit assessment of the wall, but only have local susceptibility artifact. Other such devices include atrial septal occluders deployed between the abdominal aortic wall and the IVC wall after transcaval access for transcatheter aortic valve replacement in patients with severe femoral arterial vascular disease.

Median arcuate ligament syndrome

MALS is a clinical syndrome associated with dynamic extrinsic arterial stenosis caused by a narrowed opening of the diaphragmatic crus.[35] The celiac axis, superior mesenteric artery, and/or the renal arteries can be involved. The extrinsic compression of the arterial vasculature in MALS is accentuated at end-expiration (Fig. 12). MRA is an ideal imaging technique to assess respiratory-phase-associated stenosis. Multiphase MR angiographic imaging can be obtained in inspiration and expiration with gadolinium-based contrast media or a blood pool agent. When using gadolinium-based contrast, MRA is performed in inspiration followed by pseudo–steady-state imaging with an end-expiratory-phase trigger. Blood pool contrast agents are well suited for MRA in MALS as the prolonged blood pool dwell time enables conventional unsubtracted MR angiographic techniques, 3D Dixon fat/water separation T1-weighted imaging, and 3D inversion recovery prepared bSSFP techniques. 4D flow MR imaging with an end-expiration respiratory trigger can demonstrate collateral arterial arcades, confirming

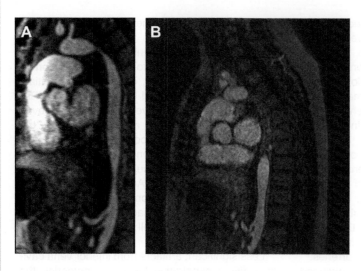

Fig. 12. Dynamic narrowing of the celiac axis. (*A*) Inspiratory-phase steady-state MR angiogram with ferumoxytol with a sagittal multiplanar reconstructionslice through the proximal celiac axis and (*B*) expiratory-phase respiratory navigator gated 3D inversion recovery prepared gradient recalled echo imaging in the same orientation demonstrating dynamic stenosis of the celiac axis with wide patency of the superior mesenteric artery throughout the respiratory cycle.

the hemodynamic significance of the dynamic arterial stenosis.

Vasculitis

MRA is an ideal imaging technique to evaluate for vasculitis in medium and larger vessels, including the mesenteric arteries.[31] In addition to evaluating for the degree of arterial stenosis, vessel wall imaging enables assessment of disease status (**Fig. 13**). Acute inflammation is identified by perivascular inflammation and edema using fat-saturated T2-weighted imaging sequences often with black blood preparation pulses. Wall enhancement is assessed with precontrast, early postcontrast, and late postcontrast T1-weighted imaging with fat suppression. Early wall enhancement is indicative of acute inflammation, whereas late wall enhancement indicates fibrosis.[32] Identification of abnormally thickened vessel walls is facilitated by the use of 3D T1-weighted pulse

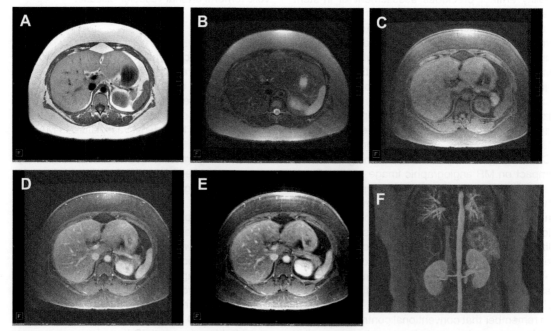

Fig. 13. Active Takayasu's arteritis. (*A*) Dark blood T1-weighted turbo spin echo imaging demonstrating wall thickening at the aortic hiatus with corresponding edema on dark blood short tau inversion recovery imaging (*B*). Mural enhancement is seen comparing precontrast (*C*) with 1-minute (*D*) and 5-minute (*E*) postcontrast T1-weighted fat-saturated imaging. These mural changes are not as apparent on first-pass MRA (*F*).

sequences with dark blood preparation.[36] Late gadolinium enhancement using inversion prepared 2D and 3D pulse sequences has been used to identify arterial fibrosis.[32] Differentiation of active atherosclerosis from active vasculitis can be difficult on imaging alone; segmental regions of abnormal wall thickening and enhancement with intervening normal-appearing vessel walls suggests vasculitis over atherosclerosis. Similarly, circumferential, symmetric vessel wall thickening favors vasculitis, although precontrast imaging is helpful in excluding an intramural hematoma. Vascular calcifications can be seen in patients after treatment or with coexistent atherosclerosis. An advantage of MRA is the lack of vascular calcification-associated artifacts. Novel pulse sequences have been developed that enable visualization of arterial calcifications at MR imaging.[37] Fusion imaging also enables overlay of noncontrast CT with MRA to highlight the location and distribution of vascular calcifications.[38] MR/PET imaging combining metabolic imaging with MRA and vessel wall imaging is an excellent modality enabling distinction of regionally active from quiescent disease.[39]

Noninflammatory vasculopathies

Fibromuscular dysplasia (FMD) and segmental arterial mediolysis (SAM) can both involve the mesenteric arterial vasculature. FMD is a nonatherosclerotic, noninflammatory disorder presenting with vascular stenosis. The vascular pathology associated with FMD can manifest in the intima, media, or adventitia with a variety of different MR angiographic appearances. Although the renal arteries are the most commonly impacted arterial bed, the mesenteric arteries are uncommonly affected (**Fig. 14**). Patients rarely present with mesenteric ischemia. Differentiation of this entity from atherosclerosis or SAM is important as patients with FMD respond to balloon angioplasty.[40] Patients with FMD present with segmental dilation alternating with webs causing stenoses (intimal subtype), smooth discrete stenoses (medial subtype), or aneurysms (adventitial subtype).[41] Identifying coexistent disease in other vascular beds, such as the iliac and/or renal arteries, is helpful in making the diagnosis of FMD.

SAM results from degeneration of the media of medium-sized muscular arteries, with dissection, occlusion, and aneurysm formation with stenosis occurring during the healing phase of the disease

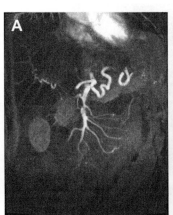
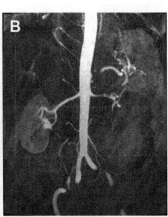
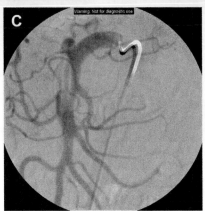

Fig. 14. Mesenteric fibromuscular dysplasia. (*A*) Thin slab maximum-intensity projection image from a first-pass MR angiogram demonstrating segmental dilation and dissection in the proximal superior mesenteric artery. The associated renal involvement with typical webs and aneurysms (*B*) is helpful in making the diagnosis of fibromuscular dysplasia. (*C*) Digital subtraction angiogram confirming fibromuscular dysplasia involvement of the superior mesenteric artery.

process (Fig. 15).[42] Patients with SAM often present with abdominal pain or bleeding. The celiac axis and superior mesenteric artery are the most commonly involved vessels. Treatment is conservative with supportive measures.[43] Coil embolization has been performed for patients with bleeding not responsive to supportive care with good outcomes. Stent placement or open surgical techniques have been associated with relatively high mortality due to the friable nature of the involved vessel segments. The primary differential diagnosis for SAM includes mycotic aneurysms, medium-vessel vasculitis, and FMD. The location of involved vascular segments, laboratory tests, and evolution of vascular changes on imaging is helpful in distinguishing these entities.

Arterial dissection

Dissections of the mesenteric arteries can be associated with propagation of a dissection flap from the abdominal aorta or can be associated with atherosclerosis or an underlying vascular disorder, including FMD or SAM. Patient presentation is related to the location of the lesion, the degree of associated stenosis of the true lumen, propagation of the dissection to involve branch vessels, and

distal embolization. Multiphase imaging enabled by MRA is well suited to characterize arterial dissection and identify complications, including distal embolization, thrombosis of the false lumen, and occlusion of branch vessels.

Arterial embolization

Thromboembolism to the mesenteric arteries is an important cause of mesenteric ischemia. Unlike in slowly progressive atherosclerosis, the sudden occlusion of a mesenteric branch does not permit adequate recruitment of arterial collaterals. Acute embolic occlusion is distinguished from underlying atherosclerosis by the location of the clot typically at a branch point in the proximal vessel, rather than at the vessel ostium (Fig. 16). Multiple emboli are commonly present; identifying other embolic events, including visceral infarctions is helpful in making the diagnosis. Treatment is focused on urgently restoring arterial flow; as such lytic therapy plays little role in management. Rather embolectomy with adjunctive balloon angioplasty or stenting is performed to re-establish flow quickly. MRA is well suited to identify the thromboembolism and can be performed efficiently by relying on multiphase imaging. Noncontrast methods can identify

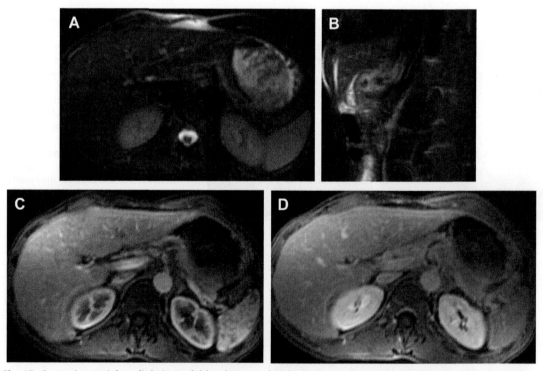

Fig. 15. Systemic arterial mediolysis. Dark blood T2-weighted imaging in the axial (A) and sagittal (B) planes demonstrates edema around the celiac axis without involvement of the abdominal aorta. Postcontrast T1-weighted imaging with fat suppression in the early arterial (C) and portal venous (D) phases of enhancement demonstrates luminal irregularity with a thrombosed dissection extending into the common hepatic and splenic arteries with progressive mural enhancement.

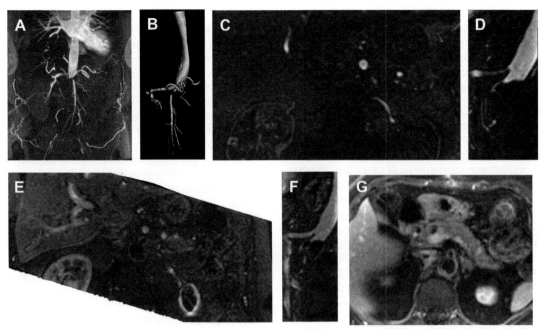

Fig. 16. Superior mesenteric arterythrombus. (*A*) Coronal 3D maximum-intensity projection, (*B*) 3D volume rendered image, (*C*) Coronal, and (*D*) oblique sagittal multiplanar reformat first-pass MR angiogram demonstrated an eccentric filling defect in the proximal superior mesenteric artery with thrombus in the abdominal aorta. (*E*) Coronal and (*F*) oblique sagittal multiplanar reformats from a venous-phase MRA showing mural enhancement and contrast along the anterior aspect of the vessel outlining the thrombus. (*G*) Postcontrast T1-weighted imaging with Dixon fat separation demonstrating the superior mesenteric artery thrombus and aortic thrombus.

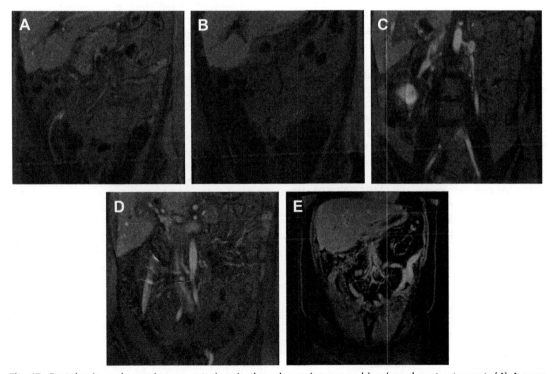

Fig. 17. Portal vein and superior mesenteric vein thrombus using a non-blood pool contrast agent. (*A*) A near-occlusive filling defect in the superior mesenteric vein is seen on coronal venous-phase MRA, the extent of which is better depicted with a minimum intensity projection technique (*B*). Main portal (*C*) with right portal extension (*A*, *D*) clot is also present with abnormal enhancement of the right lobe of the liver. Late-phase T1-weighted fat-saturated imaging demonstrates associated thrombophlebitis with avid enhancement of the wall of the superior mesenteric vein surrounding the thrombus (*E*).

the stenosis associated with the emboli; however, the characteristic appearance of a filling defect is difficult to appreciate with noncontrast techniques. In addition, noncontrast imaging approaches often take longer to perform.

Venous thrombosis

Mesenteric venous thrombosis can present with abdominal pain in a manner that mimics arterial stenosis.[44] Thrombosis of the mesenteric veins is often associated with gastrointestinal infections. Venous engorgement ensues. MR angiographic techniques are well suited to assess the presence and extent of mesenteric venous thrombosis with both blood pool and extracellular contrast agents (**Fig. 17**). Blood pool agents are ideal in this setting because both the collateral venous drainage pathway and patient portions of the thrombosed vein are well opacified. 4D flow MR imaging can be performed with blood pool contrast agents to provide hemodynamic information lacking when using a steady-state imaging approach. Unlike CT, MRA affords a longer period of time for venous-phase imaging, with extracellular contrast agents outlining the thrombus and demonstrating the venous wall enhancement associated with acute thrombus.

SUMMARY

MRA is a flexible technique in the evaluation of the mesenteric arterial and venous vasculature in patients with suspected mesenteric ischemia. The combination of anatomic imaging with MRA and vascular functional imaging at 4D flow MR imaging enables a comprehensive assessment of the mesenteric arterial and venous vasculature. Tissue characterization sequences using black blood preparation pulses can be obtained to better characterize vascular pathology. Novel blood pool Fe-based contrast media show promise to shorten the imaging time and reduce the complexity of MR angiographic protocols. MRA should be considered a primary imaging modality in the outpatient evaluation of suspected mesenteric ischemia and considered as an alternative to CT angiography in the acute setting.

DISCLOSURE

The authors have nothing to disclose.

REFERENCES

1. Prince MR, Narasimham DL, Stanley JC, et al. Breath-hold gadolinium-enhanced MR angiography of the abdominal aorta and its major branches. Radiology 1995;197(3):785–92.

2. Riedy G, Golay X, Melhem ER. Three-dimensional isotropic contrast-enhanced MR angiography of the carotid artery using sensitivity-encoding and random elliptic centric k-space filling: technique optimization. Neuroradiology 2005;47(9):668–73.

3. Gadian DG, Payne JA, Bryant DJ, et al. Gadolinium-DTPA as a contrast agent in MR imaging—theoretical projections and practical observations. J Comput Assist Tomogr 1985;9(2):242–51.

4. Menke J. Contrast-enhanced magnetic resonance angiography in peripheral arterial disease: improving image quality by automated image registration. Magn Reson Med 2008;60(1):224–9.

5. Carroll TJ, Grist TM. Technical developments in MR angiography. Radiol Clin North Am 2002;40(4):921–51.

6. Winterer JT, Blanke P, Schaefer A, et al. Bilateral contrast-enhanced MR angiography of the hand: diagnostic image quality of accelerated MRI using echo sharing with interleaved stochastic trajectories (TWIST). Eur Radiol 2011;21(5):1026–33.

7. Grist TM, Mistretta CA, Strother CM, et al. Time-resolved angiography: past, present, and future. J Magn Reson Imaging 2012;36(6):1273–86.

8. Kodzwa R. ACR manual on contrast media: 2018 updates. Radiol Technol 2019;91(1):97–100.

9. Rustogi R, Galizia M, Thakrar D, et al. Steady-state MRA techniques with a blood pool contrast agent improve visualization of pulmonary venous anatomy and left atrial patency compared with time-resolved MRA pre- and postcatheter ablation in atrial fibrillation. J Magn Reson Imaging 2015. https://doi.org/10.1002/jmri.24907.

10. Collins JD, Semaan E, Barker A, et al. Comparison of hemodynamics after aortic root replacement using valve-sparing or bioprosthetic valved conduit. Ann Thorac Surg 2015;04:109.

11. Spinowitz BS, Kausz AT, Baptista J, et al. Ferumoxytol for treating iron deficiency anemia in CKD. J Am Soc Nephrol 2008;19(8):1599–605.

12. Singh A, Patel T, Hertel J, et al. Safety of ferumoxytol in patients with anemia and CKD. Am J Kidney Dis 2008;52(5):907–15.

13. Auerbach M, Chertow GM, Rosner M. Ferumoxytol for the treatment of iron deficiency anemia. Expert Rev Hematol 2018;11(10):829–34.

14. Gastrell P, Carrera J, Batchala P, et al. Teaching NeuroImages: diffuse cerebrovascular susceptibility artifact following ferumoxytol infusion. Neurology 2019;93(17):e1662–3.

15. Nguyen KL, Yoshida T, Kathuria-Prakash N, et al. Multicenter safety and practice for off-label diagnostic use of ferumoxytol in MRI. Radiology 2019;293(3):554–64.

16. Wells SA, Schubert T, Motosugi U, et al. Pharmacokinetics of ferumoxytol in the abdomen and pelvis: a dosing study with 1.5- and 3.0-T MRI relaxometry. Radiology 2020;294(1):108–16.

17. Finn JP, Nguyen KL, Han F, et al. Cardiovascular MRI with ferumoxytol. Clin Radiol 2016;71(8):796–806.

18. Hope MD, Hope TA, Zhu C, et al. Vascular imaging with ferumoxytol as a contrast agent. AJR Am J Roentgenol 2015;205(3):W366–73.

19. Cheng JY, Hanneman K, Zhang T, et al. Comprehensive motion-compensated highly accelerated 4D flow MRI with ferumoxytol enhancement for pediatric congenital heart disease. J Magn Reson Imaging 2016;43(6):1355–68.

20. Koh DM, Miao Y, Chinn RJ, et al. MR imaging evaluation of the activity of Crohn's disease. AJR Am J Roentgenol 2001;177(6):1325–32.

21. Roldan-Alzate A, Francois CJ, Wieben O, et al. Emerging applications of abdominal 4D flow MRI. AJR Am J Roentgenol 2016;207(1):58–66.

22. Sugiyama M, Takehara Y, Kawate M, et al. Optimal plane selection for measuring post-prandial blood flow increase within the superior mesenteric artery: analysis using 4D flow and computational fluid dynamics. Magn Reson Med Sci 2020. https://doi.org/10.2463/mrms.mp.2019-0089.

23. Ward EV, Galizia MS, Usman A, et al. Comparison of quiescent inflow single-shot and native space for nonenhanced peripheral MR angiography. J Magn Reson Imaging 2013;38(6):1531–8.

24. Hodnett PA, Ward EV, Davarpanah AH, et al. Peripheral arterial disease in a symptomatic diabetic population: prospective comparison of rapid unenhanced MR angiography (MRA) with contrast-enhanced MRA. AJR Am J Roentgenol 2011;197(6):1466–73.

25. Edelman RR, Sheehan JJ, Dunkle E, et al. Quiescent-interval single-shot unenhanced magnetic resonance angiography of peripheral vascular disease: technical considerations and clinical feasibility. Magn Reson Med 2010;63(4):951–8.

26. Edelman RR, Carr M, Koktzoglou I. Advances in non-contrast quiescent-interval slice-selective (QISS) magnetic resonance angiography. Clin Radiol 2019;74(1):29–36.

27. Bley TA, Francois CJ, Schiebler ML, et al. Non-contrast-enhanced MRA of renal artery stenosis: validation against DSA in a porcine model. Eur Radiol 2016;26(2):547–55.

28. Krishnamurthy R, Cheong B, Muthupillai R. Tools for cardiovascular magnetic resonance imaging. Cardiovasc Diagn Ther 2014;4(2):104–25.

29. Lotz J, Meier C, Leppert A, et al. Cardiovascular flow measurement with phase-contrast MR imaging: basic facts and implementation. Radiographics 2002;22(3):651–71.

30. Markl M, Frydrychowicz A, Kozerke S, et al. 4D flow MRI. J Magn Reson Imaging 2012;36(5):1015–36.

31. Broncano J, Vargas D, Bhalla S, et al. CT and MR imaging of cardiothoracic vasculitis. Radiographics 2018;38(4):997–1021.

32. Kato Y, Terashima M, Ohigashi H, et al. Vessel wall inflammation of Takayasu arteritis detected by contrast-enhanced magnetic resonance imaging: association with disease distribution and activity. PLoS One 2015;10(12):e0145855.

33. Skilton MR, Celermajer DS, Cosmi E, et al. Natural history of atherosclerosis and abdominal aortic intima-media thickness: rationale, evidence, and best practice for detection of atherosclerosis in the young. J Clin Med 2019;8(8):1201.

34. Reis SP, Majdalany BS, AbuRahma AF, et al. ACR appropriateness criteria((R)) pulsatile abdominal mass suspected abdominal aortic aneurysm. J Am Coll Radiol 2017;14(5S):S258–65.

35. Goodall R, Langridge B, Onida S, et al. Median arcuate ligament syndrome. J Vasc Surg 2019. https://doi.org/10.1016/j.jvs.2019.11.012.

36. Eiden S, Beck C, Venhoff N, et al. High-resolution contrast-enhanced vessel wall imaging in patients with suspected cerebral vasculitis: prospective comparison of whole-brain 3D T1 SPACE versus 2D T1 black blood MRI at 3 Tesla. PLoS One 2019;14(3):e0213514.

37. Edelman RR, Flanagan O, Grodzki D, et al. Projection MR imaging of peripheral arterial calcifications. Magn Reson Med 2015;73(5):1939–45.

38. Yoshida T, Nguyen KL, Shahrouki P, et al. Intermodality feature fusion combining unenhanced computed tomography and ferumoxytol-enhanced magnetic resonance angiography for patient-specific vascular mapping in renal impairment. J Vasc Surg 2019. https://doi.org/10.1016/j.jvs.2019.08.240.

39. Padoan R, Crimi F, Felicetti M, et al. Fully integrated ^{18}F-FDG PET/MR in large vessel vasculitis. Q J Nucl Med Mol Imaging 2019. https://doi.org/10.23736/S1824-4785.19.03184-4.

40. Mahmud E, Brocato M, Palakodeti V, et al. Fibromuscular dysplasia of renal arteries: percutaneous revascularization based on hemodynamic assessment with a pressure measurement guidewire. Catheter Cardiovasc Interv 2006;67(3):434–7.

41. Stanley JC, Gewertz BL, Bove EL, et al. Arterial fibrodysplasia. Histopathologic character and current etiologic concepts. Arch Surg 1975;110(5):561–6.

42. Baker-LePain JC, Stone DH, Mattis AN, et al. Clinical diagnosis of segmental arterial mediolysis: differentiation from vasculitis and other mimics. Arthritis Care Res (Hoboken) 2010;62(11):1655–60.

43. Park YJ, Park KB, Kim DI, et al. Natural history of spontaneous isolated superior mesenteric artery dissection derived from follow-up after conservative treatment. J Vasc Surg 2011;54(6):1727–33.

44. Russell CE, Wadhera RK, Piazza G. Mesenteric venous thrombosis. Circulation 2015;131(18):1599–603.

Imaging of Vascular Malformations

Amira Hussein, MD, Nagina Malguria, MD*

KEYWORDS

• Vascular malformations • Capillary • Lymphatic malformations • Venous anomalies • Arteriovenous

KEY POINTS

- The latest classification from International Society for the Study of Vascular Anomalies (ISSVA) divides vascular malformations into simple, combined, vascular malformations of named major vessels and syndromic vascular malformations.
- Simple vascular malformations include high-flow and low-flow vascular malformations.
- Low-flow vascular malformations include venous malformations, capillary malformations, and lymphatic malformations.
- High-flow vascular malformations include arteriovenous malformations and arteriovenous fistulae.

INTRODUCTION

Vascular anomalies (VAs) are a group of lesions that result from errors of vascular embryogenesis.[1] VAs include vascular tumors and vascular malformations, typically present during childhood, and may involve any part of the body.[2] They often pose a diagnostic dilemma, because of the multiplicity of appearances, wide differential diagnosis, and the various classification systems that have been proposed over the years.

The International Society for the Study of Vascular Anomalies (ISSVA) provides the most standardized and accepted classification. The ISSVA classification was first introduced in 1997 and most recently updated in 2018.[3] This classification divides VAs into 2 major categories: (1) vascular tumors, and (2) vascular malformations.[3,4] Vascular tumors are true neoplasms that show rapid postnatal growth and slow regression into late childhood; these include hemangiomata and kaposiform hemangioendothelioma. In contrast, congenital vascular malformations (CVMs) do not regress or enlarge; they grow at the same rate as the child and include arteriovenous malformations (AVMs), arteriovenous fistulae (AVFs), capillary malformations (CMs), venous malformations (VMs), and lymphatic malformations (LMs). In the current version of the ISSVA classification, CVMs are divided into 4 groups: simple malformations, combined malformations, malformations of major named vessels, and malformations associated with other anomalies (syndromic vascular malformation).[3] Based on their flow characteristics, simple vascular malformations are further differentiated into high-flow lesions (AVM and AVF) and low-flow lesions (CM, VM, LM).[5] The 2018 version of the ISSVA classification emphasizes the known genetic mutations associated with CVM, reflecting a growing interest in the genetic basis of vascular malformations (**Tables 1** and **2**).

IMAGING

Gray-scale ultrasonography coupled with color Doppler imaging and spectral analysis is the initial screening imaging modality at some centers for vascular malformation given the low cost, fast and real-time information, and lack of ionizing radiation. However, ultrasonography is limited in its ability to accurately assess large and deep lesions and to detect bone involvement.[6] Contrast-enhanced ultrasonography has been suggested for evaluation of CVMs and has been used for monitoring response to therapy, including microcirculatory changes.[7]

Department of Radiology, Johns Hopkins Hospital, 601 North Caroline Street, Baltimore, MD 21287, USA
* Corresponding author.
E-mail address: nmalgur1@jhmi.edu

Radiol Clin N Am 58 (2020) 815–830
https://doi.org/10.1016/j.rcl.2020.02.003

Table 1
The International Society for the Study of Vascular Anomalies vascular anomalies 2018 classification

VAs				
Vascular Tumors		**Vascular Malformations**		
Benign	Simple	Combined	CVMs of major named vessels	Syndromic CVMs
1 Congenital hemangioma				
2 Infantile hemangioma	High flow	1 CM-VM	Anomalies of	See Table 2
3 Epithelioid hemangioma	1 AVM	2 CM-LM	1 Origin	
4 Spindle cell hemangioma	2 AVF	3 LM-VM	2 Course	
5 Tufted angioma		4 CM-AVM		
6 Pyogenic granuloma		5 CM-LM-AVM	3 Number	
7 Others		6 Others		
Locally malignant	Low flow		4 Length	
1 Kaposiform hemangioendothelioma	1 VM			
	2 LM		5 Diameter	
2 Retiform hemangioendothelioma	3 CM		6 Valves	
			7 Connection	
3 Others			8 Persistence (of embryonal vessel)	
Malignant				
1 Angiosarcoma				
2 Epithelioid hemangioendothelioma				
3 Others				

From ISSVA Classification of Vascular Anomalies ©2018 International Society for the Study of Vascular Anomalies Available at "issva.org/classification" Accessed [10/16/2018]; with permission.

Magnetic resonance (MR) imaging is the most valuable modality for imaging vascular malformation because of its high temporal and contrast resolution, which allows accurate assessment of CVMs and their relation to the surrounding structures.[8] The ability to characterize flow dynamics by MR imaging permits differentiation of high-flow and low-flow CVMs and enables discrimination between CVMs and other vascular lesions. MR imaging has also been used for

Table 2
Clinical syndromes associated with vascular malformations

Clinical Syndrome	Vascular Malformation	Other Manifestations	Mutation
Sturge-Weber	CM; face, trigeminal nerve distribution	Gyral atrophy, glaucoma	GNAQ
Klippel-Trénaunay	CM, LM, VM; cutaneous and soft tissue	Overgrowth of soft tissue and bone, usually limited to 1 limb	PIK3CA
Parkes Weber	CM, VM, AVM; cutaneous and soft tissue	Overgrowth of soft tissue and bone, usually limited to 1 limb	RASA1
Proteus syndrome	CM, VM, LM; soft tissue ± visceral	Disproportionate progressive overgrowth of hands or feet	AKT1
Maffucci syndrome	VM; soft tissue	Multiple enchondromas in the hands and feet, ±chondrosarcoma	IDHH1/IDH2
CLOVES syndrome	CM, VM, LM, AVM	Lipomatosis, nevi, scoliosis, skeletal anomalies hands and feet	PICK3CA

Abbreviation: CLOVES, congenital lipomatous overgrowth, vascular malformations, epidermal nevi, spinal/skeletal anomalies/scoliosis.
From ISSVA Classification of Vascular Anomalies ©2018 International Society for the Study of Vascular Anomalies Available at "issva.org/classification" Accessed [10/16/2018]; with permission.

treatment planning and assessment of treatment success.[9] A comprehensive MR imaging examination should include contrast-enhanced conventional MR imaging and dynamic contrast-enhanced MR angiography (MRA), such as time-resolved imaging of contrast kinetics (TRICKS) or time-resolved angiography with interleaved stochastic trajectories (TWIST). The protocol for vascular malformations at our institution includes triplanar T2-weighted images with fat saturation, precontrast axial T1-weighted images, and post-contrast triplanar T1-weighted images with fat saturation. Because flow characteristics (arterial, venous, both arterial and venous, none) are essential to the classification of vascular malformations, we obtain our dynamic contrast-enhanced images with a temporal resolution of 1 to 1.5 seconds to allow separation of arterial and venous phases. Other investigators have recommended optional three-dimensional arterial spin labeling sequences for hemangiomas and arteriovenous shunting as well, and diffusion-weighted imaging to rule out other lesions and tumors when the diagnosis is uncertain[10] (Table 3).

Radiography and contrast-enhanced computed tomography (CT) are not routinely used for the diagnosis of a vascular malformation owing to the use of ionizing radiation and the lower temporal resolution compared with MR imaging; however, radiographs and CT may detect phleboliths, calcification, and bone involvement.[11–13] CT may be used as an alternative imaging for patients who cannot undergo MR imaging.

SIMPLE VASCULAR MALFORMATIONS
Low-Flow Malformations

Capillary malformation
CMs, usually referred to as port-wine stain, are found in 0.5% of the population and affect the skin capillaries.[14] They commonly present at birth as pink or red macules that do not involute. Most of these lesions involve the face and tend to be in the trigeminal nerve distribution.[14] The lesion enlarges and darkens as a child grows older, resulting in a cobblestone appearance.[15] Central nervous system (CNS) involvement can occur, particularly in association with lesions in the V1 or midline distribution. The risk of having Sturge-Weber syndrome increases to 25% when half of the face, including the ophthalmic division of the trigeminal nerve, is involved, and increases to 33% when both sides of the face are involved.[15]

Most CMs can be diagnosed by a physical examination. With high-frequency ultrasonography transducers, CMs can appear as superficial hypoechoic areas that vary in depth from 0.2 mm to 3.7 mm,[16] with increased vascularity on color Doppler imaging.[6,16] If MR imaging is performed, the lesion may appear as subtle signal abnormality within the subcutaneous fat with skin thickening.[17] MR imaging and CT are helpful in evaluation for CNS involvement and may detect progressive gyral atrophy, gyral enhancement, enhancement of ipsilateral choroid plexus, and cortical calcification (Fig. 1). Abnormal cortical veins and contrast stasis can be seen on cerebral angiography.[15]

Lymphatic malformation
LMs consist of cystic dilated lymphatic channels and spaces without connection to the lymphatic system. They are described as macrocystic, microcystic, or combined,[15] depending on the appearance of the cystic spaces. LMs are usually apparent at birth or by 2 years of age and grow with the child. They can affect any area of the body, with about 70% of all reported cases being found in the head and neck as soft, spongy masses.[18] LMs can potentially cause functional impairment of nearby structures and disfigurement of affected areas. Generalized LM can be seen in generalized lymphatic anomaly (GLA) and Gorham-Stout disease (GSD). GLA is characterized by multifocal LMs involving several organ systems as well as the bones, whereas the LMs in GSD mainly involve the bones.[19,20] Additional features of GLA and GSD include splenic cysts, hepatic cysts, and pleural effusions.[20]

On ultrasonography, macrocystic LMs typically appear as multiple, anechoic cystic spaces with thin internal septations. Varying degrees of internal floating echoes can be seen in the cystic spaces if the lesion is complicated with hemorrhage or infection (Fig. 2). Heterogeneous echogenic clots as well as fluid-fluid levels in the lesion can be related to intralesional hemorrhage but are not pathognomonic to LMs and can be seen with VMs and other VAs.[21] On color flow Doppler imaging, macrocystic LMs often show absence of flow within the cystic spaces with no flow or low vascular density within the septa (both arterial and venous flow).[6] Microcystic LM often appears as an ill-defined echogenic mass with scant tiny cysts, or no cysts. Color Doppler imaging usually shows no or low flow within the lesion.[8] Hyperemia of the adjacent soft tissues can be present in cases of superimposed infection.[6]

CT may be used as an alternative to MR imaging if not available or contraindicated. Most LMs present on CT as homogeneous cystic lesions. Heterogeneous density within the lesion may reflect the presence of proteinaceous or hemorrhagic components within the lesion.[6]

MR is the preferred method to assess LMs and is of particular value in evaluating the anatomy of

Table 3
Magnetic resonance imaging and ultrasonography findings for simple vascular malformation

	Venous	Lymphatic	Capillary	AVM	AVF
Appearance	Serpentine tubular structures or dilated channels	Septated lobulated mass, microcytic or microcytic	Skin-thickness lesion	No well-defined mass Enlarged feeding arteries and draining vein + nidus	No well-defined mass Enlarged draining vein, no nidus
T1WI	Intermediate	Low	Low	Intermediate	Intermediate
T2WI	High	High	Slight high	High	High
GRE	Intermediate	Low, intermediate, high	—	High	High
Flow voids on SE	No	No	No	Yes	Yes
Fluid-fluid levels	Uncommon	Common	No	No	No
Enhancement	No arterial or early venous enhancement, slow gradual diffuse enhancement on delayed images	Rim and septal enhancement if macrocystic; no significant or slight diffuse enhancement if microcystic	Faint subcutaneous enhancement	Early enhancement of enlarged feeding arteries and nidus with shunting to draining veins	Early enhancement of enlarged feeding arteries with shunting to draining veins, no nidus
Ultrasonography	Heterogeneous, compressible	Variable echogenicity, noncompressible	Subtle low echogenicity	Low echogenicity	Low echogenicity
Color Doppler 1 Vascular density 2 Spectral Analysis	Low Venous flow, or sometimes no flow	No or low flow in the septa Both arterial and venous flow in the septa	Low to moderate	High Arteries: high velocity, low resistance, spectral broadening Veins: pulsatile venous flow Nidus: turbulent flow	High Arteries: high velocity, low resistance, spectral broadening Veins: pulsatile venous flow
Others	Phleboliths	—	—	Calcifications	—

Abbreviations: GRE, gradient recalled echo; SE, spin echo; T1WI, T1-weighted imaging; T2WI, T2-weighted imaging.

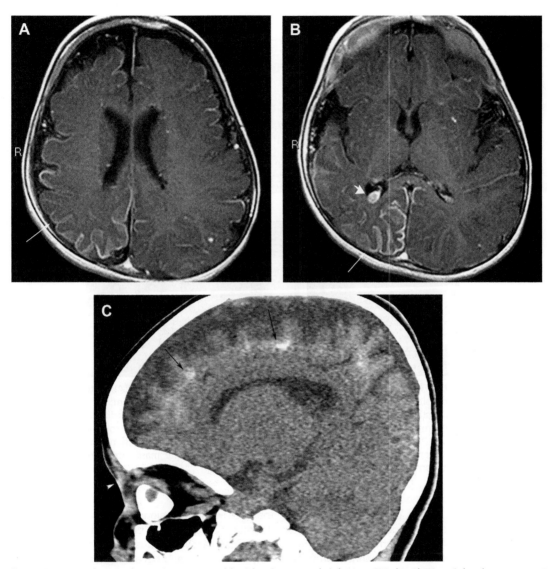

Fig. 1. Sturge-Weber syndrome in a 1-year-old with seizures and right eye CM. (*A, B*) T1-weighted postcontrast axial images reveal atrophy of the right parietal and occipital lobes with gyriform contrast enhancement (*white long arrows*). Note asymmetric enlargement of the right choroid plexus (*short white arrow*). (*C*) Sagittal CT image shows cortical atrophy and calcifications (*black arrows*). Note right scleral prosthesis and minimal skin thickening of the right eye corresponding with CM (*arrowhead*).

deep-seated and extensive lesions. The classic appearance of a macrocystic LM is a lobulated, multiloculated mass; in some lesions, involvement of multiple planes may be seen (see **Fig. 2**). These lesions show intermediate to low signal intensity on T1-weighted images and high signal intensity on T2-weighted images and short-tau inversion recovery (STIR) sequences. Fluid-fluid levels are common[9,17] (see **Fig. 2**). Faint septal and capsular enhancements are noted after gadolinium administration (see **Fig. 2**). Microcystic LM usually reveals low T1 signal and increased signal on T2-weighted imaging, with small or no perceptible

cysts and absence of or mild postcontrast enhancement (see **Fig. 2**). However, if a dense cluster of microcysts is present, the lesion may show diffuse enhancement. In cases of infection or inflammation of the LMs, edema and enhancement of the adjacent soft tissue may be present.[9,17]

Venous malformation

VMs are the most common of vascular malformations.[15] VMs result from errors in the development of the venous network, leading to dilated and dysfunctional veins that are deficient in smooth

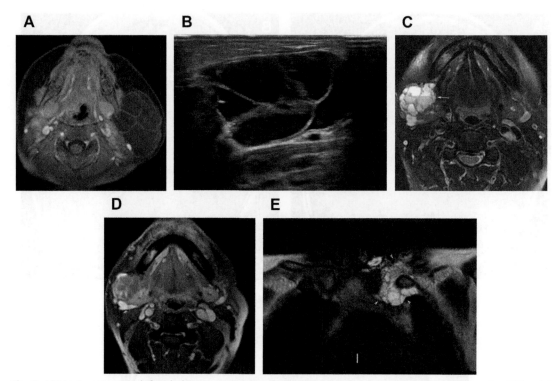

Fig. 2. LM in 3 patients. A left-sided macrocytic submandibular LM in a 1-year-old boy: (*A*) postcontrast T1 axial image shows lobulated lesion containing large cysts with septal and capsular enhancement; (*B*) ultrasonography shows a multiloculated cystic lesion with low-level echoes. A mixed LM of the right submandibular region in a 62-year-old: (*C*) T2 axial MR imaging shows multiple locules of different sizes (4 mm to 2 cm), some of which contain fluid-fluid levels (*arrow*); (*D*) axial postcontrast-enhanced T1 MR imaging shows septal enhancement. A microcytic LM in a 10 year old presenting as an infiltrative supraclavicular/retroclavicular mass containing clusters of T2 hyperintense microcysts (*arrowheads*) (*E*).

muscle cells. These lesions may be focal, multifocal, or infiltrative and are commonly found in the head and neck (40%), extremities (40%), and trunk (20%).[22,23] Based on their connection with the deep venous system, VMs were further subclassified by Dubois and colleagues[24] and Puig and colleagues[25] as (1) type I, isolated lesions without venous connection; (2) type II, lesions that drain into normal veins; (3) type III, lesions with drainage into dysplastic veins; and (4) type IV, lesions composed of venous ectasia. Type I and type II respond to local sclerotherapy and type III and type IV may need systemic treatment.[2] Although VMs are present at birth, they grow with the child and may become more evident later in life. Symptoms from VMs vary depending on their location and extension and include swelling, disfigurement, pain, bleeding, and functional impairment.[23] The superficial VMs present at clinical examination as compressible soft tissue swelling or discrete masses that increase in size with Valsalva maneuver and in dependent positioning.[26] Rapid enlargement of the lesions may

be seen with intralesional thrombosis and during hormonal changes of puberty and pregnancy. Intramuscular VMs cause greater limitation of physical activity and have a higher rate of pain as the presenting symptom because of increased risk of local intravascular coagulation and thrombosis.[11,23]

Most VMs reveal heterogeneous echotexture on gray-scale ultrasonography imaging and are hypoechoic relative to the surrounding soft tissues.[27] Fifty percent of these lesions contain hypoechoic venous channels and only 16% of cases show hyperechoic shadowing phleboliths. The focal superficial lesions are well defined and lobulated and are compressible when pressure is applied to the transducer, whereas the diffuse form of VMs manifest as multiple varicosities infiltrating various tissue planes.[6] Monophasic venous flow within the VMs is the typical finding on color Doppler imaging.[8] However, flow may not be detected in some lesions with internal thrombosis or very slow flow.[6]

CT and conventional radiography have limited roles in VM diagnosis. Phleboliths related to thrombosis and calcifications within the lesions can be detected by both CT and radiographs.[26] Bone involvement can be seen on both modalities as osteolysis, deformity, hypoplasia, and periosteal reaction. The classic appearance of VM on CT is a hypodense mass with tubular enhancement on postcontrast imaging.[26]

MR imaging is considered a valuable imaging modality for diagnosis of VMs and is particularly useful in pretreatment planning and posttreatment evaluation of the diffuse lesions. VMs are typically hypointense on T1-weighted images and hyperintense on T2-weighted images and fluid-sensitive sequences (eg, STIR) (Figs. 3 and 4). Occasionally, high T1 signal intensity can be detected within the lesion and is likely related to intralesional thrombosis, hemorrhage, or fat.[28] Fluid-fluid levels can be present but are less common compared with LMs. Phleboliths, the key finding in VMs, are shown as scattered rounded areas of low signal intensity in all pulse sequences that can be further confirmed on gradient recalled echo imaging (see Fig. 3). Phleboliths are also reported in some cases of LM and spindle cell hemangioendothelioma.[28] Absence of flow void on spin-echo (SE) sequences differentiates VMs from high-flow vascular malformations. On contrast-enhanced MRA, VMs show absence of arterial and early venous enhancement and slow gradual filling with contrast on delayed venous imaging (see Fig. 3). Diffuse enhancement of the venous channels on delayed postcontrast T1-weighted images is characteristic of VMs (see Fig. 4). Delayed postcontrast images are also helpful in treatment planning by detecting any connection between VMs and the deep venous system, which increases the risk of deep venous thrombosis.[29]

High-Flow Malformations

AVMs and AVFs form one-third of vascular malformations and result from abnormal connection or channel formation between arteries and veins during early development. In AVFs, single or multiple abnormal direct connections are present between arteries and veins without an intervening capillary bed, whereas in AVMs there is a low-resistance nidus connected to multiple feeding arteries and draining veins.[11] The fast blood shunting from the arteries to the veins that occurs in AVMs and AVFs deprives the distant soft tissues of blood supply and does not allow a gradual pressure decrease from the high arterial pressure to the low pressure on the venous side.[30] The clinical staging system by Schobinger divides AVMs into 4 phases: (1) quiescence phase, in which AVM manifests as an area of skin warmth and blush; (2) expansion phase, in which pulsatile lesions have palpable bruit; (3) destruction phase, reflecting skin ulceration and steal leading to distal ischemia and pain; and (4) decompensation phase, complicated by decompensation or high-output cardiac failure.[18] The lesions may be sporadic or multiple, particularly in hereditary hemorrhagic telangiectasia (HHT). In many

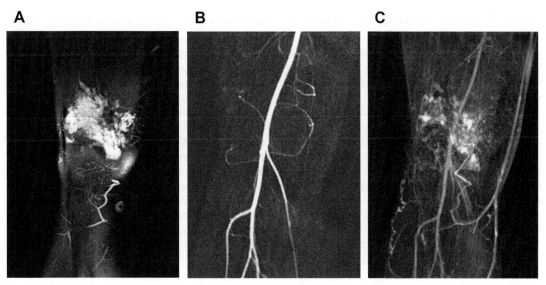

Fig. 3. VM of the lower extremity (knee) appears as a T2 hyperintense, multilobulated, septated mass (A). Dynamic time-resolved MRA (TWIST) shows no contrast enhancement on arterial phase (B) and progressive enhancement on delayed venous phase (C). Type II VM.

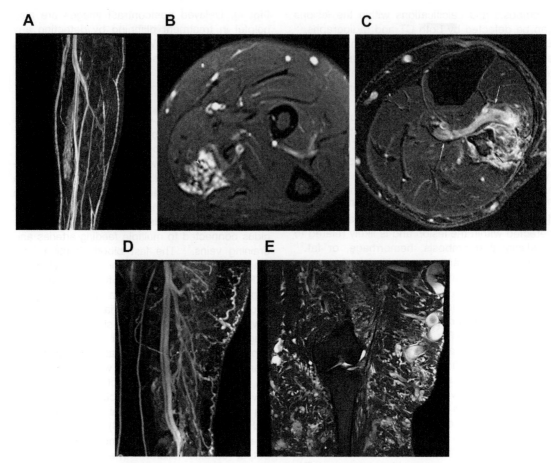

Fig. 4. Various imaging appearances of VMs in 4 different patients. Type II VM in the forearm that drains into normal veins (as shown on contrast-enhanced MRA) (*A*), and shows T2 hyperintensity and multiple phleboliths seen as signal voids in the lesion on axial STIR image (*arrowheads*) (*B*). Type III VM of the leg draining into a dysplastic vein (*white arrows*) with infiltration of multiple planes and intraosseous extension (*black arrow*) on T1 postcontrast axial image (*C*). Type IV VM in 2 different patients composed of predominantly ectatic veins, diffusely infiltrating the lower extremity on coronal contrast-enhanced MRA (*D*) and coronal T2 images (*E*).

patients with HHT, the first symptom is epistaxis. Gastrointestinal bleeding is noted in about 25% to 30% of patients. Pulmonary AVFs are present in 30% of patients.[31]

On ultrasonography, AVMs appear as conglomerates of tortuous and enlarged vascular channels with a dilated draining vein. The lesion shows high vascular density with multidirectional flow on Doppler ultrasonography. Spectral Doppler analysis reveals low resistance and spectral broadening in the supplying artery, pulsatile flow with high velocities in the draining vein, and turbulent flow at the connecting channel.[6]

CT shows serpentine and enlarged feeding arteries with early venous filling caused by shunting.[26]

AVMs and AVFs show intermediate signal on T1-weighted images and high signal on T2-weighted images. Flow voids are detected on SE sequences,

with corresponding high signal within vessels on gradient echo sequences (**Figs. 5** and **6**). Postcontrast imaging reveals arterial enhancement (see **Fig. 5**). MRA and dynamic sequences are useful in showing the high-flow nature of the malformation with early venous filling and aid in identifying the feeding artery and draining veins.[32] Time-of-flight sequences, and more recently four-dimensional-flow MRA, are used for evaluation of intracranial AVMs, in the assessment of the feeding artery, the nidus, and the draining vein, but cerebral angiography remains the definitive tool for evaluation of intracranial AVMs[33] (see **Fig. 5**).

Pitfalls and Differential Diagnosis

Peripheral nerve sheath tumors

Peripheral nerve sheath tumor (PNST) typically manifests as a low T1 and high T2 signal intensity

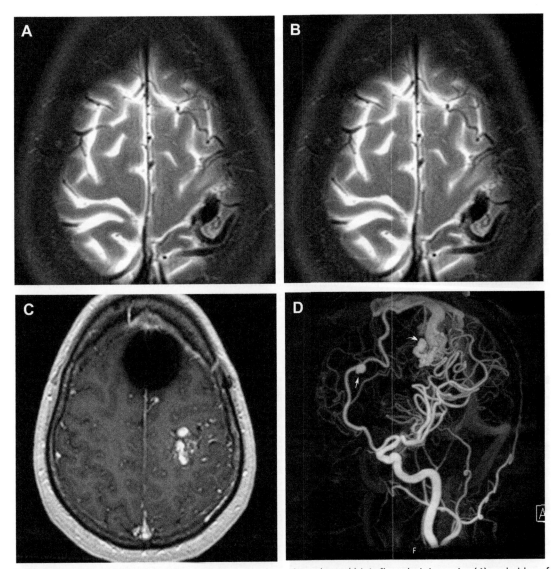

Fig. 5. Left parietal AVM. T2-weighted axial images show the enlarged high-flow draining veins (*A*) and nidus of the AVM as signal voids (*B*). Postcontrast axial T1 image reveals contrast filling of the nidus (*C*). Conventional angiography shows nidus (*curved arrow*), enlarged anterior and middle cerebral feeding arteries, draining veins, and flow-related anterior cerebral artery aneurysm (*straight arrow*) (*D*).

fusiform mass that shows internal fascicular bundles and has splayed fat tissue around it; it is located along the peripheral nerves or the nerve roots.[34] Some PNSTs share imaging characteristics with CVMs, including (1) PNSTs with internal hemorrhage or necrosis may show cystic areas with fluid-fluid levels mimicking LMs and VMs; (2) PNSTs with target sign (peripheral hyperintensity, central low intensity) on fluid-sensitive MR imaging may be confused with VMs with central hypointense thrombus (**Fig. 7**); (3) plexiform-type neurofibromas reveal bag-of-worms appearance resembling dilated vessels within CVMs on T1-weighted and fluid-sensitive MR images (see

Fig. 7); (4) diffuse-type neurofibromas may contain ectatic low-flow vessels and vivid and homogeneous contrast enhancement, as can be found in VMs.[23]

A target sign seen with PNST will reverse on postcontrast MR imaging because of delayed central enhancement that does not occur in VMs.[35] Dynamic time-resolved MR imaging and color flow Doppler provide information about the hemodynamic characteristics of the CVMs that helps in differentiating them from PNSTs. Additional differentiating criteria on MR imaging and ultrasonography include presence of phleboliths, lesion compressibility when pressure is applied to the

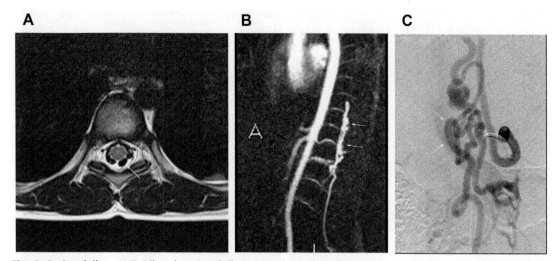

Fig. 6. Perimedullary AVF. Dilated perimedullary veins (*arrow*) as flow voids on T2-weighted axial image (*A*). Dilated intersegmental arteries and perimedullary veins (*arrows*) on MRA (*B*). Conventional angiography shows supply by the left T12 intersegmental artery and drainage through the perimedullary veins (*arrows*) (*C*).

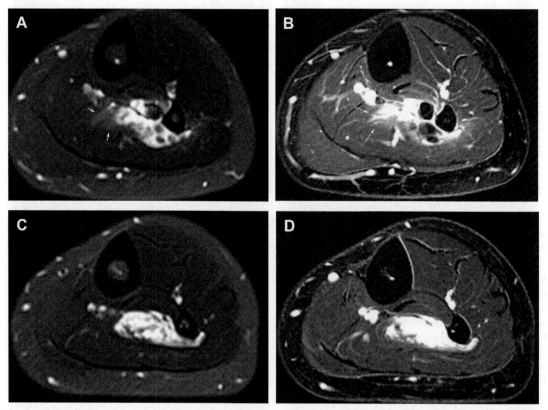

Fig. 7. VM in the lower extremity after percutaneous sclerotherapy. Axial T2-weighted MR images acquired at 3 months after treatment shows perilesional hyperintensity (*short arrow*) (*A*) as well as postcontrast enhancement (*long arrows*) (*B*) termed pseudoprogression, which disappeared on the follow-up axial T2 (*C*) and axial postcontrast T1 scan (*D*) obtained 1 year later. Note intralesional hypointensity related to sclerotherapy (*arrowhead in A*).

ultrasonography probe, and enlargement after tourniquet application in VMs, which are not features of PNSTs.[23,27]

Hemangioma and Other Vascular Tumors

Both hemangioma and high-flow vascular malformations show arterial and venous waveforms on Doppler ultrasonography, flow voids on T1-weighted and T2-weighted images, high signal within vessels on gradient echo sequences, and arterial enhancement on postgadolinium imaging. The differentiation between the 2 entities is based on a lack of associated mass in high-flow vascular malformations, which is a feature of hemangioma. Distinction between other vascular tumors (including hamartomas, hemangioendothelioma, and congenital fibrosarcoma) and vascular malformations is also based on detection of a mass in vascular tumors but not with vascular malformation. However, some investigators report cases of CVMs that presented on sonography and MR imaging with a small soft tissue mass.[36,37] This finding may be related to the presence of fibrofatty proliferation in CVMs that mimics some vascular tumors.[8] Another potential explanation is Masson tumor (intravascular papillary endothelial hyperplasia) seen in some VMs as a result of stasis and intralesional clotting, leading to intraluminal capillary ingrowth forming papillary projections in the vascular channels. On imaging, these lesions show a solid component and internal arterial and capillary flow.[6]

Cystic lesions and cystic tumors

In contrast with LMs, which are almost always multiloculated, dermoid and epidermoid cysts show a thicker capsule and contain no or minimal septations. Dermoid cysts reveal signal dropout on fat saturation sequences, a feature that differentiates it from LMs, which do not have fat. Cutaneous ciliated cysts are mainly unilocular and sometimes difficult to differentiate from LMs. Other ciliated cysts (including bronchogenic, thymic, enteric, and thyroglossal cysts) are differentiated from LMs based on their classic locations.[6,38]

The presence of fat and/or calcifications is the key for the diagnosis of a teratoma. Occasionally, some teratomas do not have macroscopic fat or calcium and may be difficult to differentiate from LMs. In other partially cystic neoplasms (eg, epithelioid sarcoma, angiomatoid fibrous histiocytoma, and synovial sarcoma), the presence of soft tissue and/or thick nodular septations is the main differentiating feature from LMs[38] (**Fig. 8**).

TREATMENT AND POSTTREATMENT IMAGING

The management of vascular malformation is mainly expectant with both noninvasive and invasive treatment of symptomatic lesions. Lesions located in the head and neck region may need special attention because they can obstruct critical structures such as the visual axis or the airway.[15]

A   **B**

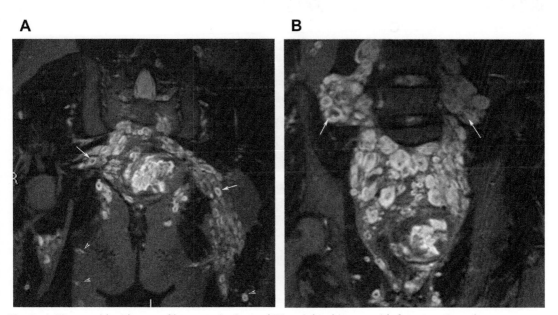

Fig. 8. A 22-year-old with neurofibromatosis. Coronal T2-weighted image with fat saturations shows numerous neurofibromas as tubular hyperintensities (bag of worms) in abdomen, pelvis, and bilateral lower extremities, many of which show target sign (*arrows*). Note multiple additional soft tissue neurofibromas (*arrowheads*) (*A, B*).

Sclerotherapy is the treatment of choice for VM (particularly types I and II) and macrocytic LM with surgical resection being the second-line therapy.[26] Sclerosing agents include STS, polidocanol, and absolute alcohol.[4,15] Access to the vascular malformation is generally acquired by direct puncture, using ultrasonography or MR imaging guidance. The process is repeated depending on the size of the malformation, and large VMs may require coil embolization or balloon occlusion, in addition to sclerotherapy. Sclerotherapy has good to excellent results depending on the size and definition of the treated lesion.[10,11]

CMs are commonly treated with ablative treatment such as pulsed-dye laser, which uses a light beam to gradually destroy the dilated blood vessels. Many CMs lighten and some (about 15%) disappear.[26] Surgery is reserved for lesions that are refractory to ablative treatment or are causing significant disfigurement.[15]

Transcatheter embolization by angiography is the treatment of choice of high-flow vascular malformation; however, it is more challenging and less

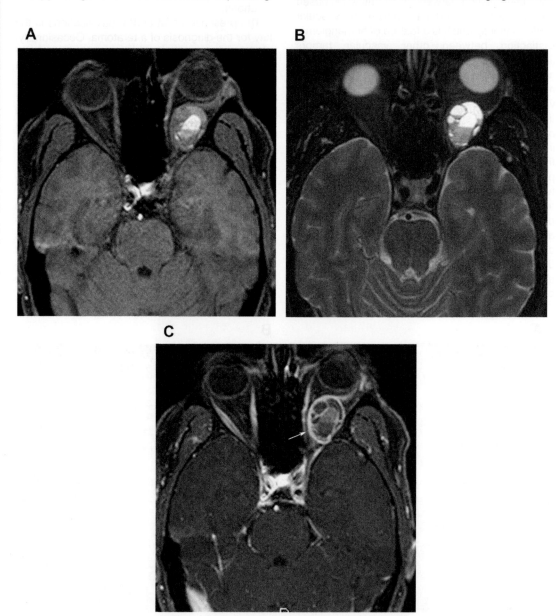

Fig. 9. Hemangiopericytoma. A 50-year-old with left orbital multicystic lesion containing blood products and fluid-fluid levels, mimicking LM on axial T1-weighted (*A*) and axial T2-weighted images (*B*) through the orbits. Note the thick capsular enhancement on T1-weighted postcontrast image, which is not a feature of LM (*arrow*) (*C*).

successful in AVM compared with AVF because of recruitment of new vessels, and resection is often required. Embolization of AVF is done by using coils or occlusion devices such as Amplatzer vascular plug. Embolization of AVM is obtained by filling the nidus with liquid embolic agent via the feeding vessels. A commonly used embolic agent is n-butyl cyanoacrylate (n-BCA), known as superglue. Alternatively, particulate agents, such as polyvinyl alcohol, may be used.[26]

MR imaging is a helpful modality for evaluation of treatment success and is useful for long-term management decisions. MR imaging of treated AVM reveals thrombosis of the nidus caused by embolization. Early venous filling related to shunting may be reduced or absent on the posttreatment scan.[9,39] Sclerotherapy causes thrombosis of the CVMs leading to heterogeneous signal intensity on both T1-weighted and T2-weighted images and lack of postcontrast enhancement (Fig. 9).

If follow-up MR imaging is performed early in the posttreatment phase, peripheral high T2 signal intensity with marked postcontrast enhancement may be observed as a result of inflammatory changes induced by the sclerotic agent (pseudoprogression) (see Fig. 9). These changes may persist for up to 3 months and disappear on the subsequent scans with progressive shrinking of the malformation.[9,39] Spectral Doppler sonography can also be used to monitor response to therapy.[40]

COMBINED VASCULAR MALFORMATION

In combined-type vascular malformation, there are 2 or more simple vascular malformations incorporated in 1 lesion. Some of these lesions are associated with a cutaneous CM and an underlying VM, LM, or AVM, or a VM with an LM (Fig. 10).[41]

VASCULAR MALFORMATION OF NAMED VESSEL

Malformations of major named vessels involve any large-caliber vessel and consist of anomalies in the origin, course, number, length, diameter (aplasia, hypoplasia, ectasia/aneurysm) or valves.

SYNDROMIC VASCULAR MALFORMATIONS

Syndromic VMs are a group of syndromes manifested by vascular malformation and caused by genetic mutations in most cases.[3] Some of the named syndromes are described later and a more comprehensive list is provided in Table 2.

Overgrowth Syndromes with Complex Vascular Malformation

These syndromes are composed of extremity overgrowth and vascular malformation.

CLOVES (congenital lipomatous overgrowth, vascular malformations, epidermal nevi, spinal/skeletal anomalies/scoliosis) syndrome presents at birth with truncal, nonprogressive lipomatous masses in association with vascular malformations, including capillary, lymphatic, venous, and arteriovenous (geographic stains). Skeletal anomalies in these patients are hand and feet deformities (macrodactyly, sandal-gap toe deformity) and scoliosis. There is increased risk of Wilms tumor in patients with CLOVES syndrome (3.3%).[42] Klippel-Trénaunay syndrome is characterized by a triad of cutaneous CM (port-wine stain), lymphatic anomalies, and VM in association with variable overgrowth of soft tissue and bone, usually limited to 1 limb (Fig. 11). Parkes Weber syndrome is similar to Klippel-Trénaunay syndrome but features formation of AVMs and no LMs.[6] Proteus syndrome is manifested by

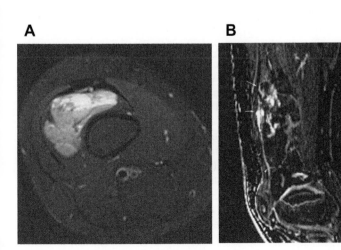

A **B**

Fig. 10. Combined VM-LM of the lower extremity consists of a lower cystic lymphatic component with fluid-fluid levels on axial T2-weighted image (*A*). Sagittal postcontrast image (*B*) shows an upper linear enhancing venous component (*arrows*) and the lower cystic lymphatic component (*arrowheads*).

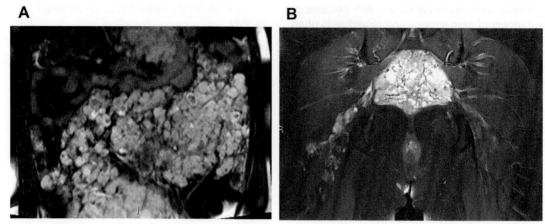

Fig. 11. Klippel-Trénaunay syndrome. Coronal T2-weighted MR images show extensive VM involvement of the abdomen, pelvis, and right lower extremity as tubular hyperintense lesions (A, B).

asymmetric and disproportionate progressive overgrowth of hands or feet. Forty-percent of patients have extensive soft tissue CMs, LMs, and VMs that may be associated with visceral vascular malformations. Other cutaneous findings include multiple nevi and lipomas.[43]

Maffucci Syndrome

Maffucci syndrome consists of multiple enchondromas in the hands and feet, combined with VMs and LMs that present at birth or at early childhood. It is associated with a substantial risk of malignant transformation of enchondroma to chondrosarcoma later in life.[11]

Sturge-Weber Syndrome

Sturge-Weber syndrome is characterized by a triad of facial CM (port-wine stain), seizures, and glaucoma. Progressive gyral atrophy and calcifications can be detected on CT scan and MR imaging[15] (see **Fig. 1**).

SUMMARY

Vascular malformation comprises a variety of lesions that share clinical and imaging features with other pathologic entities. Understanding the classification of vascular malformations, imaging features, and potentially associated syndromes helps make an accurate diagnosis and facilitates management.

DISCLOSURE

The authors have no disclosures.

REFERENCES

1. Cohen MM Jr. Vascular update: morphogenesis, tumors, malformations, and molecular dimensions. Am J Med Genet A 2006;140(19):2013–38.
2. Snyder E, Puttgen K, Mitchell S, et al. Magnetic resonance imaging of the soft tissue vascular anomalies in torso and extremities in children: an update with 2014 International Society for the Study of Vascular Anomalies Classification. J Comput Assist Tomogr 2018;42(2):167–77.
3. ISSVA Classification of Vascular Anomalies ©2018 International Society for the Study of Vascular Anomalies. Available at: issva.org/classification. Accessed October 16, 2018.
4. Mulliken JB, Glowacki J. Hemangiomas and vascular malformations in infants and children: a classification based on endothelial characteristics. Plast Reconstr Surg 1982;69:412–22.
5. Jackson IT, Carreño R, Potparic Z, et al. Hemangiomas, vascular malformations, and lymphovenous malformations: classification and methods of treatment. Plast Reconstr Surg 1993;91(7): 1216–30.
6. Johnson CM, Navarro OM. Clinical and sonographic features of pediatric soft tissue vascular anomalies part 2: vascular malformations tissue vascular anomalies. Pediatr Radiol 2017;47:1196–208.
7. Wiesinger I, Jung W, Zausig N, et al. Evaluation of dynamic effects of therapy-induced changes in microcirculation after percutaneous treatment of vascular malformations using contrast-enhanced ultrasound (CEUS) and time intensity curve (TIC) analyses. Clin Hemorheol Microcirc 2018;69(1–2): 45–57.
8. Dubois J, Alison M. Vascular anomalies: what a radiologist needs to know. Pediatr Radiol 2010;40(6): 895–905.

9. Flors L, Leiva-Salinas C, Maged I, et al. MR imaging of soft-tissue vascular malformations: diagnosis, classification, and therapy follow-up. Radiographics 2011;31:1321–40.

10. Mamlouk MD, Nicholson AD, Cooke DL, et al. Tips and tricks to optimize MRI protocols for cutaneous vascular anomalies. Clin Imaging 2017;45:71–80.

11. Nosher JL, Murillo PG, Liszewski M, et al. Vascular anomalies: a pictorial review of nomenclature, diagnosis and treatment. World J Radiol 2014;6(9):677–92.

12. Hyodoh H, Hori M, Akiba H, et al. Peripheral vascular malformations: imaging, treatment approaches, and therapeutic issues. Radiographics 2005;25(Suppl 1):S159–71.

13. Behr G, Mulliken JB, Glowacki J. Vascular anomalies: hemangiomas and beyond—part 1, fast-flow lesions. AJR Am J Roentgenol 2013;200(2):414–22.

14. Colletti G, Valassina D, Bertossi D, et al. Contemporary management of vascular malformations. J Oral Maxillofac Surg 2014;72(3):510–28.

15. Cox JA, Bartlett E, Lee EI. Vascular malformations: a review. Semin Plast Surg 2014;28(2):58–63.

16. Troilius A, Svendsen G, Ljunggren B. Ultrasound investigation of port wine stains. Acta Derm Venereol 2000;80:196–9.

17. Moukaddam H, Pollak J, Haims AH. MRI characteristics and classification of peripheral vascular malformations and tumors. Skeletal Radiol 2009;38(6):535–47.

18. Garzon MC, Huang JT, Enjolras O, et al. Vascular malformations: Part I. J Am Acad Dermatol 2007;56:353–70 [quiz: 371–4].

19. Lala S, Mulliken JB, Alomari AI, et al. Gorham-Stout disease and generalized lymphatic anomaly–clinical, radiologic, and histologic differentiation. Skeletal Radiol 2013;42:917–24.

20. Rasalkar DD, Chu WC. Generalized cystic lymphangiomatosis. Pediatr Radiol 2010;40(Suppl 1):S47.

21. Dubois J, Garel L. Imaging and therapeutic approach of hemangiomas and vascular malformations in the pediatric age group. Pediatr Radiol 1999;29:879–93.

22. Loose DA. Surgical management of venous malformations. Phlebology 2007;22:276–82.

23. Olivieri B, White CL, Restrepo R, et al. Low-flow vascular malformation pitfalls: from clinical examination to practical imaging evaluation— part 2, venous malformation mimickers. AJR Am J Roentgenol 2016;206:952–62.

24. Dubois J, Soulez G, Oliva VL, et al. Soft-tissue venous malformations in adult patients: imaging and therapeutic issues. Radiographics 2001;21:1519–31.

25. Puig S, Casati B, Staudenherz A, et al. Vascular low-flow malformations in children: current concepts for classification, diagnosis and therapy. Eur J Radiol 2005;53:35–45.

26. Mulligan PR, Prajapati HJS, Martin LG, et al. Vascular anomalies: classification, imaging characteristics and implications for interventional radiology treatment approaches. Br J Radiol 2014; 87: 20130392.

27. Trop I, Dubois J, Guibaud L, et al. Soft-tissue venous malformations in pediatric and young adult patients: diagnosis with Doppler US. Radiology 1999;212: 841–5.

28. Ernemann U, Kramer U, Miller S, et al. Current concepts in the classification, diagnosis and treatment of vascular anomalies. Eur J Radiol 2010;75(1):2–11.

29. Herborn CU, Goyen M, Lauenstein TC, et al. Comprehensive time- resolved MRI of peripheral vascular malformations. AJR Am J Roentgenol 2003;181(3):729–35.

30. Frieden I, Enjolras O, Esterly N. Vascular birthmarks and other abnormalities of blood vessels and lymphatics. In: Schacner LA, Hanson RC, editors. Pediatric dermatology. 3rd edition. St Louis (MO): Mosby Publishers; 2003. p. 833–62.

31. Dakeishi M, Shioya T, Wada Y, et al. Genetic epidemiology of hereditary hemorrhagic telangiectasia in a local community in the northern part of Japan. Hum Mutat 2002;19:140–8.

32. Navarro OM, Laffan EE, Ngan BY. Pediatric soft- tissue tumors and pseudotumors: MR imaging features with pathologic correlation. I. Imaging approach, pseudotumors, vascular lesions, and adipocytic tumors. Radiographics 2009;29(3):887–906.

33. Fujima N, Osanai T, Shimizu Y, et al. Utility of noncontrast-enhanced time-resolved four-dimensional MR angiography with a vessel-selective technique for intracranial arteriovenous malformations. J Magn Reson Imaging 2016;44(4):834–45.

34. Murphey MD, Smith WS, Smith SE, et al. From the archives of the AFIP: imaging of musculoskeletal neurogenic tumors— radiologic-pathologic correlation. Radiographics 1999;19:1253–80.

35. O'Keefe P, Reid J, Morrison S, et al. Unexpected diagnosis of superficial neurofibroma in a lesion with imaging features of a vascular malformation. Pediatr Radiol 2005;35:1250–3.

36. Dubois J, Patriquin HB, Garel L, et al. Soft-tissue hemangiomas in infants and children: diagnosis using Doppler sonography. AJR Am J Roentgenol 1998;171:247–52.

37. Patel AS, Schulman JM, Ruben BS, et al. Atypical MRI features in soft-tissue arteriovenous malformation: a novel imaging appearance with radiologic–pathologic correlation. Pediatr Radiol 2015;45: 1515–21.

38. White CL, Olivieri B, Restrepo R, et al. Low-flow vascular malformation pitfalls: from clinical examination to practical imaging evaluation—part 1, lymphatic malformation mimickers. AJR Am J Roentgenol 2016;206:940–51.

39. Hagspiel K, Stevens P, Leung D, et al. Vascular malformations of the body: treatment follow-up using MRI and 3D gadolinium-enhanced MRA. In: CIRSE 2002. Abstracts of the annual meeting and postgraduate course of the Cardiovascular and Interventional Radiological Society of Europe and the 4th Joint Meeting with the European Society of Cardiac Radiology (ESCR). Lucern, Switzerland, October 5-9, 2002. Cardiovasc Intervent Radiol 2002;25(suppl 2): S77–265.

40. Dunham GM, Ingraham CR, Maki JH, et al. Finding the nidus: detection and workup of non-central nervous system arteriovenous malformations. Radiographics 2016;36:891–903.

41. Zhang B, Ma L. Updated classification and therapy of vascular malformations in pediatric patients. Pediatr Invest 2018;2(2):119–23.

42. Martinez-Lopez A, Blasco-Morente G, Perez-Lopez I, et al. CLOVES syndrome: review of a PIK3CA-related overgrowth spectrum (PROS). Clin Genet 2017;91:14–21.

43. Kaduthodil MJ, Prasad DS, Lowe AS, et al. Imaging manifestations in Proteus syndrome — an unusual multisystem developmental disorder. Br J Radiol 2012;85:e793–9.

Peripheral Vascular Imaging Focusing on Nonatherosclerotic Disease

Christopher J. François, MD

KEYWORDS

- Peripheral vascular disease • Popliteal entrapment syndrome • External iliac artery endofibrosis
- Vasculitis

KEY POINTS

- Cross-sectional imaging with ultrasound, computed tomography angiography, and magnetic resonance angiography has an essential role in the evaluation of patients with nonatherosclerotic peripheral vascular disease.
- Magnetic resonance angiography with stress maneuvers can detect popliteal entrapment syndrome accurately.
- External iliac arterial wall thickening, stenosis, and kinking are features of external iliac artery endofibrosis.
- In advanced stages of thromboangiitis obliterans, corkscrew collateral vessels can be apparent on imaging.
- Visceral artery dissections are a hallmark of segmental arterial mediolysis.

INTRODUCTION

Although atherosclerosis, varicose veins, and deep venous thrombosis are the most common vascular disease affecting the lower extremities,[1–3] a wide variety of other chronic diseases also can affect the lower extremity arteries. This article presents examples of the more commonly encountered of these, including popliteal arterial entrapment syndrome, external iliac endofibrosis, vasculitis, connective tissue disease, and noninflammatory vascular diseases. Imaging has an essential role in the diagnosis and management of these entities. Keys to imaging nonatherosclerotic vascular diseases include visualization of the vessel wall and surrounding soft tissues in addition to imaging the vessel lumen. Cross-sectional imaging, including ultrasound (US), computed tomography angiography (CTA), and magnetic resonance angiography (MRA), are fundamental in assessing patients suspected of having one of these syndromes[4–7] and for preoperative planning.[3,8–10]

POPLITEAL ARTERY ENTRAPMENT SYNDROME

Patients with popliteal artery entrapment syndrome (PAES) frequently present with lower extremity claudication, paresthesia, or swelling with exertion. PAES commonly occurs in young adults. Complications of PAES include distal thromboembolism and formation of aneurysms.[3,8–15] PAES can be due to anatomic variants or functional entrapment that occurs during plantar flexion. There are 6 types of PAES (Table 1). Anatomic PAES (types 1–5) can be due to abnormal course of the vessel (type 1) or due to an abnormal course of the muscles or fibrous band within the popliteal fossa (types 2–4). When an anatomic type also involves the popliteal vein, it is considered type 5. Type 6 of PAES is known as functional PAES due

Department of Radiology, University of Wisconsin, 600 Highland Avenue, Madison, WI 53792, USA
E-mail address: CFrancois@uwhealth.org

Radiol Clin N Am 58 (2020) 831–839
https://doi.org/10.1016/j.rcl.2020.02.007
0033-8389/20/© 2020 Elsevier Inc. All rights reserved.

Table 1
Classification of popliteal entrapment syndrome

Type	Description
1	Popliteal entrapment due to an abnormal popliteal artery course, usually medially to the medial head of the gastrocnemius muscle
2	Popliteal entrapment due to the medial head of the gastrocnemius muscle compressing the normally located popliteal artery
3	Popliteal entrapment due to and accessory slip of the medial head of the gastrocnemius muscle compressing the normally located popliteal artery
4	Popliteal entrapment due to the popliteus muscle or fibrous band compressing the normally located popliteal artery
5	When types 1–4 involve the popliteal artery and vein
6	Functional compression of the popliteal artery (and vein) between the medial and lateral heads of the gastrocnemius

to compression of the popliteal artery between the medial and lateral heads of the gastrocnemius muscle. The etiology of functional PAES remains uncertain, but it occurs when there is popliteal artery compression despite normal anatomy. A diagnosis of PAES relies on a combination of ankle-brachial index, US, MRA, and CTA.

For the initial evaluation of patients with suspected PAES, US with duplex Doppler frequently is used because it allows for real-time visualization of popliteal artery compression. Occasionally, the popliteal artery is completely compressed. During plantar flexion, Doppler pressure measurements increase in the affected extremity and are essential in establishing the diagnosis.[12,14] In patients with functional PAES (Figs. 1 and 2), detection of these changes in pressure with provocation can be crucial in making a diagnosis because this may be the only finding in the absence of anatomic abnormalities on CTA and MRA.[14]

The need to apply pressure with the transducer during the evaluation, which can artificially increase velocities, is a limitation of US for the evaluation of PAES.[10] Furthermore, the popliteal vessels can move out of the region of interest of the Doppler during plantar flexion resulting in an apparent occlusion.[3,10] Athletes are a particular

group of patients in whom duplex Doppler US can have a high false-positive rate in the initial assessment of PAES.[8] In patients with a positive duplex Doppler US examination or in patients with a negative duplex Doppler US examination with a high pretest probability of PAES, MRA should be performed for confirmation.

As with duplex Doppler US, contrast-enhanced MRA with time-resolved acquisitions (Fig. 3) can be performed without and with dynamic plantar flexion.[12] Although MRA frequently is used as a confirmatory test after duplex Doppler US, the long MRA acquisitions during plantar flexion can lead to motion artifacts that lower the quality of the study.[3,10,11] Even with these potential limitations, MRA recently was shown superior to digital subtraction angiography (DSA) for PAES diagnosis.[9] This is probably because the assessment of the anatomy within the popliteal fossa is an essential component of the evaluation and is best accomplished using a combination of T1-weighted and T2-weighted sequences.[10,11]

CTA can be used to confirm the presence of PAES in a similar fashion as MRA, with dynamic acquisitions during plantar flexion and at rest (see Fig. 2). CTA can be performed with a single, long contrast bolus administration.[11] Abnormal muscular and tendinous structures within the popliteal fossa also can be detected with CTA.[8,15] Due to the ionizing radiation with CTA, MRA and duplex Doppler US remain the preferred imaging studies in patients with PAES.

Invasive catheter x-ray angiography (XA) is considered the reference standard for identifying the dynamic vascular deviation and obstruction in patients with PAES.[8,10,11] XA, however, is not able to assess the extravascular anatomy and determine the exact type of PAES.

EXTERNAL ILIAC ARTERY ENDOFIBROSIS

External iliac artery endofibrosis (EIAE) is an uncommon cause of lower extremity claudication. As implied by its name, the external iliac artery affected is most commonly. The common iliac artery also can be involved, however, in up to 15% of patients.[16] EIAE frequently is associated with long-distance cycling but has been reported in other types of high-performance endurance athletes. Patients with EIAE suffer from performance-limiting lower extremity pain and weakness that is relieved with rest.[17] The exact cause of EIAE is not known but may be related to the repetitive trauma the hypertrophied psoas muscles exert on the external iliac artery during flexion, causing vasospasm[18] and arterial kinking.[19] The initial

A

	Rest	Planta	Dorsi
R Ankle (DP):	165	16	170
L Ankle (DP):	174	135	201
L Brachial:	144	144	144
R ABI:	1.15	0.11	1.18
L ABI:	1.21	0.94	1.40

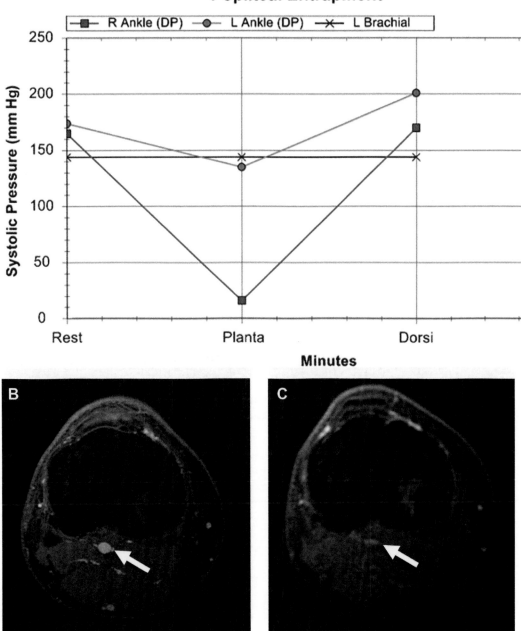

Fig. 1. MRA in a 24-year-old man with functional popliteal entrapment syndrome. (*A*) Ankle-brachial index in the right lower extremity decreased dramatically with plantar flexion. (*B*) The popliteal artery has a normal course and is widely patent in the neutral (rest) position (*arrow*). (*C*) The popliteal artery is completely compressed with plantar flexion between the medial and lateral heads of the gastrocnemius muscle (*arrow*). ABI, ankle-brachial index; DP, dorsalis pedis; L, left; R, right.

A

	Rest	Planta	Dorsi
R Ankle:	139	0	137
L Ankle:	152	136	138
L Brachial:	137	137	137
R ABI:	1.01	0.00	1.00
L ABI:	1.11	0.99	1.01

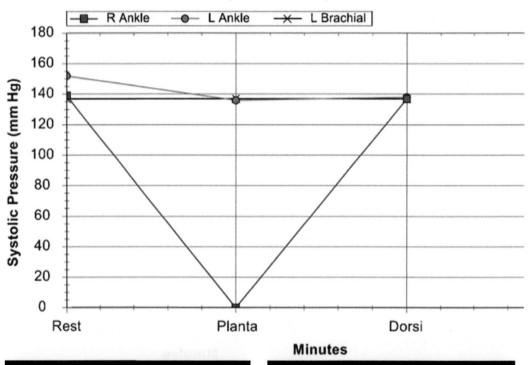

Popliteal Entrapment

Legend: — ■ — R Ankle   — ● — L Ankle   — ✕ — L Brachial

Y-axis: Systolic Pressure (mm Hg) — 0, 20, 40, 60, 80, 100, 120, 140, 160, 180

X-axis: Rest, Planta, Dorsi

Minutes

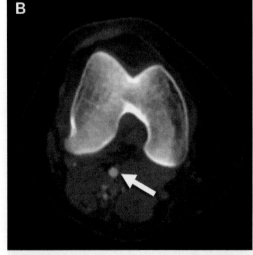

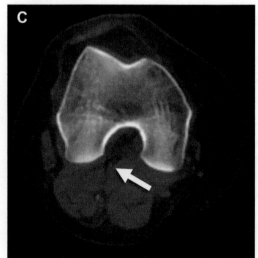

Fig. 2. CTA in a 31-year-old woman with functional popliteal entrapment syndrome. (*A*) Ankle-brachial index in the right lower extremity decreased dramatically with plantar flexion (*arrow*). (*B*) The popliteal artery has a normal course and is widely patent in the neutral (rest) position. (*C*) The popliteal artery is completely compressed with plantar flexion between the medial and lateral heads of the gastrocnemius muscle (*arrow*).

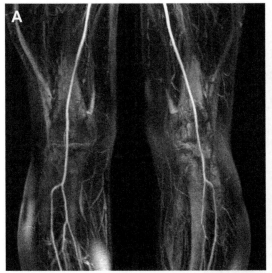
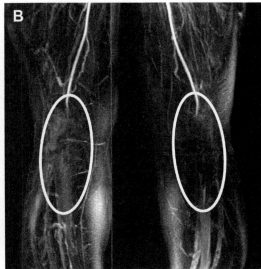

Fig. 3. MRA in a 36-year-old woman with functional popliteal entrapment syndrome. (*A*) The popliteal arteries have a normal course and are widely patent in the neutral (rest) position. (*B*) The popliteal arteries are completely compressed with plantar flexion between the medial and lateral heads of the gastrocnemius muscles bilaterally (*ellipses*).

evaluation of patients with EIAE includes assessment of ankle-brachial pressure indices at rest and during exercise. Patients with EIAE have decreased ankle-brachial pressure indices with exercise.[17]

US, CTA (**Figs. 4 and 5**), and MRA can be used to assess the patency of the external iliac arteries in patients with EIAE. Findings of EIAE include arterial wall thickening, stenosis, and kinking. US duplex Doppler US has the advantage of being able to assess flow and vessel morphology in real time during provocative maneuvers in patients with suspected EIAE.[18,19] duplex Doppler US should be performed with the hip flexed and extended to try to detect changes in anatomy and flow typical of EIAE.[18–20] Catheter angiography can be used to measure pressure changes in the external iliac artery during maneuvers[16,20] and to treat EIAE noninvasively with stent placement.

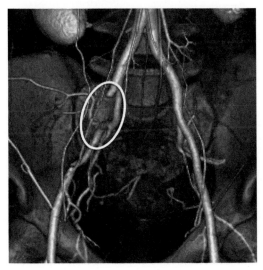

Fig. 4. CTA in a 36-year-old male competitive runner with EIAE. The right external iliac artery is occluded (*ellipse*).

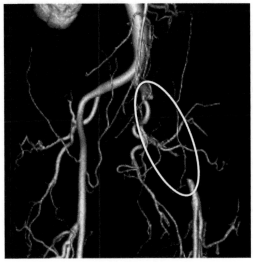

Fig. 5. CTA in a 49-year-old female competitive cyclist with EIAE. The left external iliac artery is occluded (*ellipse*).

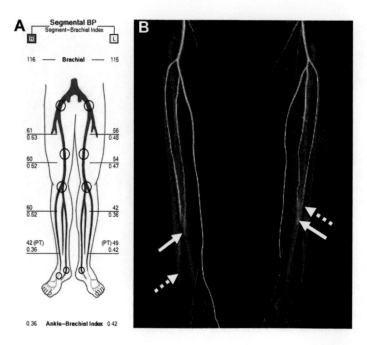

Fig. 6. CTA in a 37-year-old woman with thromboangiitis obliterans. (*A*) Ankle-brachial indices are abnormally low in both lower extremities. (*B*) The posterior tibial (*dashed arrows*) and peroneal (*solid arrows*) are occluded distally in both lower extremities.

VASCULITIS AND CONNECTIVE TISSUE DISEASES

Vasculitis and connective tissue diseases affect the lower extremity vessels less frequently than other vascular territories. Of the vasculitides, thromboangiitis obliterans is an inflammatory vasculitis that affects the medium-sized and small-sized arteries of the distal upper and lower extremities. A vast majority of patients with thromboangiitis obliterans are smokers and are younger adults (25–45 years of age). The incidence in North America is approximately 126 per 1 million. Clinically, patients with thromboangiitis obliterans present with worsening claudication, paresthesia, ulcerations, superficial thrombophlebitis, and rest pain. The classic finding on imaging in patients with thromboangiitis obliterans is related to the occlusion of vessels (**Fig. 6**), which results in the development of collateral flow through the vasa vasorum, giving a corkscrew appearance to the runoff vessels.[5,21]

For small vessel vasculitis, such as thromboangiitis obliterans, the utility of duplex Doppler US, CTA, and MRA is less than that of invasive catheter angiography, which is regarded as the gold standard.[5] Frequent findings of vasculitis on these noninvasive vascular imaging studies include vessel wall thickening, stenosis, and occlusion. In the advanced stages (**Fig. 7**), the typical corkscrew collateral vessels may be apparent.[22] Nonvascular complications, including osteomyelitis or arthritis, can occur as well.[5]

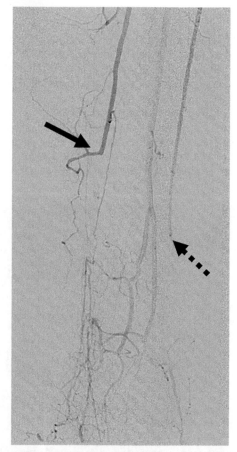

Fig. 7. Catheter XA in a 47-year-old man with thromboangiitis obliterans. (*A*) The anterior tibial (*dashed arrow*) and posterior tibial (*solid arrow*) are occluded distally. BP, blood pressure; PT, posterior tibial.

Connective tissue diseases, such Marfan syndrome (MS), vascular Ehlers-Danlos syndrome (vEDS), and Loeys-Dietz syndrome (LDS), more frequently affect the aorta and central vasculature than the peripheral arteries. MS and vEDS are autosomal dominant (AD) connective tissue disorders caused by mutations in genes responsible for fibrillin-1 and type III collagen production, respectively. LDS also is an AD connective tissue disease that is due to defects in the genes that part of the transforming growth factor β pathway. Aortic aneurysms and dissections are the vascular abnormalities encountered most frequently in patients with MS, vEDS, and LDS.[4,6,7,23] Involvement of the lower extremity arteries is less frequent but can occur.

CTA (Fig. 8) and MRA (Fig. 9) are performed routinely in patients with MS, vEDS, and LDS to monitor for the development and growth of aneurysms typical in these patients.[4,6,7] Due to the need for lifelong monitoring, MRA is preferred to minimize exposure to ionizing radiation. In patients with MS and LDS, imaging to assess the size of the vessels is recommended at least every 2 years[4] and 1 year,[6] respectively. In patients with suspected lower extremity involvement, MRA and CTA are both appropriate, although CTA may offer higher routine spatial resolution than typical MRA techniques. Catheter angiography is not considered routinely for diagnostic imaging in patients with connective tissue diseases due to the higher risk for complications.[4,7]

NONINFLAMMATORY VASCULAR DISEASES

Fibromuscular dysplasia (FMD) is a noninflammatory vascular disease, which usually causes stenosis and aneurysms of the carotid and renal arteries. Lower extremity arterial involvement is uncommon but can be present. In patients with lower extremity FMD, symptoms can include pain, pallor, claudication, and critical limb ischemia due to microembolization.[24,25] Segmental arterial mediolysis (SAM) is another noninflammatory vascular disease that usually affects the visceral arteries within the abdomen. SAM can, unusually, affect the iliac arteries as well.[26] Degradation of the medial layer of the vessel wall leads to arterial dissection, aneurysm, stenosis, or occlusion in patients with SAM. Rarely, patients with SAM can present with extensive hemorrhage from rupture of the vessel.[27–29] Cystic adventitial disease (Fig. 10) is a rare noninflammatory vascular disease that occurs in otherwise healthy young men. The popliteal artery is the most commonly affected vessel in patients with cystic adventitial disease and is associated

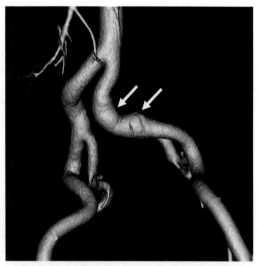

Fig. 8. CRA in a 29-year-old man with vEDS. The left common iliac artery is aneurysmal (*arrows*).

with claudication or sudden onset of pain within the popliteal fossa.

Invasive catheter angiography remains the reference standard for the diagnosis of FMD, SAM, and cystic adventitial disease.[24,25,30–33] CTA and MRA, however, are important in the initial evaluation of these patients.[7,24,30,34] As with the small-vessel vasculitides, noninvasive imaging is less sensitive for milder disease.[30] Because many patients diagnosed with SAM present with acute abdominal pain, initial diagnosis frequently is made with CTA.[27,28] Follow-up of the aneurysms and dissections in patients with SAM can be performed with CTA or MRA.[26] Cystic adventitial disease patients

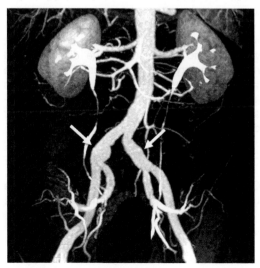

Fig. 9. MRA in a 25-year-old man with LDS. The common iliac arteries are aneurysmal bilaterally (*arrows*).

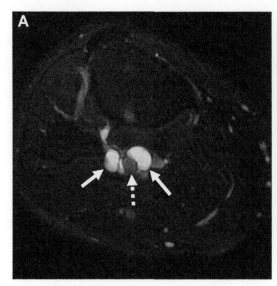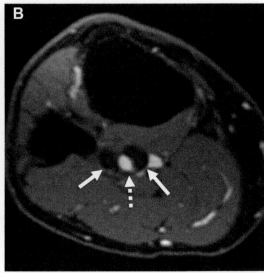

Fig. 10. MRA in a 34-year-old woman with cystic adventitial disease. (*A*) Fat-suppressed, T2-weighted, and (*B*) fat-suppressed, T1-weighted, postcontrast images reveal thin-walled cysts (*solid arrows*) along the wall of the popliteal artery (*dashed arrows*).

have small cysts on CTA and MRA. With MRA, additional T1-weighted and T2-weighted imaging should be acquired to confirm the presence of adventitial cysts and differentiate them from other potential cystic lesions in the popliteal fossa.[35] duplex Doppler US can be used to detect the anechoic adventitial cysts in patients with cystic adventitial disease.[35]

SUMMARY

In summary, a variety of nonatherosclerotic diseases can affect the arteries of the pelvis and lower extremities. These include chronic repetitive traumatic conditions, such as popliteal entrapment and external iliac artery fibroelastosis, vasculitis and connective tissue diseases, and noninflammatory vascular diseases. Noninvasive vascular imaging with US, CTA, and MRA plays an essential role in the initial assessment and management of patients with peripheral vascular disease.

DISCLOSURE

GE Healthcare provides research support to the University of Wisconsin Department of Radiology.

REFERENCES

1. Diehm N, Kickuth R, Baumgartner I, et al. Magnetic resonance angiography in infrapopliteal arterial disease: prospective comparison of 1.5 and 3 Tesla magnetic resonance imaging. Invest Radiol 2007; 42(6):467–76.
2. Kalva SP, Mueller PR. Vascular imaging in the elderly. Radiol Clin North Am 2008;46(4):663–83, v.
3. Pillai J, Levien LJ, Haagensen M, et al. Assessment of the medial head of the gastrocnemius muscle in functional compression of the popliteal artery. J Vasc Surg 2008;48(5):1189–96.
4. Chu LC, Johnson PT, Dietz HC, et al. CT angiographic evaluation of genetic vascular disease: role in detection, staging, and management of complex vascular pathologic conditions. AJR Am J Roentgenol 2014;202(5):1120–9.
5. Dimmick SJ, Goh AC, Cauzza E, et al. Imaging appearances of Buerger's disease complications in the upper and lower limbs. Clin Radiol 2012; 67(12):1207–11.
6. Kalra VB, Gilbert JW, Malhotra A. Loeys-Dietz syndrome: cardiovascular, neuroradiological and musculoskeletal imaging findings. Pediatr Radiol 2011;41(12):1495–504 [quiz: 616].
7. Zilocchi M, Macedo TA, Oderich GS, et al. Vascular Ehlers-Danlos syndrome: imaging findings. AJR Am J Roentgenol 2007;189(3):712–9.
8. Goh BK, Tay KH, Tan SG. Diagnosis and surgical management of popliteal artery entrapment syndrome. ANZ J Surg 2005;75(10):869–73.
9. Ozkan U, Oguzkurt L, Tercan F, et al. MRI and DSA findings in popliteal artery entrapment syndrome. Diagn Interv Radiol 2008;14(2):106–10.
10. Pillai J. A current interpretation of popliteal vascular entrapment. J Vasc Surg 2008;48(6 Suppl):61S–5S [discussion 5S].

11. Anil G, Tay KH, Howe TC, et al. Dynamic computed tomography angiography: role in the evaluation of popliteal artery entrapment syndrome. Cardiovasc Intervent Radiol 2011;34(2):259–70.

12. Causey MW, Quan RW, Curry TK, et al. Ultrasound is a critical adjunct in the diagnosis and treatment of popliteal entrapment syndrome. J Vasc Surg 2013; 57(6):1695–7.

13. Kim SY, Min SK, Ahn S, et al. Long-term outcomes after revascularization for advanced popliteal artery entrapment syndrome with segmental arterial occlusion. J Vasc Surg 2012;55(1):90–7.

14. Lane R, Nguyen T, Cuzzilla M, et al. Functional popliteal entrapment syndrome in the sportsperson. Eur J Vasc Endovasc Surg 2012;43(1):81–7.

15. Zhong H, Gan J, Zhao Y, et al. Role of CT angiography in the diagnosis and treatment of popliteal vascular entrapment syndrome. AJR Am J Roentgenol 2011;197(6):W1147–54.

16. Rouviere O, Feugier P, Gutierrez JP, et al. Arterial endofibrosis in endurance athletes: angiographic features and classification. Radiology 2014;273(1): 294–303.

17. INSITE Collaborators (INternational Study group for Identification and Treatment of Endofibrosis). Diagnosis and management of iliac artery endofibrosis: results of a Delphi Consensus Study. Eur J Vasc Endovasc Surg 2016;52(1):90–8.

18. Shalhub S, Zierler RE, Smith W, et al. Vasospasm as a cause for claudication in athletes with external iliac artery endofibrosis. J Vasc Surg 2013;58(1): 105–11.

19. Falor AE, Zobel M, de Virgilio C. External iliac artery fibrosis in endurance athletes successfully treated with bypass grafting. Ann Vasc Surg 2013;27(8): 1183.e1-4.

20. Peach G, Schep G, Palfreeman R, et al. Endofibrosis and kinking of the iliac arteries in athletes: a systematic review. Eur J Vasc Endovasc Surg 2012;43(2): 208–17.

21. Fujii Y, Soga J, Nakamura S, et al. Classification of corkscrew collaterals in thromboangiitis obliterans (Buerger's disease): relationship between corkscrew type and prevalence of ischemic ulcers. Circ J 2010; 74(8):1684–8.

22. Bas A, Dikici AS, Gulsen F, et al. Corkscrew collateral vessels in buerger disease: vasa vasorum or vasa nervorum. J Vasc Interv Radiol 2016;27(5): 735–9.

23. Dormand H, Mohiaddin RH. Cardiovascular magnetic resonance in Marfan syndrome. J Cardiovasc Magn Reson 2013;15:33.

24. Ketha SS, Bjarnason H, Oderich GS, et al. Clinical features and endovascular management of iliac artery fibromuscular dysplasia. J Vasc Interv Radiol 2014;25(6):949–53.

25. Plouin PF, Perdu J, La Batide-Alanore A, et al. Fibromuscular dysplasia. Orphanet J Rare Dis 2007;2:28.

26. Kalva SP, Somarouthu B, Jaff MR, et al. Segmental arterial mediolysis: clinical and imaging features at presentation and during follow-up. J Vasc Interv Radiol 2011;22(10):1380–7.

27. Michael M, Widmer U, Wildermuth S, et al. Segmental arterial mediolysis: CTA findings at presentation and follow-up. AJR Am J Roentgenol 2006;187(6):1463–9.

28. Shenouda M, Riga C, Naji Y, et al. Segmental arterial mediolysis: a systematic review of 85 cases. Ann Vasc Surg 2014;28(1):269–77.

29. Slavin RE. Segmental arterial mediolysis: course, sequelae, prognosis, and pathologic-radiologic correlation. Cardiovasc Pathol 2009; 18(6):352–60.

30. Blondin D, Lanzman R, Schellhammer F, et al. Fibromuscular dysplasia in living renal donors: still a challenge to computed tomographic angiography. Eur J Radiol 2010;75(1):67–71.

31. Meuse MA, Turba UC, Sabri SS, et al. Treatment of renal artery fibromuscular dysplasia. Tech Vasc Interv Radiol 2010;13(2):126–33.

32. Mousa AY, Campbell JE, Stone PA, et al. Short- and long-term outcomes of percutaneous transluminal angioplasty/stenting of renal fibromuscular dysplasia over a ten-year period. J Vasc Surg 2012;55(2):421–7.

33. Sabharwal R, Vladica P, Coleman P. Multidetector spiral CT renal angiography in the diagnosis of renal artery fibromuscular dysplasia. Eur J Radiol 2007; 61(3):520–7.

34. Bolen MA, Brinza E, Renapurkar RD, et al. Screening CT angiography of the aorta, visceral branch vessels, and pelvic arteries in fibromuscular dysplasia. JACC Cardiovasc Imaging 2017;10(5): 554–61.

35. Paravastu SC, Regi JM, Turner DR, et al. A contemporary review of cystic adventitial disease. Vasc Endovascular Surg 2012;46(1):5–14.

Moving?

Make sure your subscription moves with you!

To notify us of your new address, find your **Clinics Account Number** (located on your mailing label above your name), and contact customer service at:

Email: journalscustomerservice-usa@elsevier.com

800-654-2452 (subscribers in the U.S. & Canada)
314-447-8871 (subscribers outside of the U.S. & Canada)

Fax number: 314-447-8029

Elsevier Health Sciences Division
Subscription Customer Service
3251 Riverport Lane
Maryland Heights, MO 63043

ELSEVIER

Moving?

Make sure your subscription moves with you!

To notify us of your new address, find your Clinics Account Number (located on your mailing label above your name), and contact customer service at:

Email: journalscustomerservice-usa@elsevier.com

800-654-2452 (subscribers in the U.S. & Canada)
314-447-8871 (subscribers outside of the U.S. & Canada)

Fax number: 314-447-8029

Elsevier Health Sciences Division
Subscription Customer Service
3251 Riverport Lane
Maryland Heights, MO 63043

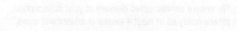

To ensure uninterrupted delivery of your subscription, please notify us at least 4 weeks in advance of move.

Printed and bound by CPI Group (UK) Ltd, Croydon, CR0 4YY

08/05/2025

01864691-0020